Diseases of bone and joints

SECOND EDITION

Diseases of bone and joints

Louis Lichtenstein, M.D.

Clinical Professor of Pathology, University of California, San Francisco
Professor Extraordinario, National University of Mexico
Honorary Fellow, Royal College of Pathologists of Australia
Honorary Member, Spanish Orthopedic Society (SECOT)
Honorary Member, Western Orthopedic Association
Fellow, New York Academy of Medicine
Consultant in Pathology, Children's Hospital, San Francisco
Consultant in Pathology, U. S. Naval Hospital, Oakland
Consultant in Orthopaedic Pathology, St. Joseph's Hospital and
  Mt. Zion Hospital and Medical Center, San Francisco

with 332 illustrations

THE C. V. MOSBY COMPANY
Saint Louis   1975

Second edition

Copyright © 1975 by The C. V. Mosby Company

All rights reserved. No part of this book may be reproduced in any manner without written permission of the publisher.

Previous edition copyrighted 1970

Printed in the United States of America

Distributed in Great Britain by Henry Kimpton, London

Library of Congress Cataloging in Publication Data

Lichtenstein, Louis, 1906-
  Diseases of bone and joints.

  Includes bibliographies.
  1. Bones—Diseases.   2. Joints—Diseases.
I. Title. [DNLM: 1. Bone diseases. 2. Joint diseases. WE200 L696d]
RD684.L49 1975   616.7'1   74-14781
ISBN 0-8016-3007-X

VH/VH/VH 9 8 7 6 5 4 3 2 1

*To all my students over the years
who have provided me with as much
stimulation as I hope
I have given them.*

Preface

The format of the first edition has been maintained, but a major part of the book has been revised to make it more informative and to incorporate recent advances in the field of bone and joint disease. Thus, the important chapters on osteoporosis and on the skeletal changes in renal disease have been amplified and completely rewritten. Similarly, the chapters on infections, endocrine disorders, metabolic disorders, and the chemical and radiation effects on bone have been substantially revised and brought up to date. Among the specific subjects dealt with more fully are some of the infections, particularly brucellosis, syphilis, tuberculosis, and maduromycosis; the effects of pituitary growth hormone; hyperparathyroidism; the mucopolysaccharidoses, particularly gargoylism and its variants; the lipoidoses; sickle cell anemia; fluorosis; radiation osteitis and radiation-induced neoplasms; intraosseous ganglia; degeneration and rupture of intervertebral discs; hypertrophic osteoarthropathy; and pseudogout. In the process, many new references have been cited, especially the significant recent ones, and more than 50 new illustrations, both roentgenograms and photomicrographs, have been introduced to emphasize some of the points made in the text. Finally, many of the legends have been amplified to enhance the usefulness of the illustrations.

The new photomicrographs were prepared by Lloyd Matlovsky and the roentgenograms by Ruth Cordish of Los Angeles, who did many of the illustrations for the first edition of *Bone Tumors*. I also wish to acknowledge the courtesy of Georg Thieme Verlag, Stuttgart, in permitting the use of several illustrations from the monograph of Schmorl and Junghanns on the vertebral column, pertaining to osteoporosis and Paget's disease.

In keeping with my own background and interest, the emphasis throughout remains on pathology, although every effort has been made, without going too far afield, to integrate basic pathologic data with essential clinical information and with relevant observations in genetics, molecular biology, biochemistry, and other fields, with a view to presenting a well-rounded, comprehensive picture of skeletal disease.

Louis Lichtenstein
4016 Farm Hill Blvd., Redwood City, Calif. 94061

Preface TO FIRST EDITION

For some years now I have been urged repeatedly by my colleagues to write a book that would cover skeletal disease in general, apart from neoplasms, and that might serve as a companion volume to *Bone Tumors*. If I have not done so sooner, it is because the task appeared to be so formidable, crossing as it does ever so many specialty boundary lines. Skeletal tissues are very labile, despite their mineralized structure. There is constant new bone formation and resorption in progress, even in adults, and these processes may be accelerated and otherwise thrown out of balance under certain abnormal regulatory conditions. Furthermore, as the table of contents indicates, the structure, function, and pathologic alterations of bone and joints may reflect in many obvious and subtle ways what is going on elsewhere in the body—genetic abnormalities, altered renal function, metabolic disorders, vitamin imbalances, endocrine malfunction, neurotrophic disorders, blood diseases, and many other disease states.

This monograph is intended to provide a concise yet informative comprehensive survey for basic orientation, with emphasis on pathology, and, as such, to help meet the needs of orthopedists, general surgeons, radiologists, pathologists, pediatricians, internists, and other men in medicine and its allied sciences who have an interest in diseases of bone and joints, for whatever reason. It makes no pretense of being an encyclopedic treatise covering in detail every aspect of every conceivable subject in the field. That might require half a professional lifetime and, after all, teaching and consultation work are time consuming. There are relatively few existing books of comparable scope, in the English language at least, and their approach is somewhat different. In addition, I am not always in agreement with the views they express.

In the preparation of certain chapters I have perforce drawn upon the collective wisdom and published experience of my friends in internal medicine and endocrinology, some of them brilliant investigators who know far more than I do in these areas. Illustrative roentgenograms have been freely utilized as invaluable tools in graphically depicting many conditions. With few exceptions these have been selected from my own teaching files. Many of the observations on

Preface to first edition

pathologic conditions are based upon articles that my associates and I have published (on such subjects as aneurysmal bone cyst, fibrous dysplasia, eosinophilic granuloma of bone, histiocytosis X, gout, hereditary ochronosis, and pigmented villonodular synovitis, among others), as well as upon unpublished data that have accrued over the past 20 years or more. Relevant physiologic, genetic, immunologic, and biochemical data have been integrated at every opportunity with clinical and pathologic findings.

Louis Lichtenstein

Contents

1. Fractures and their sequelae, 1
2. Systemic anomalies of skeletal development, 16
3. Infections of bone, 52
4. Skeletal changes in vitamin deficiencies and excesses, 83
5. Skeletal changes in endocrine disorders, 100
6. Skeletal changes in metabolic disorders, 118
7. Skeletal changes in renal disease, 137
8. Osteoporosis, 145
9. Skeletal changes in neurotrophic disorders, 156
10. Skeletal changes in certain blood diseases, 164
11. Paget's disease of bone (osteitis deformans), 173
12. Histiocytosis X (eosinophilic granuloma, Letterer-Siwe disease, and Schüller-Christian disease), 196
13. Chemical and radiation effects on bone, 210
14. Pathology of some common and unusual orthopedic conditions, 218
15. Disorders of synovial joints, 265

Diseases of bone and joints

chapter 1

Fractures and their sequelae

It seems appropriate to lead off with a discussion of fractures because of the disability that fractures may produce and because they constitute by far the most commonly encountered skeletal lesion.

A fracture may be defined broadly as any break in the continuity of a bone, from whatever cause. An important practical distinction is generally made between fractures that are closed (simple) and those that are open (compound) and hence prone to infection. Numerous additional qualifying designations are also employed clinically to indicate further the particular location, type, and extent of various fractures, and especially their degree of fragmentation, the direction of the break, and the displacement of the affected bone. Terms such as incomplete (Fig. 1-1), comminuted, greenstick, fissure, stress (Fig. 1-2), subperiosteal, and epiphyseal, among many others (see Fig. 1-12), are used, not to mention literally dozens of eponyms referring to specific situations.

A fracture through a bone area that has been weakened by some antecedent lesion is commonly referred to as a pathologic fracture; some of the major predisposing causes of this fracture will be discussed later.

Actually, many surgical procedures, such as drilling, reaming, the insertion of nails, screws, and plates, and the collection of bone for grafting, inflict injuries on bone that are technically fractures, but we are not particularly concerned with these here.

In this brief discussion emphasis will be placed upon the basic pathologic aspects of the healing of fractures in general and upon failure to achieve satisfactory bony union. For comprehensive consideration of surgical management and of the practical problems entailed in dealing effectively with special situations, the reader may have recourse to the available clinical monographs on fractures, among which the standard reference treatises of Watson-Jones and Campbell are particularly informative.

Although the healing of a fracture is a continuous process,[2] it appears to be conventional, by way of didactic exposition,[3] to postulate three distinct stages: (1) organization of hematoma at the fracture site (by granulation tissue and

1

Diseases of bone and joints

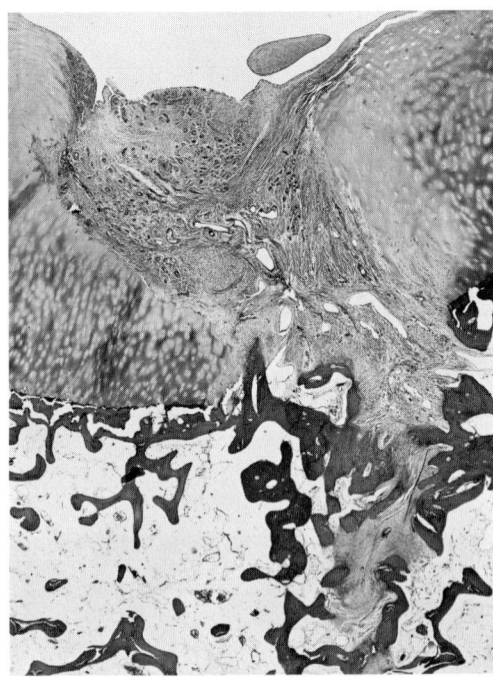

Fig. 1-1. Fibrous repair of an incomplete fracture extending through articular cartilage and into subchondral bone for a short distance. The articular cartilage at the fracture site has not regenerated, and the defect is filled by organizing granulation tissue.

fibrous connective tissue), leading to so-called procallus; (2) conversion of procallus to fibrocartilaginous callus, which fills the gap between the fracture ends; and (3) replacement in turn by osseous callus, resulting in most instances in bony union. While this neat sequence is calculated to appeal to the orderly mind of the anatomist, one does not usually observe such clear-cut stages in pathologic specimens showing recent fracture. Instead, one finds the various phases of the healing of fractures—specifically, the organization of blood clot, disposal of necrotic bone debris, fibrous replacement of resorbed bone, and exuberant formation of both cartilage and bone, representing callus—going on more or less simultaneously. It would seem more realistic, therefore, to relate what happens at a fracture site in terms of actual observation rather than as a schematized hypothesis.

To interpret the sequence of events following a fracture, it is essential to be familiar with the timetable of the changes outlined above. According to Watson-Jones and others, continuity by granulation tissue is achieved ordinarily within a few weeks, union by primary callus in 2 to 3 months, and consolidation and maturation of callus in 4 to 5 months, whereas complete restoration of structure and tubulation requires almost a year. These estimates represent convenient averages and may need revision in any individual case, depending on the location and the extent of the fracture and the age and condition of the patient, among other

Fractures and their sequelae

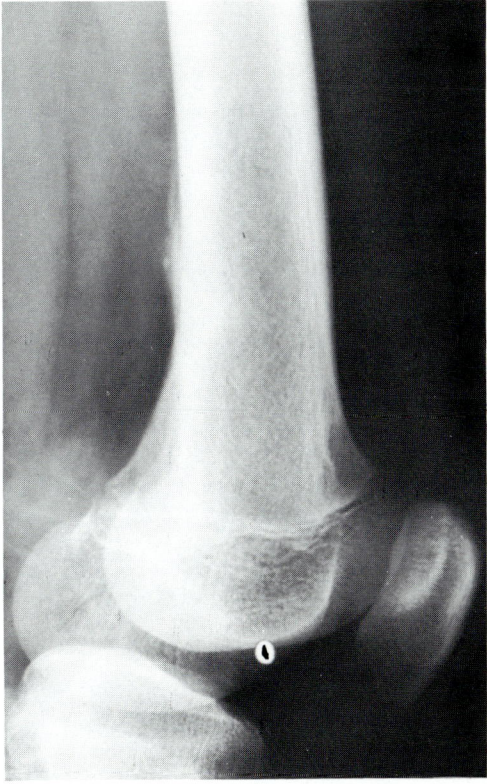

Fig. 1-2. Roentgenogram showing callus formation at the site of a stress fracture in a lower femur. Biopsy was done because of concern over the possibility of osteogenic sarcoma. As is now well known,[1] comparable stress (fatigue) or march fractures may be encountered in metatarsal bones and in the tibia and fibula as well.

factors. For example, children may deposit abundant callus with surprising rapidity compared with adults. Then too, the time intervals cited do not apply to instances in which there is appreciably delayed union or eventual nonunion, for whatever reason.

The pathologic picture at the site of a fresh fracture is characterized by two cardinal features: (1) necrosis of bone of variable extent at the fracture site, reflecting loss of blood supply, and (2) hemorrhage resulting from rupture of blood vessels. Thus if one examines sections of a fracture fragment (from a patella or a head of a radius, for example) removed in the course of open repair several days after an injury, one may readily perceive that the bone is substantially if not completely dead, as evidenced by loss of osteocytes within the lacunae. If the time interval is less than a week, the extent of necrosis may be substantially greater than is apparent, for it may take 7 to 10 days or even longer for the classical histologic sign of dead bone, the empty lacunae, to develop. It may also be found that there has been extensive extravasation of blood along the fracture line that extends into the contiguous spongy bone for an appreciable distance

Diseases of bone and joints

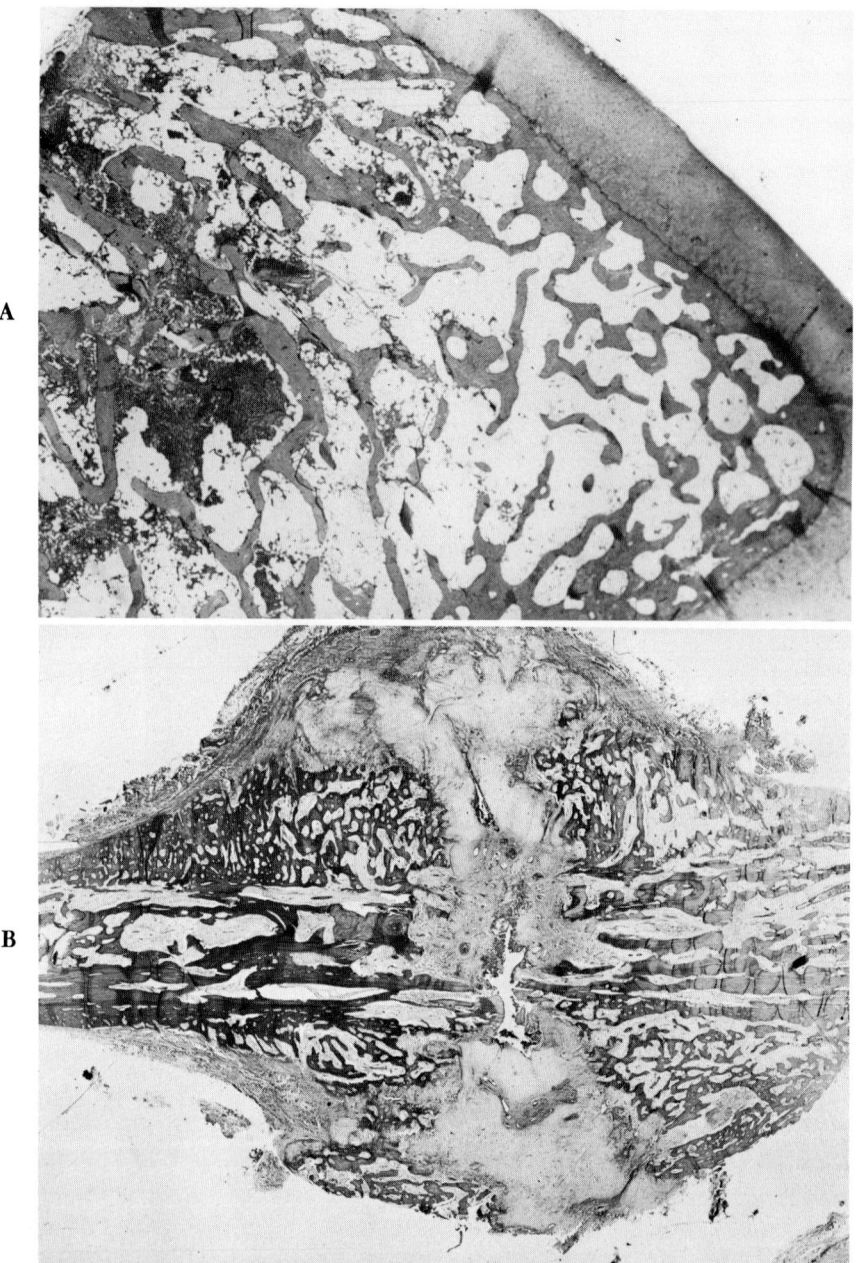

Fig. 1-3. A, Photomicrograph of surgically removed patellar fragment showing the effects of a recent (5-day-old) fracture. There is obvious hemorrhage along the fracture line (on the left). The spongy trabeculae showed avascular necrosis not readily discernible at this low magnification. The articular cartilage on its surface was unaltered. **B,** Photomicrograph of cartilaginous and bony callus at the site of a 3-week-old fracture of a rib. The callus at this stage is still relatively bulky and contains abundant cartilage (in the whitish areas of the low-power illustration). This cartilage is subsequently converted to bone.

Fractures and their sequelae

(Fig. 1-3, *A*). Concomitantly, there is extravasation and seepage of blood into the periosteum and adjacent soft parts, particularly the muscles, although reference to this hemorrhage as a hematoma in the conventional sense of a circumscribed tumorlike swelling may be somewhat inaccurate. In any event, the presence of diffused blood helps to provide a favorable medium for relatively rapid and intensive ossification. Specifically, it favors the rapid development of granulation tissue; also, organizing fibrin in proximity to bone can serve as as substrate for the formation of osteoid and new bone.

Furthermore, biochemical investigations have indicated that there is a greatly increased concentration of calcium and phosphorus at a fracture site for the first several weeks at least. This increment may well be related to vascular resorption and demineralization of the fractured bone ends. Of comparable importance is the observation[4] that phosphatase activity at a fracture site becomes strikingly increased within several days and that this heightened activity persists for some 2 months.

The formation of cartilage and bone at a fracture site, constituting what is conventionally referred to as primary callus, likewise sets in relatively early, to judge by clinical as well as experimental material.[2,5] If one examines sections of a healing fracture in a rib, for example, several weeks after injury (Fig. 1-3, *B*),

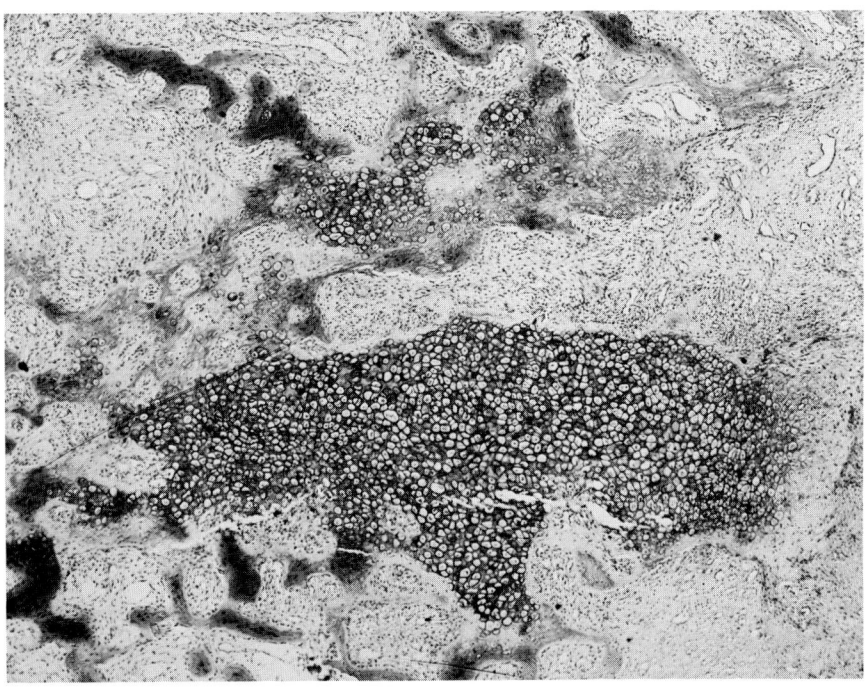

Fig. 1-4. Photomicrograph showing abundant active formation of cartilage at the periphery of a fracture site. Pathologists unfamiliar with pictures such as this are sometimes unduly concerned over the possibility of chondrosarcoma, although tumor cartilage does not look anything like this.

one observes irregular fields of actively growing cartilage undergoing osseous transformation intermingled with heavy-set trabeculae of new bone covered by proliferating osteoblasts. The early abundant formation of cartilage (Fig. 1-4), presumably by the active cambium layer of the torn periosteum, may well be a result of local anoxia. This cartilage component of the callus extends into the medullary cavity, where it merges with richly vascularized, young connective tissue containing organizing fibrin and bits of necrotic bone debris. The new bone seems clearly to be of periosteal origin, for the most part, and is deposited as a tapered thick layer on the surface of the rib, extending like cantilevers to either side of the fracture line. At this stage, however, only the scaffold has been erected, while the defect in the interior has not yet been bridged by bone.

Within the next few months, barring delayed union or nonunion, internal as well as external bony union is accomplished. This is reflected pathologically in fairly complete osseous transformation of cartilage, resorption of residual necrotic bone, and condensation and remodeling of the peripheral callus. Finally reconstruction of the medullary cavity and restoration of the bone marrow (commonly referred to as tubulation) are gradually brought about. A more detailed account of this process of healing and reconstruction may be found in the lucid description of Ham in his textbook of histology.[2] For an informative exposition in pathologic terms, one may have recourse to the discussion by Collins.[6]

Although most appropriately treated fractures go on to uneventful solid bony union in essentially the manner described, with only minor or no residual disability, an appreciable number (notably, in the shaft of the tibia, the forearm bones, and the femoral neck) fail to heal for one reason or another. There are many causes of nonunion, some of them preventable, and much attention is devoted to them in clinical texts.

Inadequate immobilization or immobilization for too short a time is one of the major causes of nonunion. As Watson-Jones has strongly admonished, meticulous attention to adequate immobilization of the affected part is of the utmost importance in attaining a good union. Extensive loss of bone substance, leaving too large a defect to be successfully bridged, may be the factor responsible in some instances. Poor apposition or malposition of fracture fragments, resulting from faulty surgical technique and failure to overcome distraction due to torsion and other powerful muscle stresses, are also common predisposing factors. Interposition of muscle, fascia, and other soft tissues is still another. Inadequate blood supply resulting from rupture or thrombosis of nutrient vessels may result not only in nonunion but also in avascular necrosis of the affected bone (for example, of the femoral head after fracture of the neck). Excessive resorption of fractured bone ends may likewise be responsible for nonunion (Fig. 1-5). Finally, old age, faulty nutrition, serious systemic disease, and a variety of other unfavorable constitutional factors may militate against the production of adequate bony callus on schedule.

In this connection, one may broadly stress the following general requirements:
1. Adequate protein for osseous matrix

Fractures and their sequelae

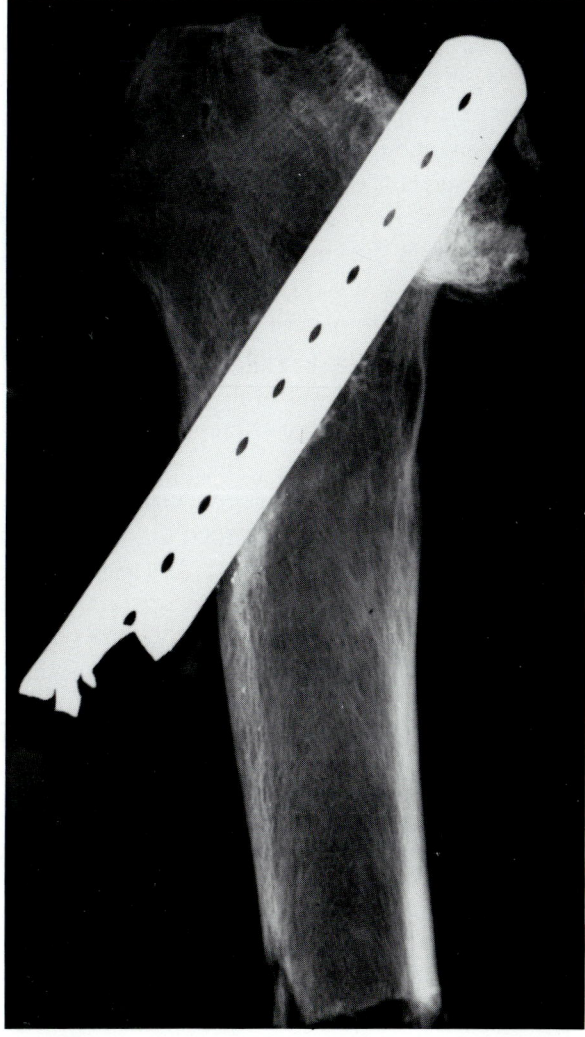

Fig. 1-5. Roentgenogram of an autopsy specimen showing virtually complete resorption of the femoral head following insertion of a nail for transcervical fracture.

  2. Enough vitamin C for adequate deposition of collagen (the connective tissue substrate of osteoid)
  3. Sufficient vitamin D for calcification of osteoid and its conversion to bone
  4. Essential concentrations of readily available calcium and phosphorus (the necessary mineral ingredients)
  5. Adequate phosphatase activity for the effective utilization of calcium and phosphorus at the fracture site
  6. Endocrine activity and interplay conducive to positive calcium balance and active ossification in general

The role of a local tissue inductor substance in promoting osteogenesis has been stressed by Urist, Mazet, and McLean,[7] although their inferences are drawn from transplantation studies in experimental animals.

Another important factor responsible for delayed union, and often for eventual nonunion of open or compound fractures particularly, is *infection.* The problem of healing may be enormously complicated by osteomyelitis with its sequelae of extensive vascular resorption of bone, sequestrum formation and draining sinuses, stiffness of neighboring joints, circulatory impairment of the affected part, and loss of good overlying skin. The practical obstacles entailed in coping with a comminuted infected fracture (in the tibia, for example, following a motorcycle accident) are all too familiar to experienced orthopedic surgeons. By the time the infection has fully subsided, the loss of bone substance may be sufficiently great to raise a formidable problem in surgical reconstruction. It is not unusual in such cases to spend several years in futile attempts to salvage a damaged lower limb.

Whatever the factors responsible for nonunion, if one examines relevant pathologic specimens removed in the course of corrective surgical procedures, one regularly observes that the gap between the fractured bone ends is filled by vascularized fibrous connective tissue (Fig. 1-6, *A* and *B*). Although this fibrous tissue is rich in capillaries and sometimes contains small inactive foci of cartilage, as a rule it shows little or no tendency to active bone formation. The impression one gains is that the process of internal bony bridging has come to an abortive standstill and that, in the absence of surgical intervention (such as grafting or shingling) calculated to stimulate osteogenesis anew, it is likely to remain dormant indefinitely. In time, certain secondary changes may take place within the fibrous connective tissue at a site of nonunion. Specifically, focal deposition of fibrinoid material may be noted, as well as myxoid degeneration and cystic softening, often leading to the formation of a sinuous cleftlike space commonly referred to as a *pseudoarthrosis,* or false joint (Fig. 1-6, *C*). The lining of a pseudoarthrosis may actually come to resemble synovium.

The question of what happens eventually to a necrotic fracture fragment is pertinent here. Basically, this depends upon whether there is an available source of blood supply, which is always an essential requisite for osseous reconstruction. Thus a loose intraarticular fracture fragment (joint body) that has no attachment to the capsule retains its dead bony core indefinitely, although it may

Fig. 1-6. A, Photomicrograph of a specimen from a site of nonunion showing two fracture fragments separated by a tract of fibrous connective tissue. This is permeated by capillaries and contains an occasional small bit of inactive cartilage, but it shows no indication whatsoever of osteogenesis. **B,** Photomicrograph of another comparable specimen showing fibrous union. **C,** Photomicrograph (low magnification) showing pseudoarthrosis at a site of fibrous union of a fracture. Note the sinuous cleft (on the left) within fibrous tissue, which is permeated by capillaries. One fracture fragment is seen on the right; only a small part of the other fragment (on the extreme left) is included in the picture.

Fractures and their sequelae

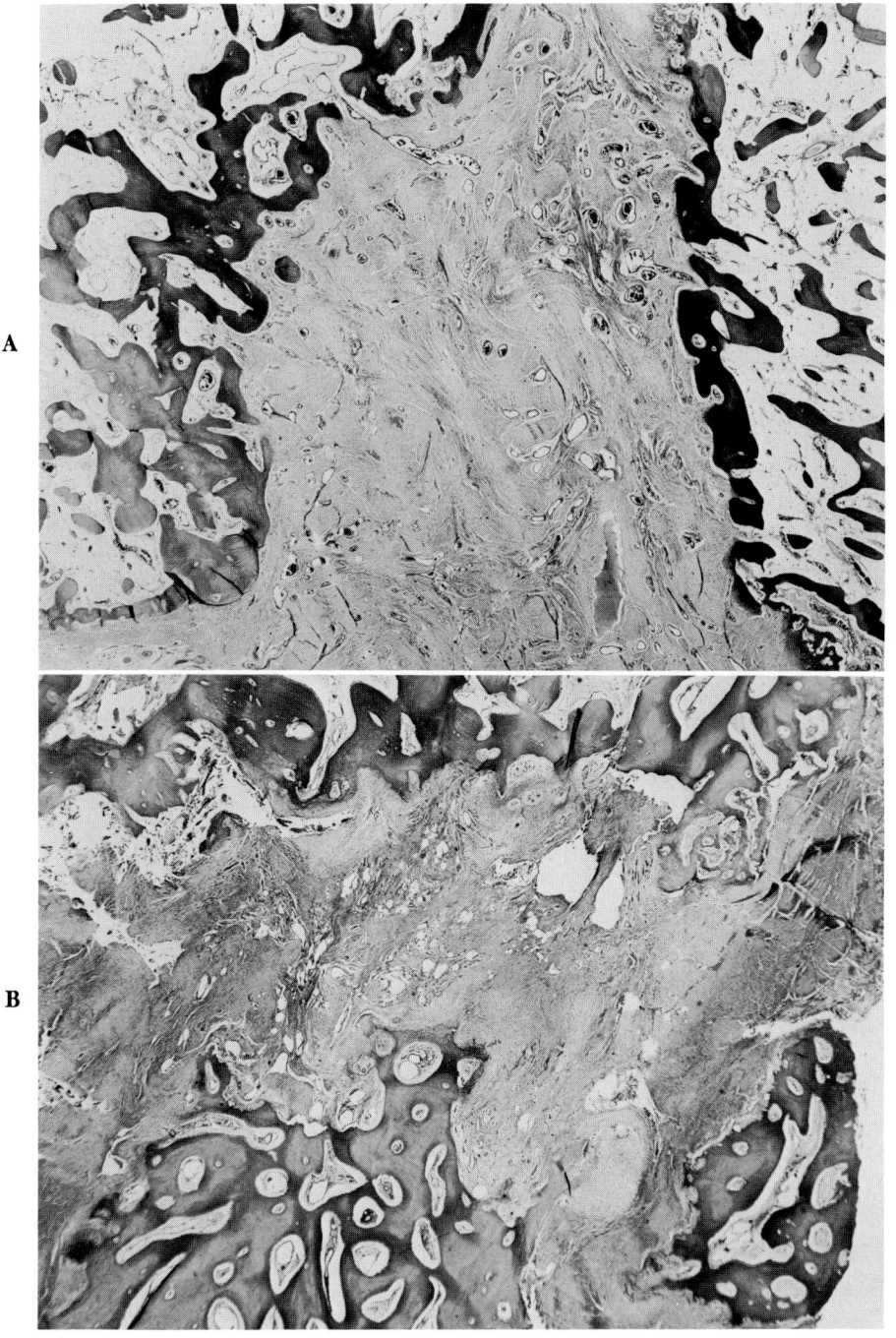

Continued.

Fig. 1-6. For legend see opposite page.

Diseases of bone and joints

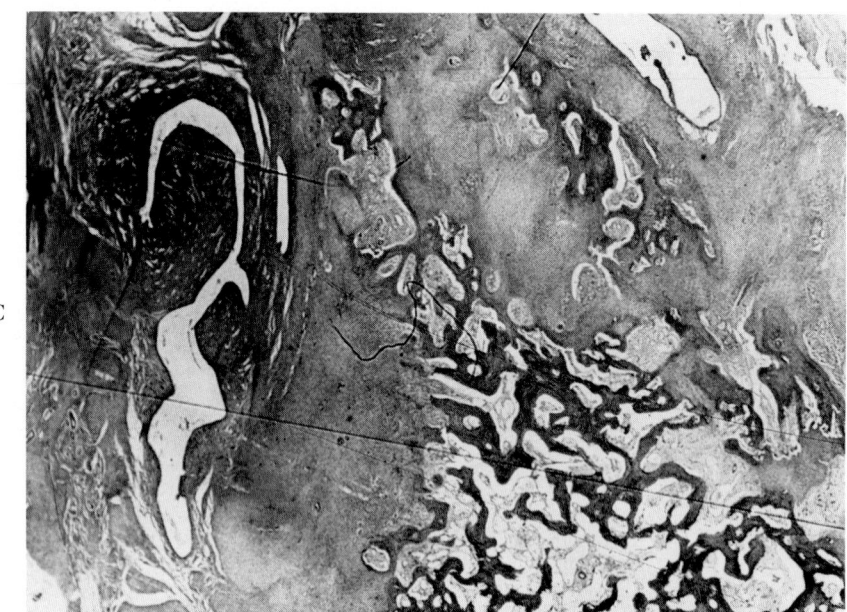

C

Fig. 1-6, cont'd. For legend see p. 8.

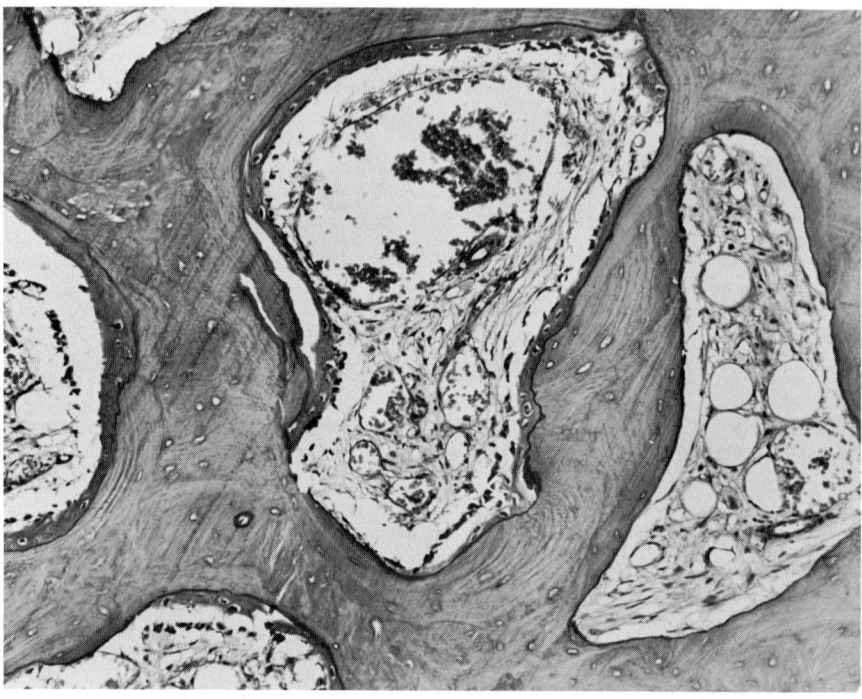

Fig. 1-7. Selected field of a fracture fragment showing avascular necrosis (the lacunae are devoid of osteocytes) and beginning creeping substitution. Note the layer of proliferating osteoblasts and the thin strips of new bone they deposit on top of the dead bone. The marrow shows congestion and some organizing fat necrosis.

Fractures and their sequelae

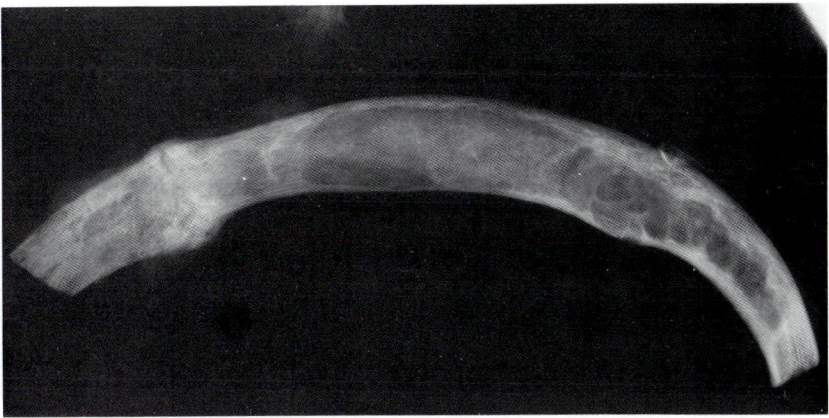

Fig. 1-8. Roentgenogram of an autopsy specimen of a rib containing myeloma and showing a healed pathologic fracture (on the left). The callus has been substantially remodeled.

slowly increase in size through the accretion of cartilage upon its surface (see Figs. 15-4 and 15-5). On the other hand, a necrotic area of bone that is not displaced and that has retained its blood supply (for example, in the femoral head) undergoes reconstruction through gradual creeping replacement or substitution; that is to say, trabeculae of new bone are deposited upon the original dead bone through osteoblastic activity (Fig. 1-7). While this process of osseous reconstruction may be relatively rapid in a child (as in Legg-Perthes' disease), it is likely to be quite slow in an adult, often requiring many years for substantial repair of a sizable area.

As noted, a fracture occurring at the site of a preexisting lesion that has attenuated the bone or otherwise rendered it more vulnerable to injury is generally referred to as a *pathologic fracture*. It is not at all unusual for a break to occur in the thinned cortex overlying a bone tumor, which may be either benign or malignant (Figs. 1-8 and 1-9). Thus the initial clinical manifestation of an enchondroma in a finger phalanx or of a nonosteogenic fibroma in a lower limb bone may be pain referable to cortical infraction. Similarly, fracture may direct attention to a focus of metastatic carcinoma.

Fracture through the attenuated expanded cortex of a bone cyst in the metaphysis, or upper shaft, of a humerus is a fairly common occurrence (Fig. 1-10). A focus of eosinophilic granuloma of bone is very likely to break through the cortex rapidly and extend into the adjacent muscle tissue.

Granulomatous infections, too, may sometimes be responsible for pathologic fracture. In severe rickets and scurvy one may observe epiphyseal separation as a complication. In osteomalacia (the adult counterpart of vitamin D rickets), symmetrical transverse fissure fractures may develop in the lower limb bones and at other sites, giving rise to the picture of Milkman's syndrome (see Fig. 4-7). Transverse fissure fractures may also be observed occasionally in lesions of Paget's

Diseases of bone and joints

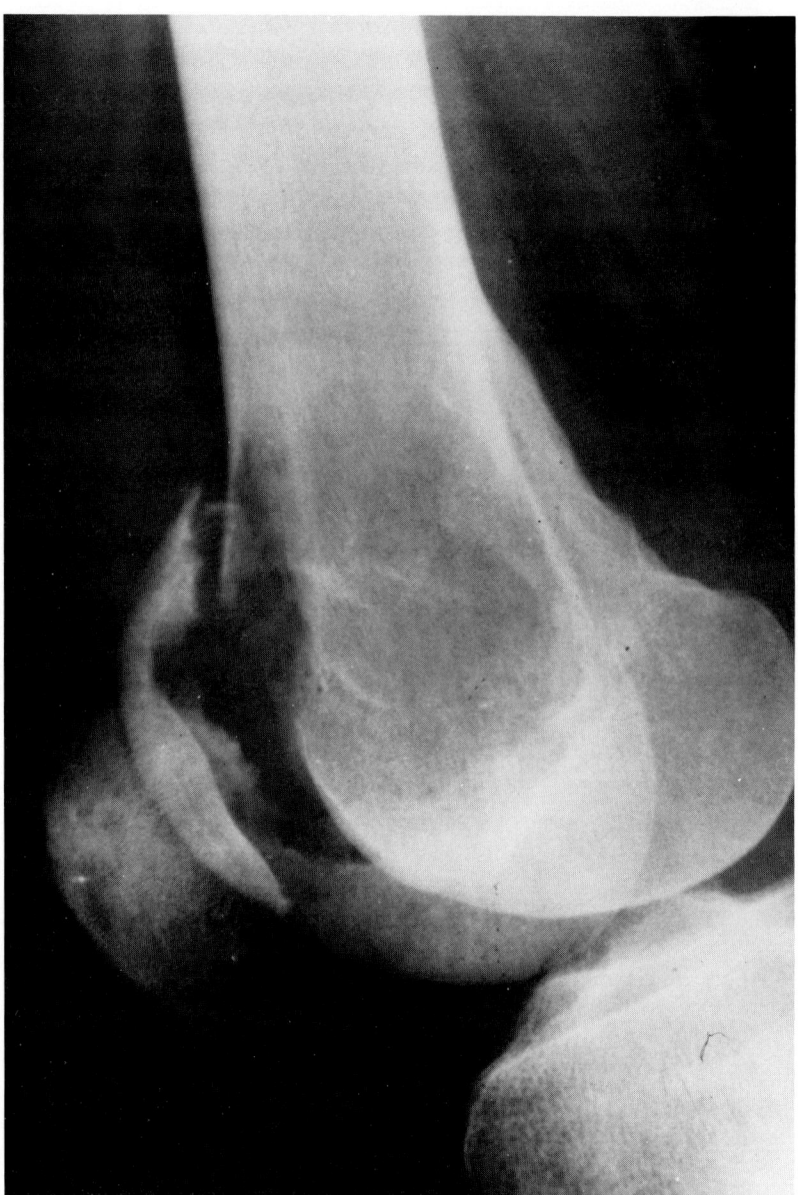

Fig. 1-9. An unusual pathologic fracture—apparently an avulsion fracture—through a lytic lesion in the distal femur, which proved to be a giant cell tumor. The tumor developed insidiously, and the fracture was its initial clinical manifestation.

Fractures and their sequelae

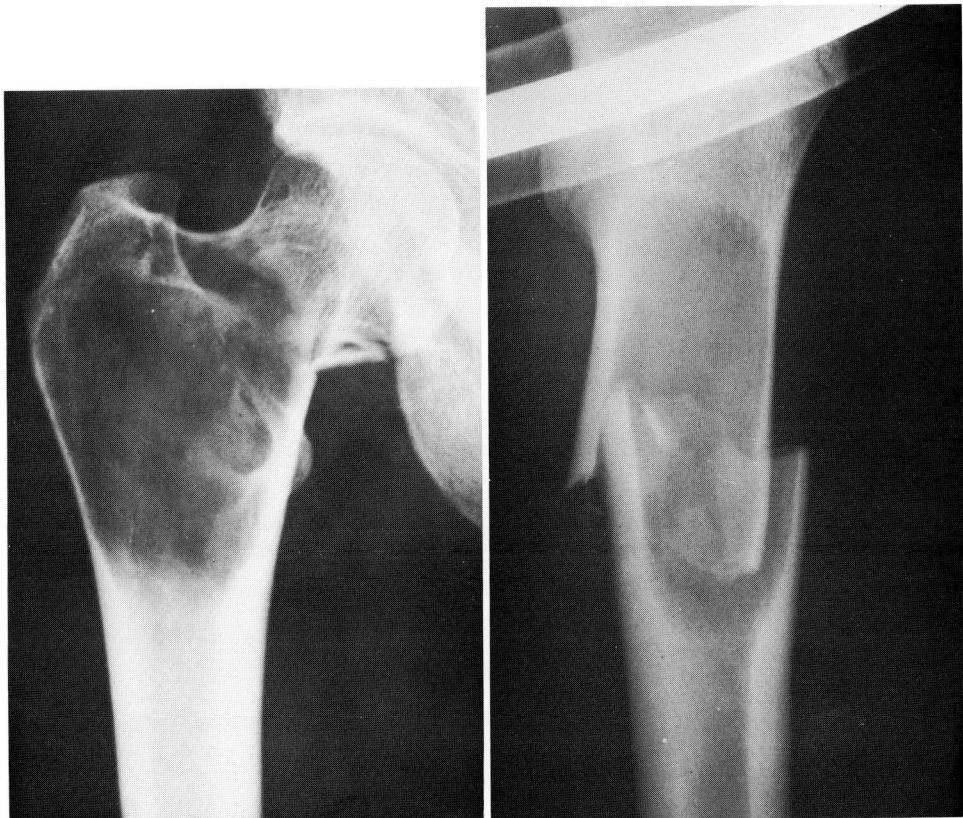

Fig. 1-10　　　　　　　　　　　　　Fig. 1-11

Fig. 1-10. Roentgenogram showing pathologic fracture of the cortex of the neck of the femur (of a young woman, age 22) at the site of a latent solitary unicameral bone cyst. In comparable cysts in the upper humerus, their most common site, such fractures are frequently encountered.

Fig. 1-11. Pathologic fracture through a solitary lesion of fibrous dysplasia in the upper shaft of a femur, where the cortex has become markedly attenuated. Prior to tissue examination, a solitary focus of fibrous dysplasia such as this may be mistaken for a tumor.

Diseases of bone and joints

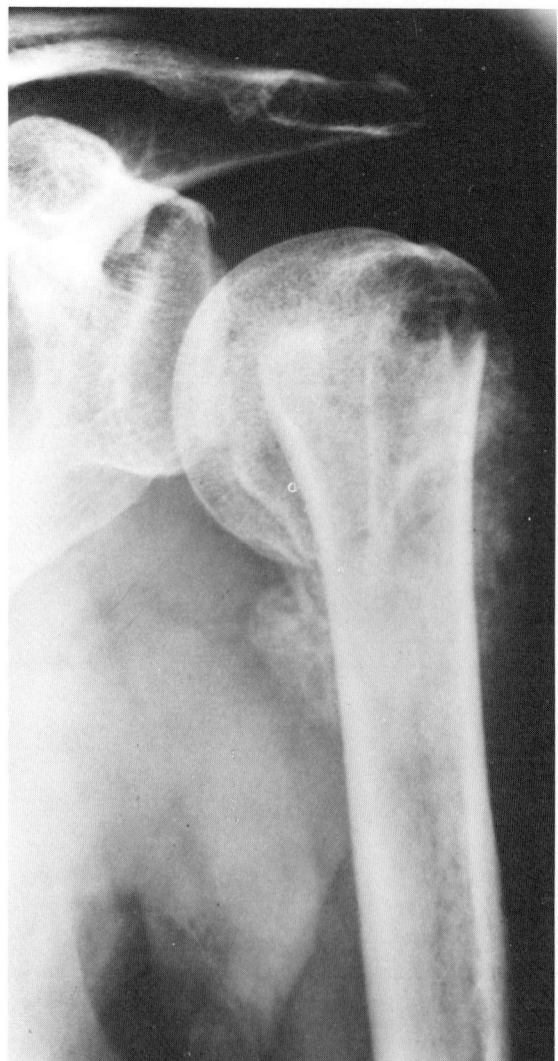

Fig. 1-12. Roentgenogram of an uncommon fracture of the upper humerus in which the distal fragment, represented by the upper shaft, has telescoped into the head and neck of the humerus (this was demonstrated in other views). The distal fragment is surrounded by callus.

disease, especially in the tibia. Extensively resorbed bones in hyperparathyroidism are likewise predisposed to fracture. As for the vertebral column in particular, compression fractures may be a result of any condition leading to advanced demineralization, be it metastatic carcinoma, multiple myeloma, osteoporosis, or sprue.

The articular bone ends in a neuropathic joint are particularly susceptible to multiple fractures. This is true also in hereditary ochronosis, an inbred metabolic disorder. To cite still another instance in point, lesions of bone in certain of the systemic anomalies of skeletal development, especially osteogenesis imperfecta and sometimes fibrous dysplasia (Fig. 1-11), are likewise vulnerable to minor injury. Also, in marble bone disease, the affected bones, though abnormally dense, are brittle. There are many other conditions in which pathologic fracture may occur, but it is not feasible in this brief discussion to list every circumstance.

REFERENCES

1. Morris, J. M.: Fatigue fractures; a clinical study, Springfield, Ill., 1967, Charles C Thomas, Publisher.
2. Ham, A. W.: Histology, ed. 6, Philadelphia, 1969, J. B. Lippincott Co.
3. Maximow, A. A., and Bloom, W.: A textbook of histology, ed. 9, Philadelphia, 1968, W. B. Saunders Co.
4. Botterell, E. H., and King, E. J.: Phosphatase in fractures, Lancet **228**:1267-1270, 1935.
5. Cohen, J., and Lacroix, P.: Bone and cartilage formation by periosteum, J. Bone Joint Surg. **37A**:717-730, 1955.
6. Collins, D. H.: Pathology of bone, London, 1966, Butterworth & Co. (Publishers) Ltd.
7. Urist, M. R., Mazet, R. Jr., and McLean, F. C.: Pathogenesis and treatment of delayed union and non-union, J. Bone Joint Surg. **36A**:931-968, 1954.

chapter 2

Systemic anomalies of skeletal development

When one considers that there are more than 200 bones in the skeleton and that their embryologic development is inherently complex both genetically and biochemically, it is not surprising that the number of congenital anomalies of all kinds is great. With reference to the hand, for example, arachnodactyly, brachydactyly, syndactyly, hypodactyly, and polydactyly are only some of the developmental aberrations observed. Similarly, a wide range of congenital deformities is known to occur also in the foot, hip, knee, vertebral column, and skull, as well as in other skeletal parts. Everthing that may possibly go wrong apparently does so at one time or another. While these localized anomalies are of practical moment, especially to geneticists, pediatricians, and orthopedic surgeons, we are concerned here more particularly with widespread or systemic developmental disorders of the skeleton.

There are more than a dozen well-recognized systemic developmental anomalies, and there are undoubtedly many others that, because of their comparative rarity or the paucity of available biopsy material, have not yet been clearly delineated pathologically. The pertinent conditions that will be surveyed briefly in this chapter are fibrous dysplasia of bone, hereditary multiple exostosis, skeletal enchondromatosis, osteopetrosis, osteogenesis imperfecta, achondroplasia, Morquio's disease, osteopoikilosis, cleidocranial dysostosis, gargoylism, melorheostosis, progressive diaphyseal dysplasia, and monomelic medullary osteosclerosis.

Some of these conditions vary in extent and severity and, accordingly, may affect a single bone (monostotic), several bones (which may or may not comprise a functional unit), one or more limb buds, or the major part of the skeleton. Others are universal in their skeletal effects. In several anomalies listed—fibrous dysplasia, skeletal enchondromatosis, osteogenesis imperfecta, and gargoylism—the inborn error of development, while predominantly skeletal in its impact, is genetically complex and may have its reflection in certain extraskeletal anomalies as well. In others, it is well known from study of family pedigrees that there is a significant hereditary factor. Thus the genetic defect is transmitted as a mendelian dominant in achondroplasia, cleidocranial dysostosis, osteogenesis imperfecta, and multiple exostosis. Familial incidence has also been noted in gargoylism and osteopetrosis.

As for the time of appearance of the anomalies, in some the skeletal alterations may already be clinically obvious in the neonate, as in achondroplasia, osteogenesis imperfecta, and osteopetrosis. In others the abnormalities may not become manifest for some years after birth, as in multiple exostosis, Morquio's disease, and the milder expressions of fibrous dysplasia of bone.

A few general remarks concerning nomenclature seem to be indicated in the interest of clarity. For virtually all of the conditions under consideration, several, if not many, designations have been employed by various authors. While one of necessity must be preferred for the purpose of discussion, the more common alternative names will be mentioned for convenient orientation. I do not favor the use of eponyms, although in dealing with a disorder like Morquio's disease (in which the eponym enjoys general usage, whereas the suggested alternatives are not even well known) there is little choice.

Further, the use of vague, broad categories such as chondrodystrophy or dyschondroplasia will be avoided, since their use impedes general understanding of the conditions in question. Dyschondroplasia is another name for cartilage dysplasia, but it must be recognized that there are at least six common skeletal developmental anomalies that may be regarded as cartilage dysplasias of various types: multiple exostosis, skeletal enchondromatosis, osteopetrosis, achondroplasia, Morquio's disease, and (sometimes) fibrous dysplasia. For one to speak, therefore, of dyschondroplasia (or chondrodystrophy) without specifying the particular disorder he is describing is likely to be more confusing than helpful.

It is hardly possible within the limited scope of this monograph to describe the full picture of each of the disorders considered. (For convenient clinical orientation, the reader may have recourse to the splendidly illustrated atlas of Sir Thomas Fairbank.[1]) In this concise survey, the emphasis will be upon the essential pathologic features, insofar as they are recognized, as a basis for better understanding of the condition. Where roentgenograms are helpful in graphic illustration, they will be freely utilized.

FIBROUS DYSPLASIA OF BONE

With the possible exception of hereditary multiple exostosis, fibrous dysplasia is probably the most frequently encountered anomaly of skeletal development. Considerable interest has been evinced in the condition, and the pertinent literature of the past 30 years has grown too voluminous to be catalogued here.

In 1938, I directed attention to the distinctive pathologic character of the skeletal lesions and introduced the name "polyostotic fibrous dysplasia" to designate this appropriately.[2] The qualifying adjective "polyostotic" was later dropped when it became increasingly evident that often only a single bone or a portion of one bone is involved (monostotic).

Diseases of bone and joints

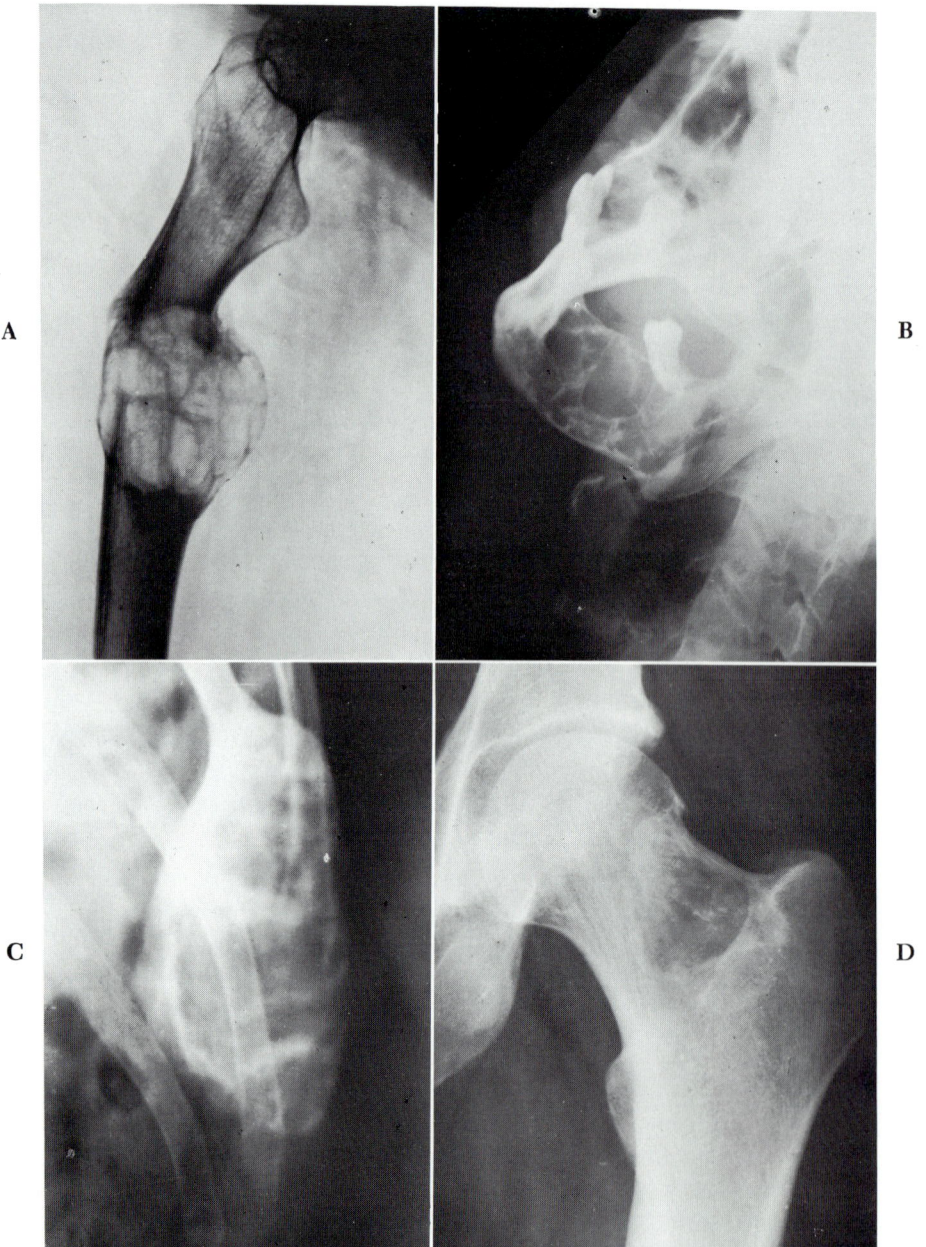

Fig. 2-1. Roentgenograms illustrating the appearance of monostotic lesions of fibrous dysplasia in various common locations. The lesions in **A** and **C** were thought clinically to be tumors and were resected as such. The lesion in the mandible, **B**, was the only one recognized as fibrous dysplasia prior to tissue examination.

Systemic anomalies of skeletal development

Such solitary foci are much more common than is generally appreciated.[3] They are encountered mainly in the ribs, the large limb bones, and the jaw and skull bones. Solitary foci are often clinically silent; they may be discovered following an injury or in the course of roentgenographic examination of the part for some other reason (Fig. 2-1). The gross and microscopic appearance of such solitary lesions is not essentially different from that of comparable lesions in cases showing more extensive involvement, and there is every reason to believe that monostotic and polyostotic lesions of fibrous dysplasia are quantitatively different expressions of the same disorder.

When more than one focus of fibrous dysplasia is present, the involved bones are likely to be solely or predominantly on one side of the body and are often confined to a single lower or upper limb bud. Occasional patients may exhibit the severe expression of the disorder in which a major part of the skeleton is affected, and the resulting deformities and disability then become manifest early in childhood (Fig. 2-2). The occurrence in such cases of associated extraskeletal changes, particularly blotchy cutaneous hyperpigmentation and certain endocrine abnormalities (notably pubertas praecox in females), was noted in the 1930's by Goldhamer, Borak and Doll, McCune and Bruch,[4] and Albright and his colleagues.[5,6] The last group particularly publicized these more dramatic cases in children, presenting various extraskeletal abnormalities in addition to widespread severe skeletal alterations. In fact, this clinical picture came to be designated by many, both in the United States and abroad as *Albright's syndrome*, although Albright himself subsequently recommended that the name "fibrous dysplasia" be generally adopted to apply to all instances of the disorder, irrespective of their severity.

In regard to those extraskeletal abnormalities, I had occasion in 1942, in a discussion of the steadily expanding literature on the subject,[7] to point out that in a number of instances hyperthyroidism, ephemeral premature skeletal growth and maturation, and cardiorenal congenital defects had also been observed. This survey is still useful for general orientation, as are the excellent reviews by Falconer, Cope, and Robb-Smith,[8] Jaffe,[9,10] and others. The recent literature contains case reports of fibrous dysplasia in both males and females who also had a wide variety of endocrine abnormalities including thyrotoxicosis, acromegaly, Cushing's syndrome, and pleuriglandular disorders.[11]

When one considers the condition as a whole, there is much to support the view that fibrous dysplasia has its basis in a genetically complex defect of development in which the clinical picture reflecting the skeletal lesions may be amplified at times by various extraskeletal abnormalities. The skeletal lesions result apparently from perverted activity of the bone-forming mesenchyme. This is manifested in replacement of the spongiosa and in filling of the medullary cavity of affected bone sites by a peculiar fibrous tissue in which trabeculae (or spherules or curlicues) of poorly calcified fiber bone are formed by osseous metaplasia (Fig. 2-3). Changus[12] has demonstrated that the dysplastic connective tissue contains abundant alkaline phosphatase, which is what one might expect.

Diseases of bone and joints

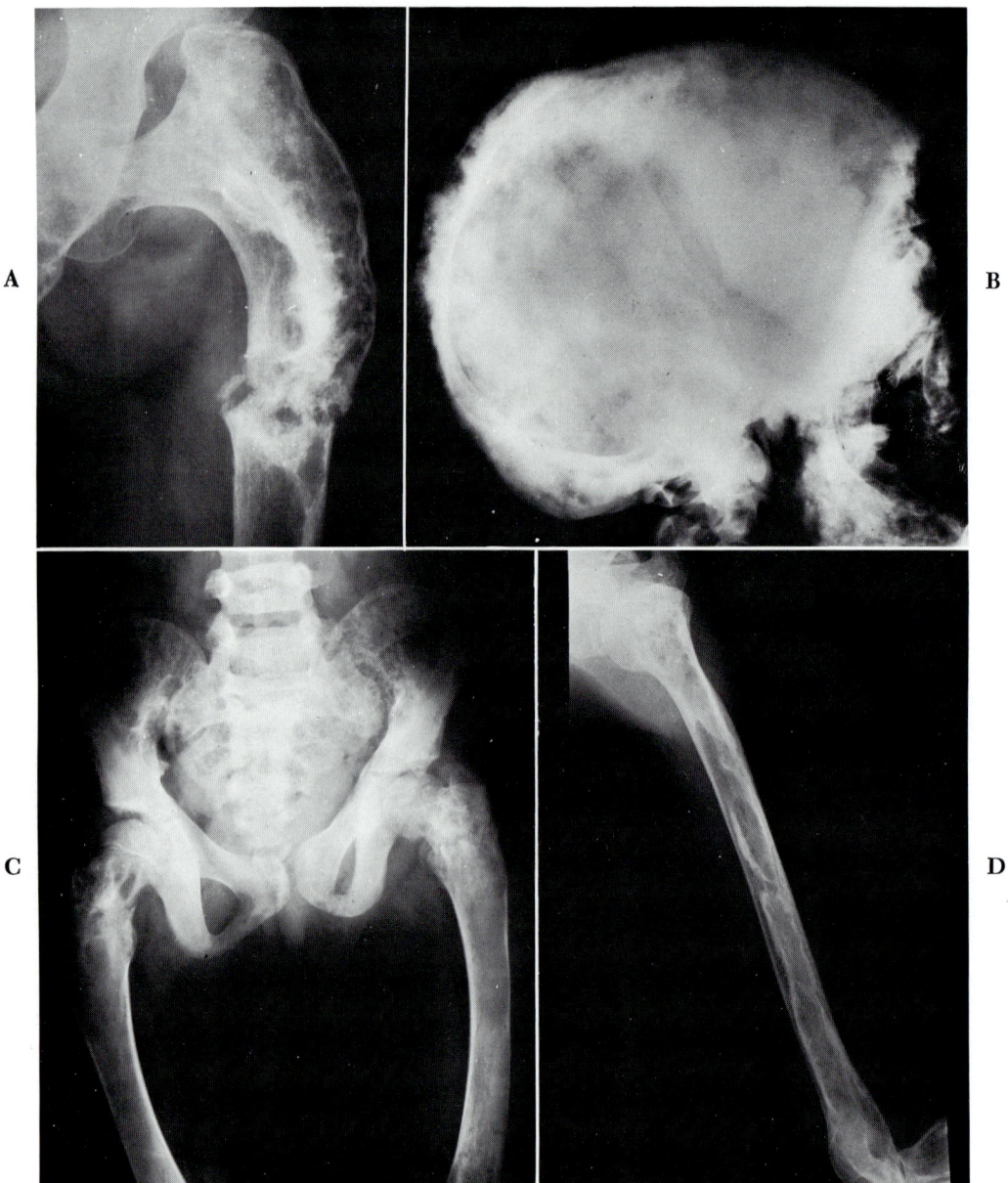

Fig. 2-2. Roentgenograms illustrating polyostotic fibrous dysplasia. If one is familiar with their appearance, the lesions in the femur, **A** and **C**, can be readily identified as fibrous dysplasia. The lesion in the humerus, **D**, might suggest enchondromatosis. The changes in the skull, **B**, while consistent with fibrous dysplasia, could conceivably suggest Paget's disease or leontiasis ossea.

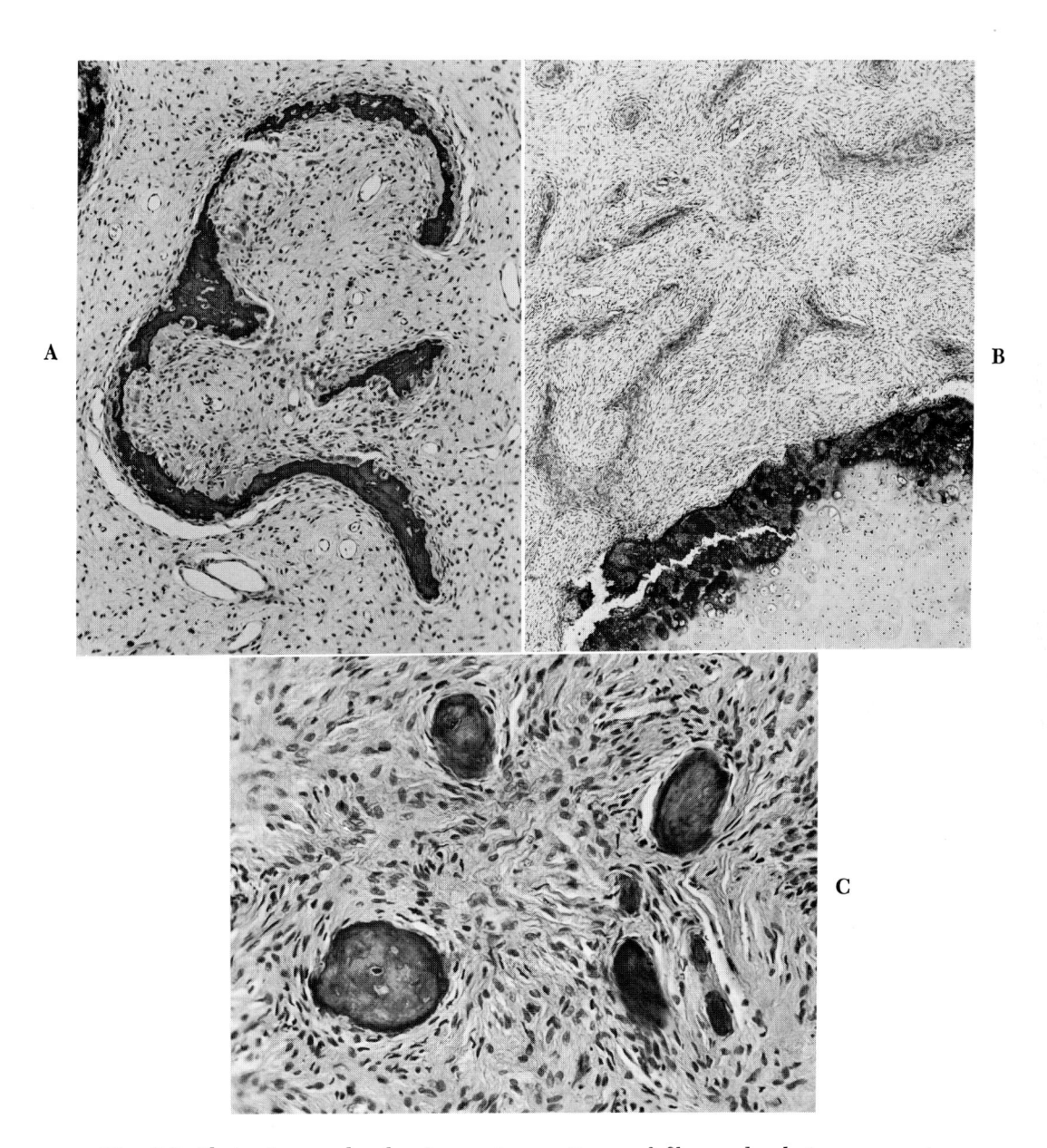

Fig. 2-3. Photomicrographs showing various patterns of fibrous dysplasia, as seen in biopsy specimens. **B** also presents an island of hyaline cartilage, calcified at its periphery (lower right). Note the delicate spindle connective tissue cells and the fact that none of the curlicues (trabeculae or spherules) of bone are rimmed by osteoblasts.

This osteogenic potential is not always realized, however, and some fields may be predominantly collagenous and manifest comparatively little deposition of new bone.

In occasional instances of fibrous dysplasia, more or less prominent islands of hyaline cartilage (remote from cartilage plate regions) may also be observed (Fig. 2-3, B). This finding suggests a possible genetic relationship between fibrous dysplasia of bone and skeletal enchondromatosis.

In cases showing polyostotic involvement, the long bones of the lower extremity are most frequently affected, but those of the upper extremity and the skull, ribs, pelvis, phalanges, and other bones may also be involved. Extensively involved, weight-bearing bones like the femurs tend to become expanded, bowed, appreciably shortened, and otherwise deformed; they are then vulnerable to pathologic fracture (Fig. 2-2, A). Extensive calvarial involvement may lead eventually in some instances to Paget-like thickening (Fig. 2-2, B), and comparable involvement of the facial bones may occasionally give rise to a clinical picture resembling leontiasis ossea. Epiphysioid bones (carpals and tarsals) and bones preformed in membrane may likewise be affected. The aforementioned changes result, as noted, in more or less prominent widening of affected bones, thinning of their cortices, and replacement of the cancellous bone and bone marrow by a peculiar, rubbery, whitish, somewhat gritty connective tissue, which may show partial cystic softening as a secondary degenerative change, especially in lesions of long standing. At times, small nests of foam cells or foci of giant cell reaction to blood extravasation may be encountered.

By way of differential diagnosis, it should be noted that the literature records instances of adult patients with fairly extensive fibrous dysplasia of bone who were thought to have hyperparathyroidism and who were subjected to exploration for parathyroid tumor. Solitary foci, on the other hand, may be mistaken clinically for tumors and, as such, treated more vigorously than necessary, for example, by block excision (Fig. 2-1, A). I have observed material from instances of involvement of the maxilla in children and teen-agers in which the upper jaw was widely resected in the mistaken belief that a neoplasm was present (Fig. 2-4, A). The surgical removal of monostotic lesions is usually elective rather than mandatory. If such a lesion, however, is still expanding (in a jaw bone, for example), painful, cosmetically deforming, or prone to pathologic fracture, it may be desirable to curet it thoroughly and to pack the defect with bone chips.

The incidence of sarcomatous change in skeletal lesions of fibrous dysplasia should be noted. Many case reports[13] have now amply confirmed the old observation of Coley and Stewart[14] that this may happen, and these observations have been compiled by Schwartz and Alpert.[15] Malignant change may develop without prior irradiation, it may be observed in monostotic as well as polyostotic lesions, and it apparently occurs most often in bones of the craniofacial region and in large limb bones. It should be emphasized, however, that this complication is less common than it is in Paget's disease and that its overall incidence appears to be on the order of a fraction of 1%. I have observed only a single in-

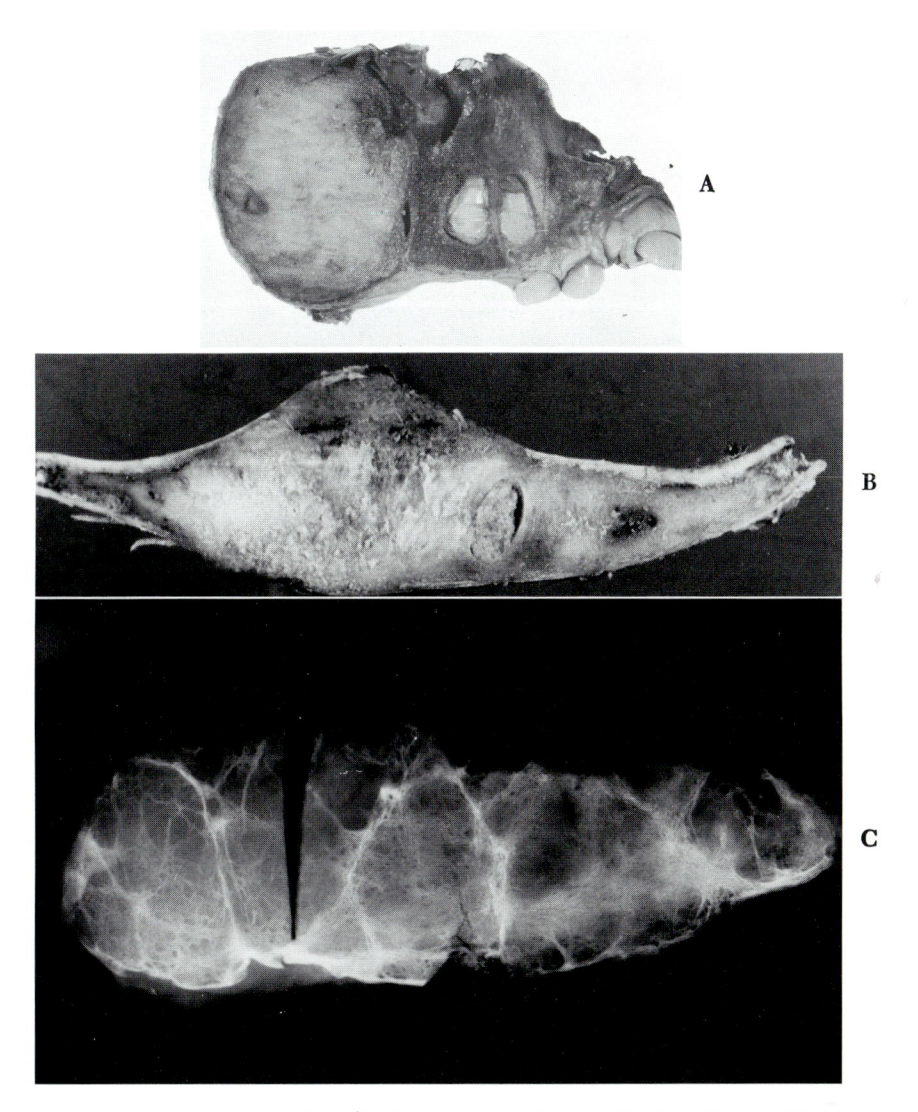

Fig. 2-4. **A**, Photograph (actual size) of a portion of a maxilla in a 7-year-old boy, resected (apparently without frozen section) on the premise that a tumor was present. Review of the sections showed the lesion to be a focus of fibrous dysplasia. **B**, Photograph (actual size) of a lesion of fibrous dysplasia in a rib of a 35-year-old man, which was discovered as an incidental finding in the course of roentgenographic examination of the chest. **C**, Roentgenogram of another resected specimen of a rib showing fibrous dysplasia. Note the expansion and thinning of the cortex. The pseudotrabeculation reflects the projection of ridges on the inner aspect of the cortical shell.

Diseases of bone and joints

stance of spontaneous malignant change in fibrous dysplasia in recent years. This tumor developed insidiously in a femur, and proved to be an osteogenic sarcoma.

HEREDITARY MULTIPLE EXOSTOSIS
(multiple cartilaginous exostoses; diaphyseal aclasis)

Hereditary multiple exostosis is one of the best known and most common systemic anomalies of skeletal development.[1,16] Detailed information in regard to its pathologic features dates back to Virchow and von Recklinghausen. Recognition of a factor of inheritance through the study of family pedigrees goes back even further, although it was not until 1925 that the genetic pattern of hereditary transmission was fully elucidated on a large scale by Stocks and Barrington.[17] Some of the other names under which relevant case material has been reported are multiple cartilaginous exostoses, multiple exostoses, hereditary deforming chondrodysplasia, and diaphyseal aclasis. The last designation is preferred by British investigators following the lead of Keith.[18] The term "hereditary multiple exostosis" is recommended by Jaffe,[19] whose detailed discussion of the distinctive pathologic changes of the disorder and of its clinical problems is still valuable for basic orientation.

The characteristic feature of hereditary multiple exostosis is the presence of numerous, often widespread, knobby cartilage-capped bony protrusions. These are most prominent in the metaphyseal regions of the long bones (Fig. 2-5) but may appear also on the ribs, scapulae, vertebrae, and even hand and foot bones. These osteocartilaginous exostoses apparently have their basis in abnormal foci of cartilage formation by the cambium layer of the periosteum.[20] At these sites, the cortex of the affected bone is defective. At the same time, as Keith[18] has emphasized, the ends of the affected limb bones tend to become broadened and blunted, apparently from defective remodeling by the periosteum (Fig. 2-5, *B*). Severely affected patients show appreciable shortening of their limb bones, and often a characteristic bowing deformity of the forearms is noted (Fig. 2-6).

Detailed information in regard to the gross and microscopic appearance of osteocartilaginous exostoses (osteochondromas) and their manner of growth may be found in discussions by Jaffe[19] and Bethge,[21] and in Chapter 4 of my monograph, *Bone Tumors*.[22] The last deals mainly with solitary osteochondroma, which may be regarded as the common, limited expression of hereditary multiple exostosis.

An osteocartilaginous exostosis is covered by thickened fibrous periosteum, beneath which there is a cap of hyaline cartilage several millimeters in thickness (Fig. 2-7). The lesion grows by endochondral ossification and ceases to enlarge when its growth zone is closed off by a thin plate of bone. Subsequently, the cartilage cap tends to involute, but remnants of it may persist. These retain a latent capacity for reactivated growth, affording an explanation for the occasional development of peripheral chondrosarcoma.

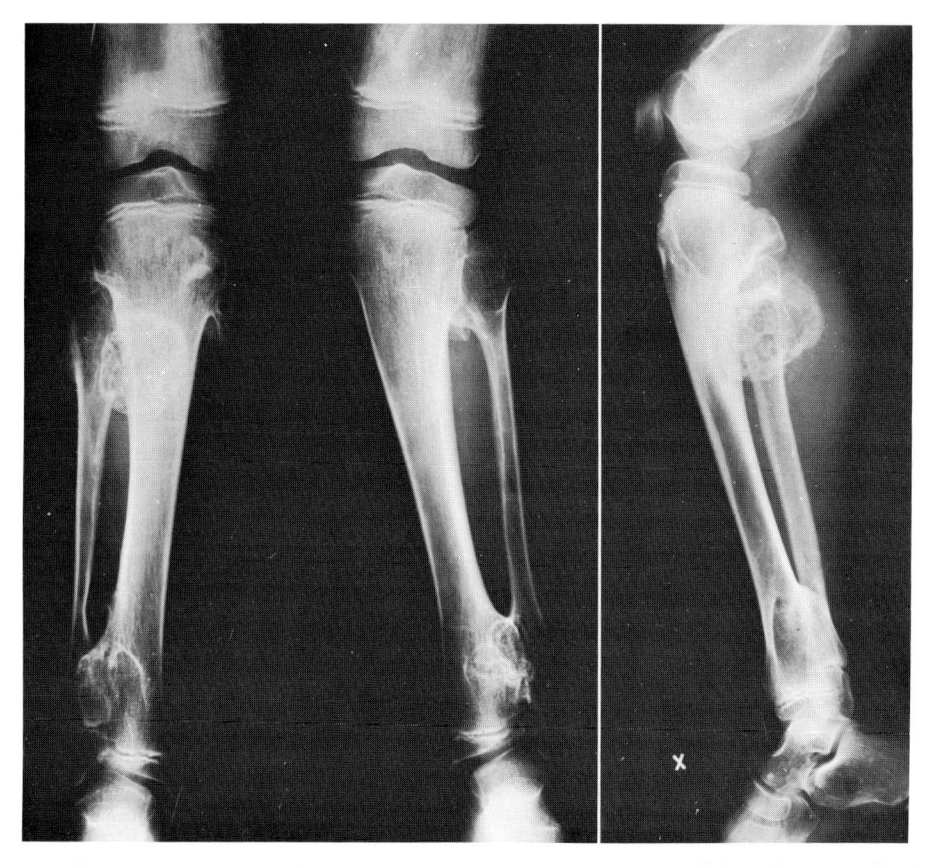

Fig. 2-5. Roentgenograms from two representative instances of hereditary multiple exostosis.

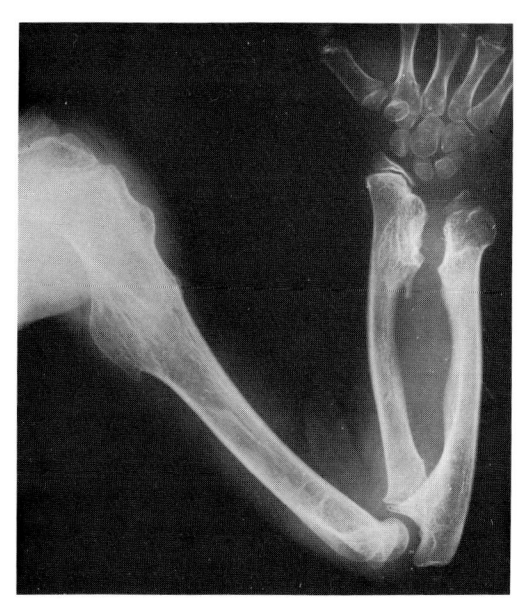

Fig. 2-6. Roentgenogram of an involved upper limb in multiple exostosis. Note the characteristic bowing deformity of the forearm bones.

Diseases of bone and joints

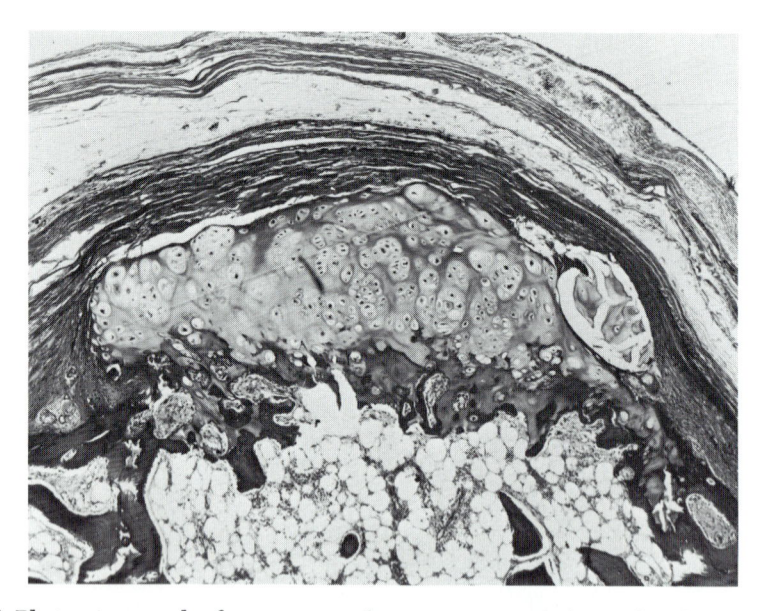

Fig. 2-7. Photomicrograph of an osteocartilaginous exostosis (osteochondroma) showing a portion of its cartilage cap. (×40.) The connective tissue covering the cartilage cap was continuous with the periosteum of the affected bone. The cartilage cap, only a few millimeters in thickness, is closed on its undersurface by a plate of bone, effecting cessation of growth of the exostosis (by endochondral ossification). The marrow in this instance is fatty, although a few small myeloid nests are present.

A

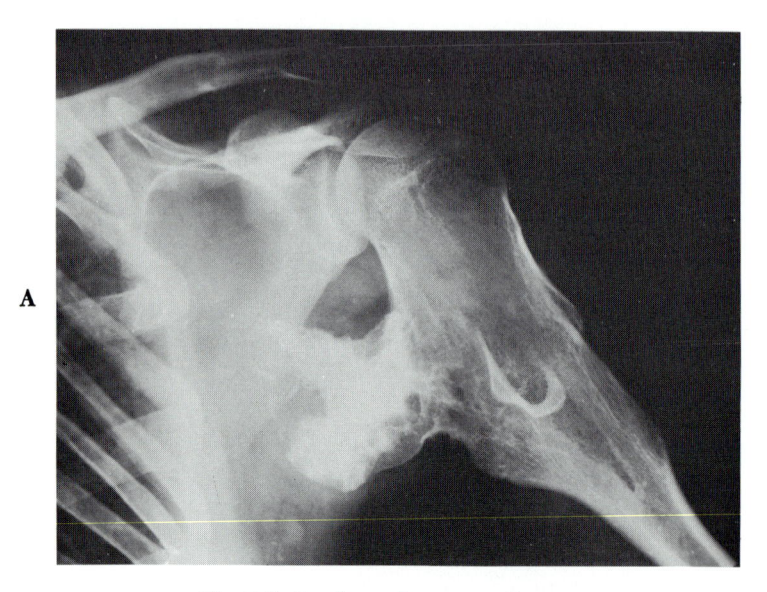

Fig. 2-8. For legend see opposite page.

Systemic anomalies of skeletal development

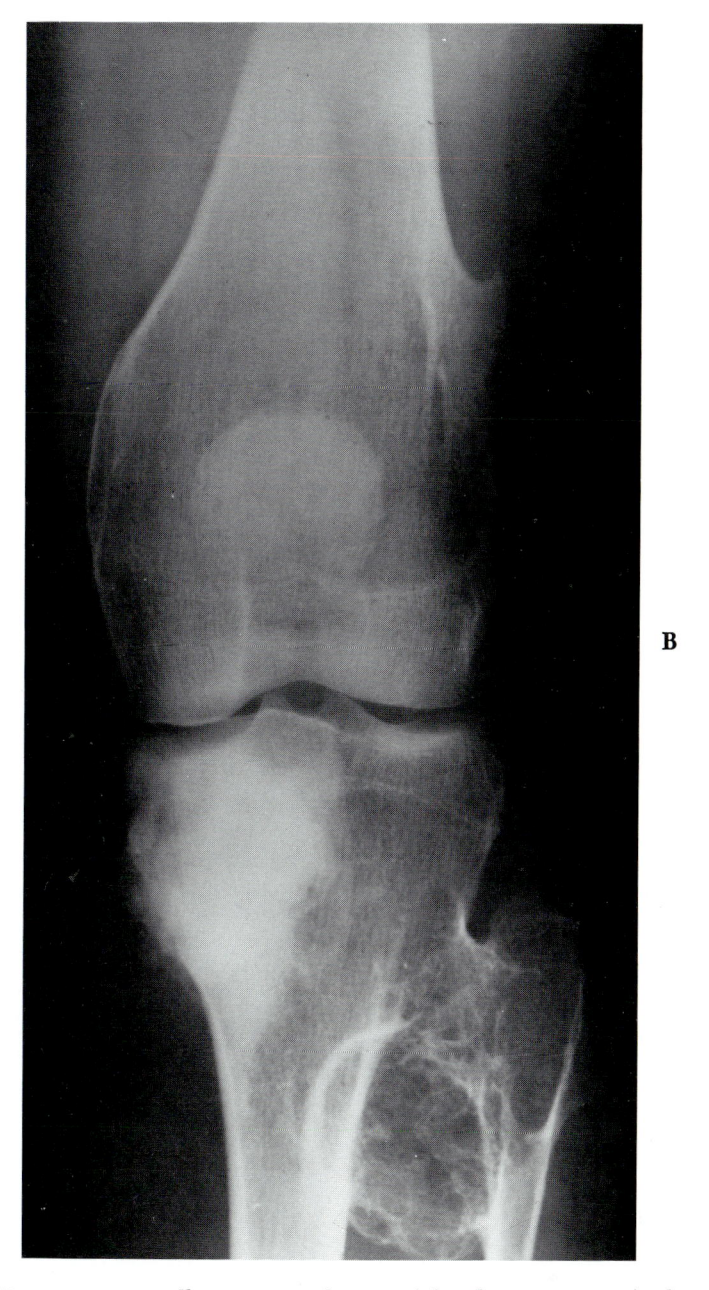

Fig. 2-8. A, Roentgenogram illustrating malignant (chondrosarcomatous) change in an exostosis on the upper humerus. The actively growing cartilage of the tumor is heavily calcified and ossified. The ostrocartilagenous exostosis was known to have been present for many years (note the broadening and blunting of the upper humerus). **B,** Roentgenogram of the knee region of an adult woman who had been followed for multiple exostosis for many years. She developed an osteogenic sarcoma in the upper tibia (for which above-knee amputation was performed). This tumor, unlike the chondrosarcoma illustrated in **A,** was fortuitous and unrelated to hereditary multiple exostosis.

Diseases of bone and joints

The incidence of malignant (chondrosarcomatous) change in multiple exostosis through activated growth of the cartilage caps of one or more protuberances is sufficienty high to be of some concern (Fig. 2-8, A). A precise long-term statistical estimate of this hazard is not available, but it apparently exceeds 10%. In dealing with solitary exostoses, on the other hand, this complication is seldom encountered, and its incidence is probably less than 1%.

SKELETAL ENCHONDROMATOSIS *(Ollier's disease)*

In skeletal enchondromatosis, central hyaline cartilage tumors are found in multiple sites. Clinical manifestations of this disease often appear early in childhood, although no hereditary factor has been demonstrated. The skeletal lesions are occasionally associated with hemangiomas of the skin (so-called Maffucci's syndrome). An informative account of the condition may be found in a survey of some eighteen instances by Carleton, Elkington, Greenfield, and Robb-Smith.[23] These authors called attention also to the incidence of anomalies other than vascular hamartomas: vitiligo (in two instances) and facial asymmetry (in six). Another well-documented report is that of Hunter and Wiles,[24] which is useful for its extensive bibliography of the older literature.

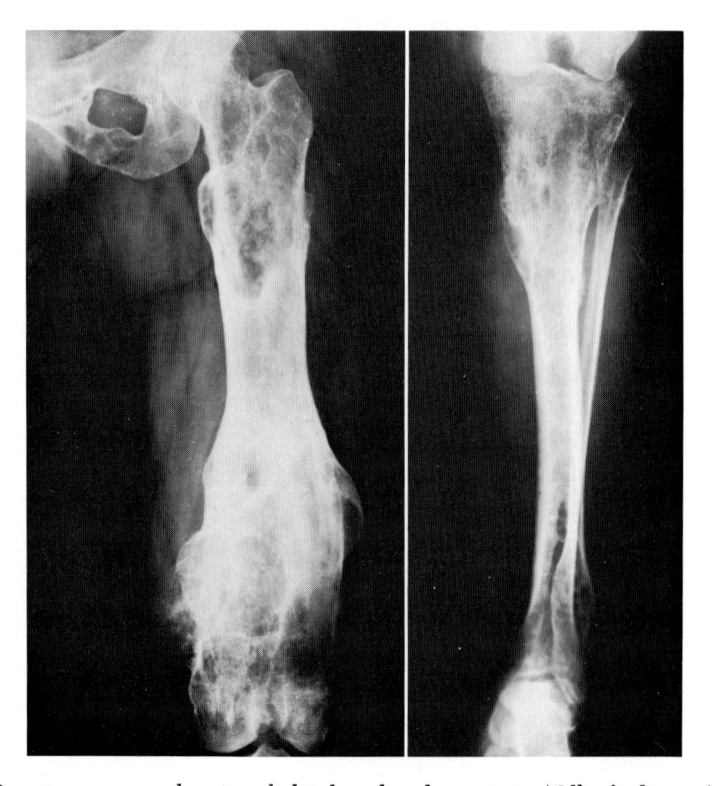

Fig. 2-9. Roentgenograms showing skeletal enchondromatosis (Ollier's disease) involving a lower limb. The patient was a young adult who had been aware of the condition since early childhood. Biopsy of the expanded lower femur failed to show evidence of malignant change.

Systemic anomalies of skeletal development

Depending upon the severity of the condition, the enchondromas may be confined to the bones of a single digit, to several or all of the digits of one or both hands, or to the bones of a single limb (usually a lower limb); or, if more extensive, they may involve many bones in both upper and lower limbs (Figs. 2-9 to 2-11). With widespread skeletal involvement, one often observes unilateral or predominantly unilateral distribution, and these instances are often referred to as *Ollier's disease*. There is also a strong tendency to appreciable, if not marked, shortening of affected limbs, much more so than is usually observed in fibrous dysplasia. The areas of cartilage growth may be limited to the ends of the long bones or may involve the entire shaft. These areas present roentgenographically as peculiar, broadened, rarefied defects. As a rule there is little tendency to calcific stippling or ossification before adolescence. For further details of the roentgenographic picture, the reader is referred to the exquisite illustrations in Fairbank's atlas.[1]

If one examines a biopsy of an individual lesion in skeletal enchondromatosis, it appears more cellular, as a rule, than a solitary enchondroma. This reflects a greater growth potential, and so it is not unusual to observe malignant change

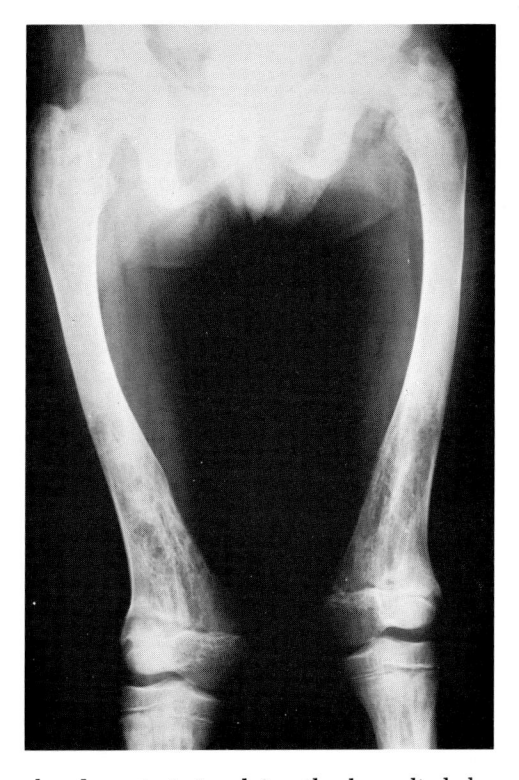

Fig. 2-10. Skeletal enchondromatosis involving the large limb bones of both lower extremities of a child. Note the symmetrical involvement, with bowing of the femora and flaring of their lower metaphyses. These alterations must be distinguished from those of fibrous dysplasia.

Diseases of bone and joints

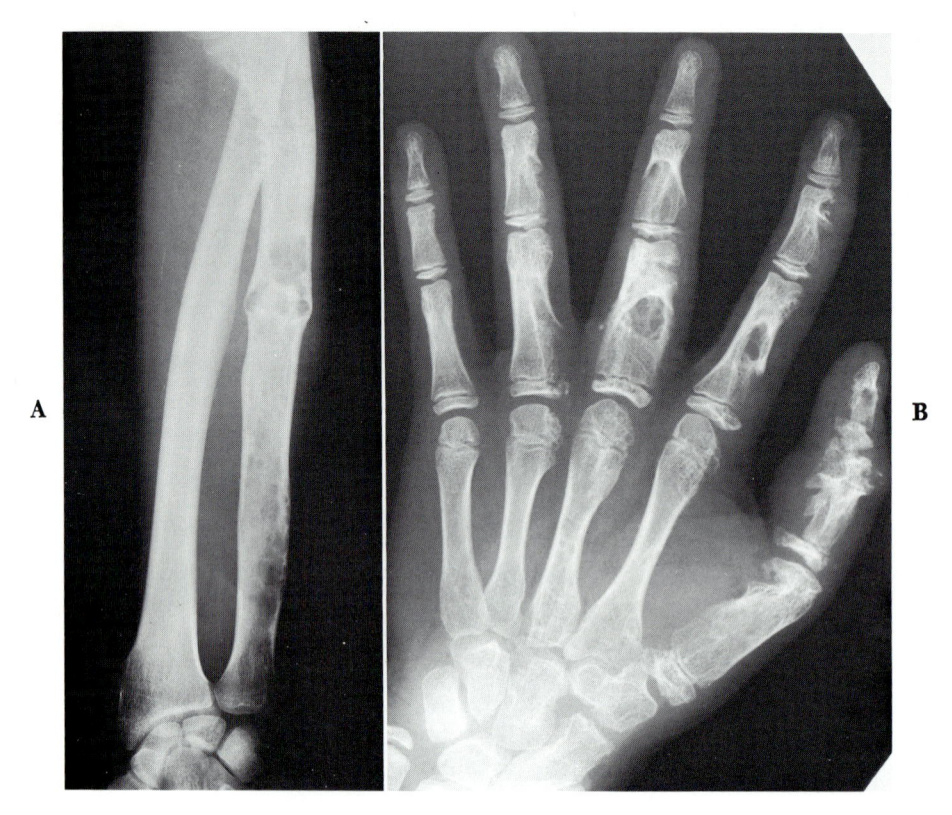

Fig. 2-11. **A,** Extensive involvement of an ulna in enchondromatosis. Some of the hand bones (not shown) were also affected. **B,** Skeletal enchondromatosis (Ollier's disease) affecting the bones of a hand. In such cases, one must be on the alert for possible malignant change in one or more foci.

during adolescence or early adult life. Thus, of the eighteen cases surveyed by Carleton and his associates,[23] sarcomatous change had occurred in four, and in three others this was "possibly true." While statistically valid estimates are difficult to arrive at, it is obvious that the hazard of chondrosarcoma in patients with skeletal enchondromatosis, even of moderate extent, is sufficiently great so that one has to be constantly on the alert for it.[22] The grotesque pictures in the older literature of patients with enchondromatosis exhibiting large protruding cartilage tumor masses on the hands, feet, or other sites furnish a striking demonstration of the spontaneous tendency to malignant change.

OSTEOPETROSIS *(marble bone disease; Albers-Schönberg disease; osteosclerosis fragilis)*

As its name implies, osteopetrosis is characterized by abnormal density of most or all of the bones of the skeleton, as first described by the German radiologist, Albers-Schönberg[25] in 1904. It was Karshner,[26] a radiologist at the Children's Hospital in Los Angeles, who in 1926 proposed the commonly employed

Systemic anomalies of skeletal development

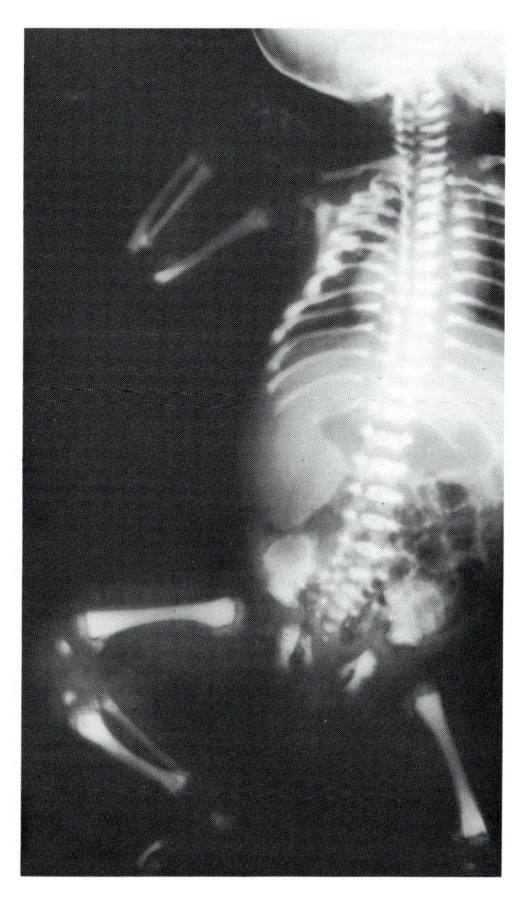

Fig. 2-12. Roentgenogram of an entire skeleton affected by osteopetrosis (marble bone disease) at 7 months' gestation. The increased density of the bones is obvious, as is clubbing of the metaphyses of the limb bones.

designation "osteopetrosis." As in many of the other skeletal anomalies, a familial and hereditary tendency has been noted.

The severity of osteopetrosis may vary within rather wide limits. Milder forms are not incompatible with longevity. In the severest expression, on the other hand, death may ensue in fetal life before term (Fig. 2-12). Children with outspoken involvement who survive may ultimately develop myelophthisic anemia (from encroachment of the compacted densified spongiosa upon the myeloid marrow) and hepatosplenomegaly (reflecting pronounced compensatory extramedullary hematopoiesis). Abnormal thickening and density of the base of the skull and sometimes of the facial and maxillary bones may be responsible for optic atrophy, facial palsy, and, occasionally, other neurologic manifestations. Since affected dense bones may also be brittle, a tendency to fractures may be a prominent feature in some cases. Occasionally, osteomyelitis or coxitis may develop, as well as other manifestations of infection.

Diseases of bone and joints

The roentgenographic recognition of the condition is not usually difficult. In addition to widespread striking radiopacity of affected bones, there is a tendency to clubbing of the metaphyses of limb bones and to the development of transverse bands of varying density producing a zebralike effect (Fig. 2-12). The only other conditions that might conceivably be considered by way of differential diagnosis are heavy metal poisoning, endemic fluorosis, and (in adults) sclerosing carcinoma extensively metastatic to the skeleton.

Pathologically, affected bones appear whitish and obviously dense. They may be substantially solid as a result of partial obliteration of the medullary cavity and fibrosis of the residual marrow. Microscopic examination of such bones from dead neonates show the presence of persistent cores of cartilage within spongy trabeculae even at a great distance from the plate regions, pointing to a defect in the normal mechanism of resorption and remodeling (Fig. 2-13). Deposition of new bone upon these unreconstructed dense trabeculae would seem to afford an adequate explanation for the abnormal bone density characterizing the disorder.

OSTEOGENESIS IMPERFECTA *(fragilitas ossium; brittle bones; osteopsathyrosis; Lobstein's syndrome; van der Hoeve's syndrome)*

Osteogenesis imperfecta is one of the more complex developmental anomalies and is characterized in fully developed cases by morphologic alterations in the skeletal tissues, the eye (sclera), and the skin. The complete clinical syndrome is featured essentially by multiple fractures, blue sclerae, deafness, and loose-jointedness, as well as by other related manifestations such as scoliosis, dwarfism, hernia, "thin skin," and stunting and discoloration of the teeth, especially the lower incisors.[1,27] Abnormal aminoaciduria (familial) and low serum creatinine and uric acid levels have also been noted.[28] The disorder may be inherited from either parent and can be traced back through several generations.

The condition apparently results from a specific defect in connective tissue development or maturation. The studies of Follis[29,30] have demonstrated failure of argyrophilic reticulin fibrils in the corium to become transformed to adult collagen fibers. Presumably a comparable defect is present in the connective tissue of the sclerae, joints, and other affected structures. The essential change in the skeleton predisposing to delicate, bent, and otherwise deformed bones prone to fracture (Figs. 2-15 and 2-16) is deficient formation of bone by osteoblasts, both in the periosteum and at sites of endochondral ossification (Fig. 2-17).

Severely affected fetuses *(osteogenesis imperfecta fetalis)* may die at birth,[31] or the infant may survive only a few days or weeks, although multiple fractures at birth are not incompatible with survival. In such subjects, so-called caput membranaceum with multiple wormian bones may be observed in the calvarium.[27] According to Stern,[32] recessive lethal or sublethal alleles are responsible for these severe cases with multiple fractures before birth.

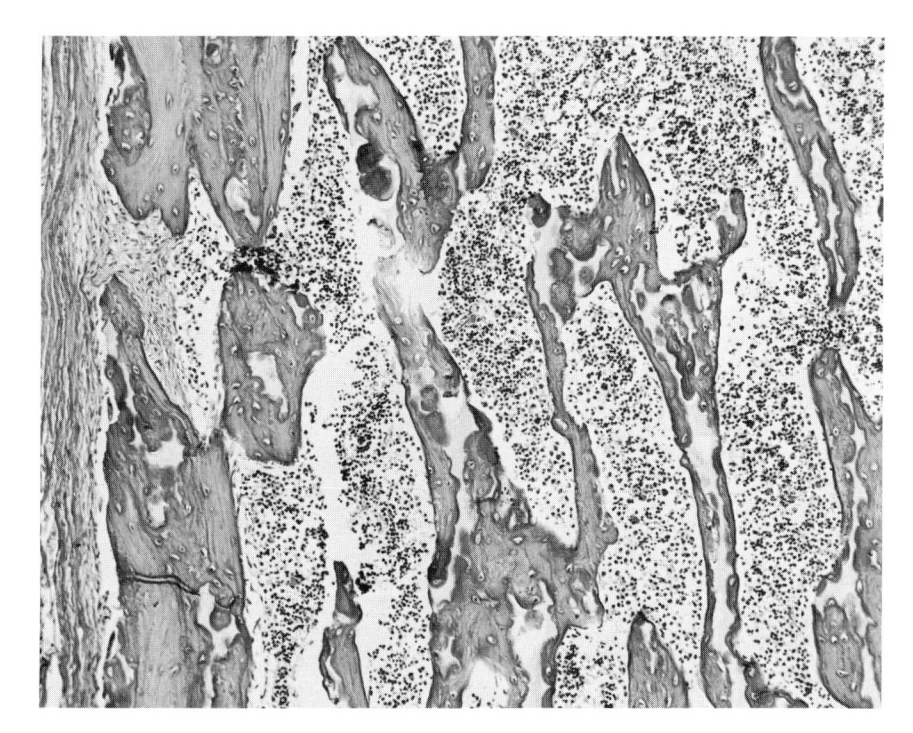

Fig. 2-13. Photomicrograph of a portion of a vertebra of a dead neonate with ostopetrosis (marble bone disease), showing unresorbed cartilage cores within spongy trabeculae (at a considerable distance from the plate region).

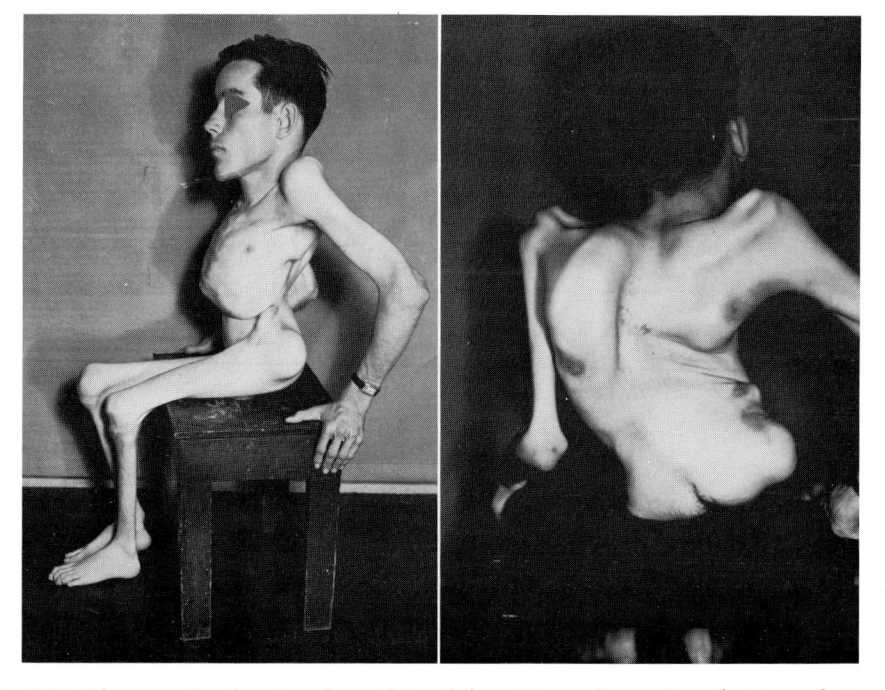

Fig. 2-14. Photographs showing the striking deformities and stunting of stature that may ensue in severe osteogenesis imperfecta.

Fig. 2-15.

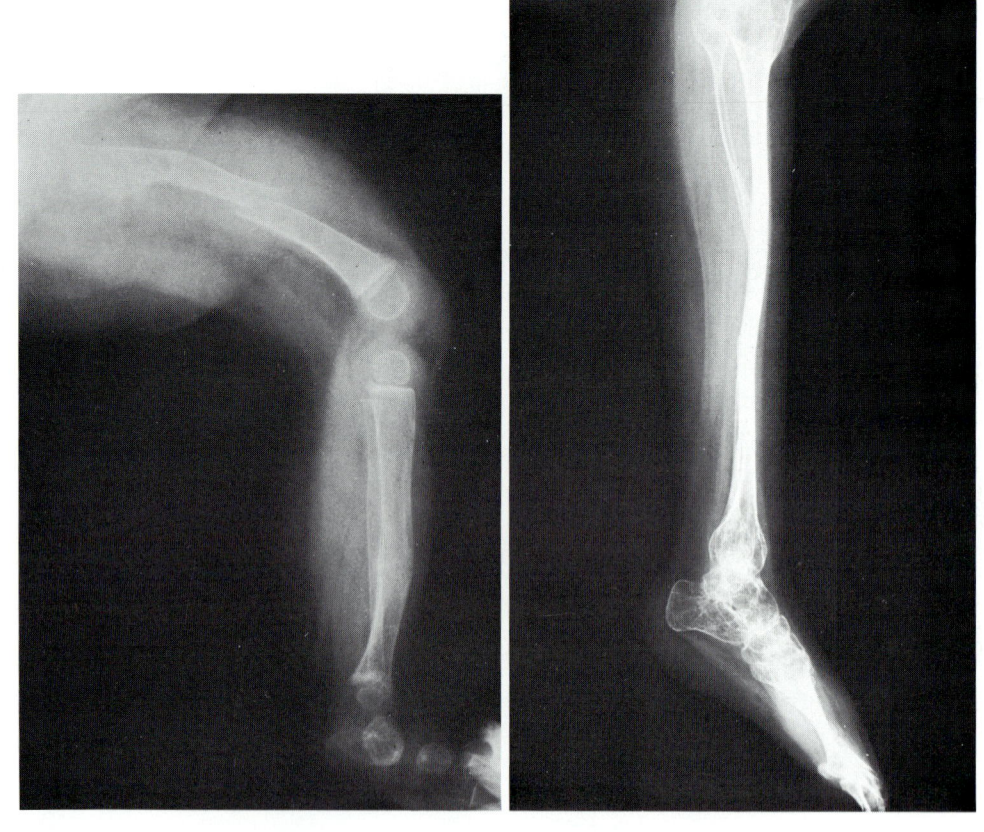

Fig. 2-16.

Fig. 2-15. Roentgenogram showing recent and healing fractures in the lower limb bones of a child with osteogenesis imperfecta.

Fig. 2-16. Roentgenogram showing strikingly thinned and otherwise deformed bones in the leg of a patient with osteogenesis imperfecta.

Osteogenesis imperfecta tarda is a term sometimes used to designate the condition in which there is a delay in the appearance of fractures, for example, in a child with blue sclerotics who does not sustain the first of many fractures until the age of 7. For that matter, blue sclerotics may be present in members of affected families without concomitant bone changes; this is ascribed by Stern[32] to a dominant gene with incomplete penetrance. The number of fractures sustained varies greatly from case to case, but in severe instances there may be as many as 100 or more. After the onset of puberty one may anticipate fewer fractures. These fractures tend to heal readily, and occasionally the callus may be so abundant as to give rise to tumorlike excrescences radiographically simulating osteogenic sarcoma. Among other skeletal changes present in many but by no means all affected patients are otosclerosis leading to progressive deafness in those who survive past 20 years of age, scoliosis (which is often severe),

Systemic anomalies of skeletal development

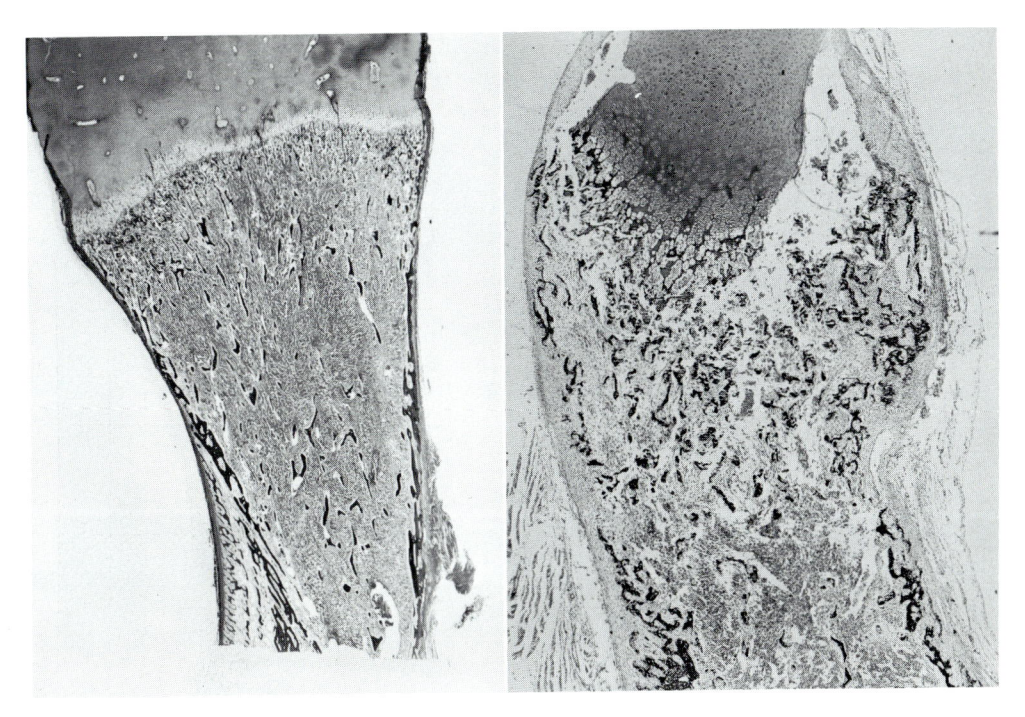

Fig. 2-17. Photomicrographs of a tibia and rib respectively from an instance of osteogenesis imperfecta congenita illustrating strikingly deficient formation of bone, both in the cortex and at the epiphyseal cartilage plates.

broadening of the skull with bulging in the temporal regions, and dwarfing of stature in the most severe cases (Fig. 2-14).

ACHONDROPLASIA *(chondrodystrophic dwarfism; chondrodystrophia fetalis; micromelia)*

Achondroplasia results from inadequacy of cartilage cell proliferation and premature closure of the growth plates of bones preformed in cartilage. It is characterized clinically by dwarfism of the short limb type associated with a large head and, in many cases, so-called trident hands (Fig. 2-18). It is the most common type of dwarfism and perhaps the most ancient—the traditional court jester is gone, but the circus dwarf lingers on. The relative frequency of the condition may be judged from the fact that Caffey[33] observed as many as forty-three cases at Babies Hospital in New York in the course of some 15 years. Meticulously compiled family pedigrees indicate that the condition results genetically from a dominant mutation that may be transmitted to all succeeding generations.[32] Many severely affected fetuses die in utero or soon after birth (which is often premature). On the other hand, survivors may live to an advanced age and be singularly sturdy and robust, as well as mentally alert.

As noted, it is particularly the bones preformed in cartilage that are fore-

Diseases of bone and joints

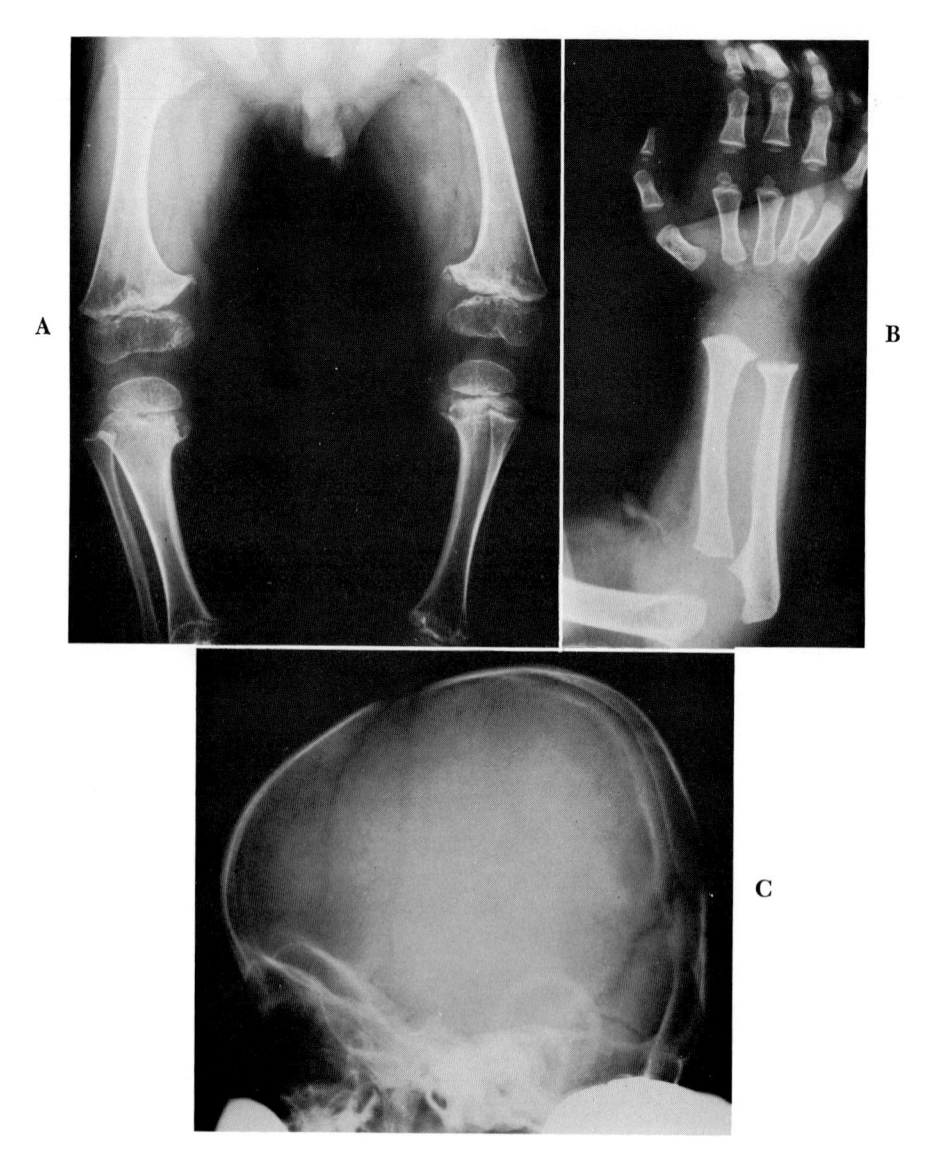

Fig. 2-18. **A,** Roentgenogram showing striking shortening of the long bones of the lower limbs in a child with achondroplasia. **B,** Roentgenogram illustrating so-called trident hand in an achondroplastic child. **C,** The skull of the same patient, showing a large calvarium, with distinct foreshortening of the base (which is largely preformed in cartilage).

shortened. Thus the size of the trunk and head of affected patients is not appreciably reduced, but the limbs are very short (like those of a dachshund). Also, since many of the bones at the base of the skull develop from cartilage anlage (in contradistinction to the calvarial vault, which is preformed in membrane), one observes characteristically a sunken bridge of the nose and foreshortening of the base of the skull (Fig. 2-18, C).

Systemic anomalies of skeletal development

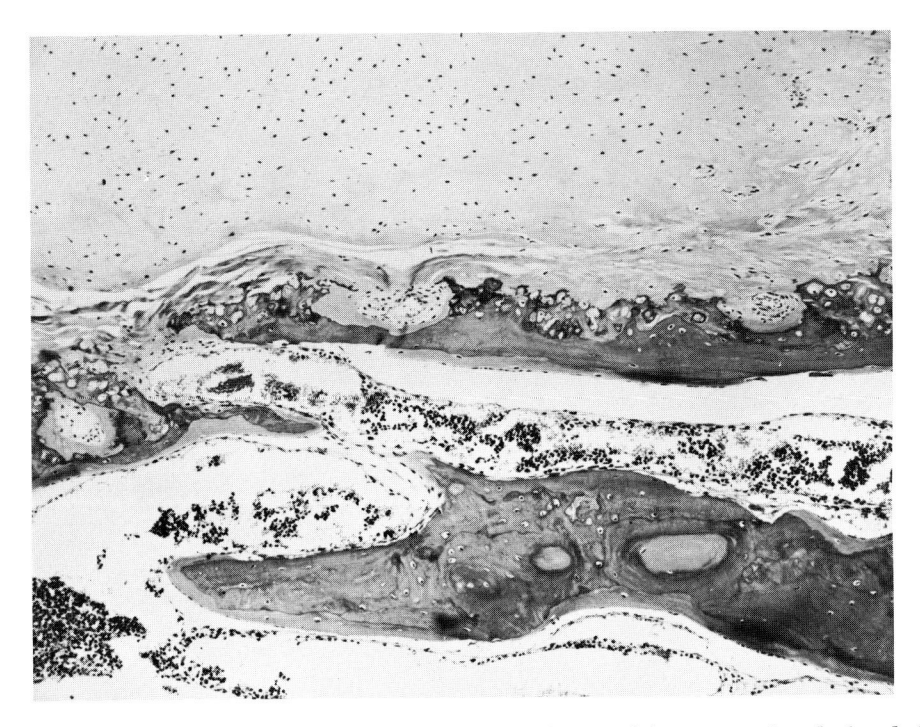

Fig. 2-19. Photomicrograph showing failure of cartilage proliferation and endochondral ossification, with premature closure of the growth plate in a young achondroplastic subject.

Available pathologic studies,[34-36] some of them quite old, show that failure of normal ossification of long bones is apparent in the fetus as early as 2 to 3 months' gestation and that the large limb bones especially may be strikingly foreshortened. There appears to be a relative aplasia of cartilage at the ends of the bones, and growth of the cartilage cells of the epiphysis is disorderly. More particularly, there is an absence of a normal orderly zone of provisional calcification, leading to premature closure of epiphyseal cartilage plates (Fig. 2-19).

MORQUIO'S DISEASE
*(chondroosteodystrophy [Morquio-Brailsford type];
eccentroosteochondrodysplasia [Morquio];
osteochondrodystrophia deformans)*

Morquio's disease is one of the more unusual anomalies of skeletal development; only a limited number of cases have been recorded since Morquio's account[37] in 1929. Its manifestations[37-43] apparently result from a congenital defect in the ossification and development of epiphyses. A tendency to familial incidence has been demonstrated in relevant pedigrees.[37] Jacobsen,[40] for example, has noted the incidence of the disorder in twenty members of a family group followed for five generations. The condition is apparently inherited as an autosomal recessive, and its incidence is estimated[43] as no more frequent than 1 in

Diseases of bone and joints

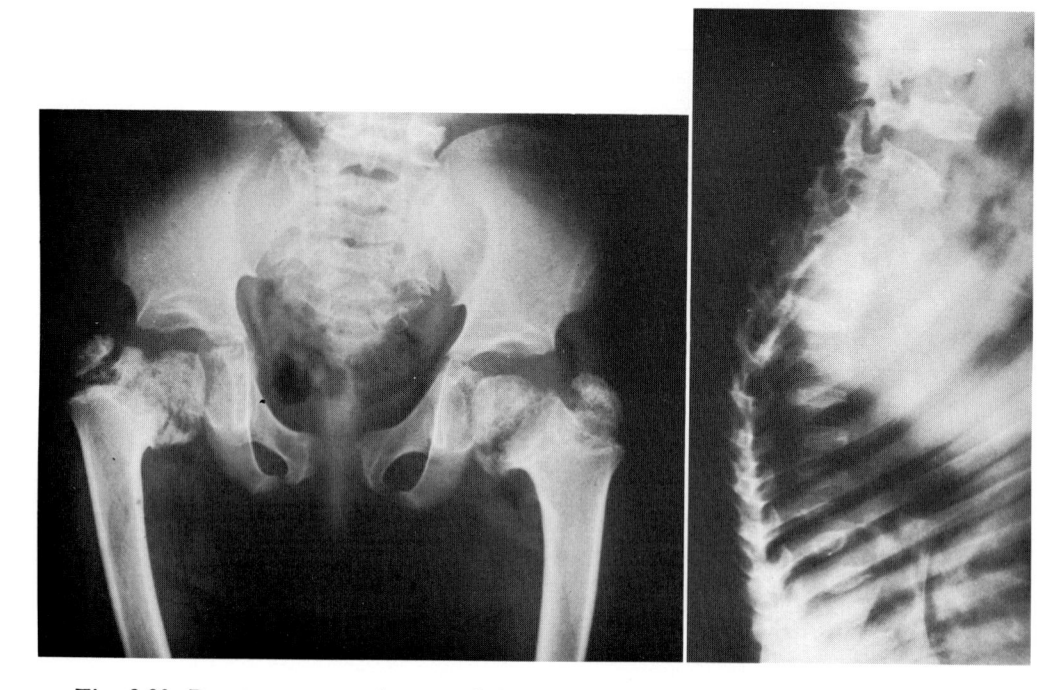

Fig. 2-20. Roentgenograms showing skeletal abnormalities in the spine and hip joints of a child, aged 6, with Morquio's disease.

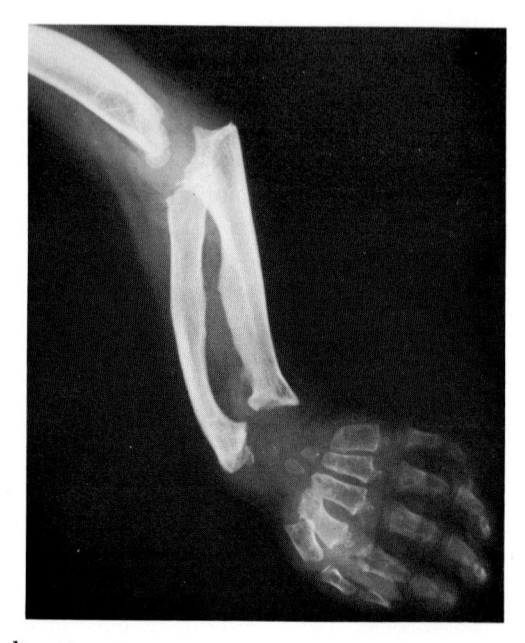

Fig. 2-21. Skeletal alterations in an upper extremity, including the hand, of a 6-year-old child with Morquio's disease.

40,000 births. There is a paucity of available pathologic data, although there is some evidence to suggest that affected epiphyses manifest anomalous eccentric centers of ossification, fusion of which leads eventually to deformity.

Morquio's disease is characterized clinically and radiographically by stunting of stature, flattening or shallowness of the vertebral bodies (universal vertebra plana), marked kyphosis, sometimes angular increase of the spinal curve at the dorsolumbar junction, and progressive changes in the articular bone ends, notably in the femoral head and acetabulum (Figs. 2-20 and 2-21). Although roentgenographic changes may be present in infancy,[42] the developmental error is usually not apparent until the affected child begins to walk, and sometimes not until the age of 4 or later. The whole skeleton may be affected to a varying extent, except for bones of the skull and face. Intelligence may be normal, in contrast to gargoylism, from which Morquio's disease must be distinguished. A subject with the fully developed disorder presents, as Fairbank[1] has aptly stated, as a "round-back, knock-kneed, flat-footed child who stands with hips and knees flexed (crouch), head thrust forward and sunk between high shoulders, and walking with a waddling duck-like gait." There is often stiffness of the hip joints, less often of other joints, although the ligaments at the joints may show increased laxity.

From a biochemical standpoint, an appreciable number of articles have appeared in recent years indicating that Morquio's disease (like gargoylism and Morquio-Ullrich disease) reflects an abnormality of mucopolysaccharide metabolism. This literature has been surveyed by Robins, Stevens, and Linker,[42] who directed attention particularly to the abnormal urinary excretion of keratosulfate and the finding of acid mucopolysaccharide cytoplasmic granules in leukocytes (Reilly bodies). It may well be, as Robins and his associates intimate, that there is a small family of related, and sometimes overlapping, hereditary disorders of mucopolysaccharide metabolism resulting from specific enzyme defects that are characterized chiefly by bone and joint abnormalities. In their classification of the genetic mucopolysaccharidoses (MPS), McKusick and his associates[43] list the Morquio syndrome as MPS IV, a variant of Hurler's syndrome or gargoylism (p. 43).

OSTEOPOIKILOSIS (spotty bones; osteopathia condensans disseminata)

Osteopoikilosis is one of the less common anomalies of skeletal development.[44-45] It is a pathologic curiosity characterized by the presence of small, spotty dense bones islands[46] mainly within the limb bones, including those of the hands and feet (Fig. 2-22). These enostoses do not ordinarily give rise to any apparent clinical symptoms. Familial incidence of this disorder has been noted by many observers. I have seen an unusual instance in which osteopoikilosis was associated with vertical striations in affected bones (so-called Voorhoeve's disease[47]; Fig. 2-23). Spotty bones may also be associated at times with unusual

Diseases of bone and joints

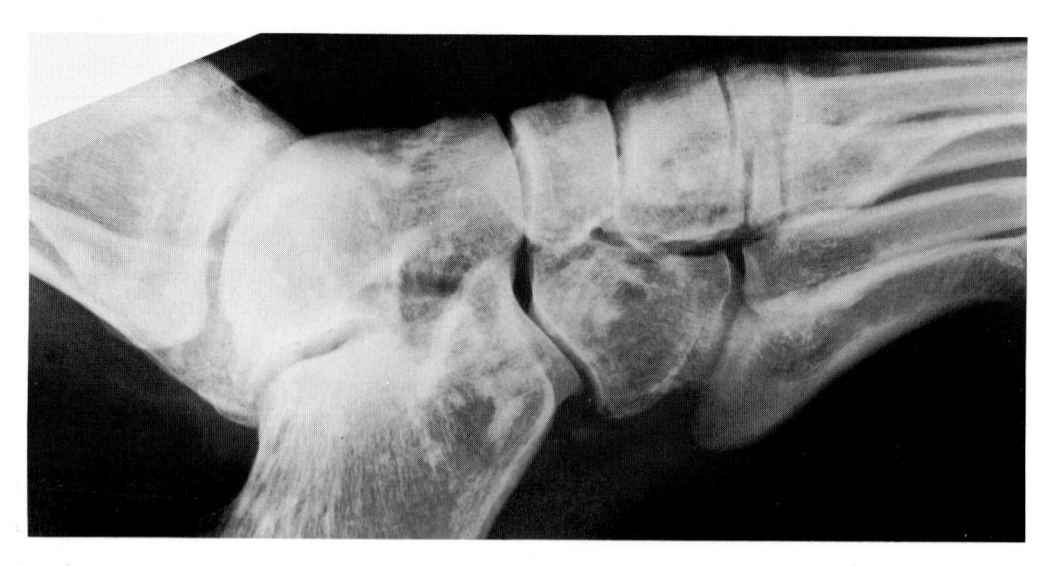

Fig. 2-22. Roentgenogram showing spotty enostoses, or bone islands, in the foot bones in osteopoikilosis.

hyperostotic changes in limb bones and kyphosis, as well as a peculiar dermatologic disease designated dermatofibrosis lenticularis disseminata. For a detailed and comprehensive discussion of the disorder in all its aspects, the comparatively recent paper by Bethge and Ridderbush[48] is recommended.

CLEIDOCRANIAL DYSOSTOSIS

Cleidocranial dysostosis is a well-known but rather uncommon congenital anomaly characterized by deficient formation of one or both clavicles, especially at the outer ends, associated with delayed and imperfect ossification of the calvarium (Fig. 2-24). Clinical reports of the condition date back as far as 1897.[49] In some instances they may be other developmental abnormalities as well. For detailed consideration of these unusual manifestations, the reader is referred to informative reviews of the subject by Fitzwilliams,[50] Fitchet,[51] and Soule.[52]

The hereditary and familial incidence of cleidocranial dysostosis has been well documented, and in particular, Stocks and Barrington[17] pointed out that in more than half of the cases collected the condition was inherited from one or the other parent.

GARGOYLISM (Hurler's syndrome; Hurler-Pfaundler disease; dysostosis multiplex)

Gargoylism is another hereditary (familial) disorder about which we have learned a great deal in recent years. It is rather serious in its implications,[1,53-55] and many affected subjects fail to survive beyond the period of completion of growth. The condition may be characterized as a genetically acquired muco-

Systemic anomalies of skeletal development

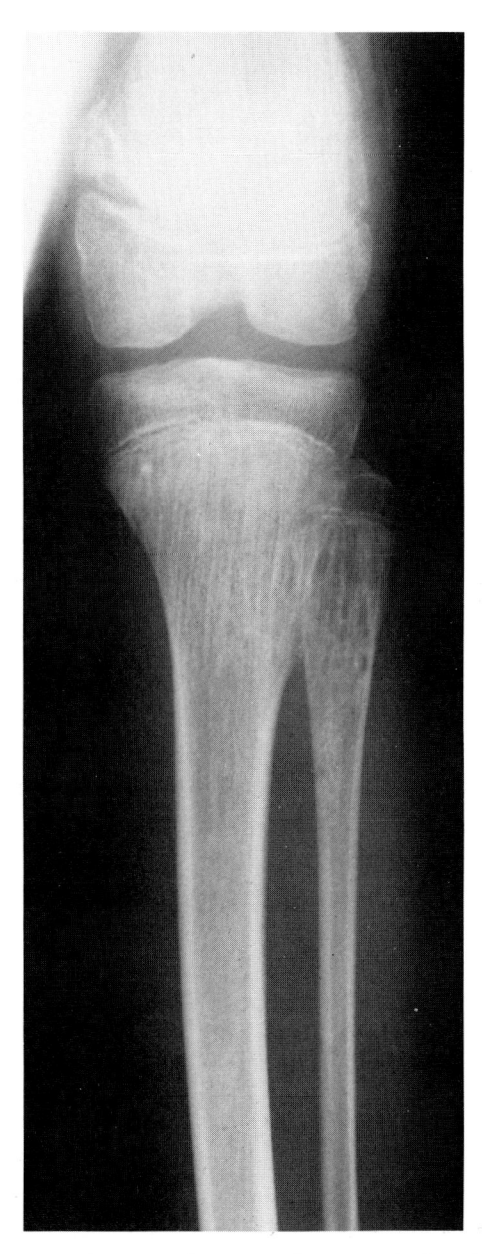

Fig. 2-23. Roentgenogram showing the anomalous vertical striations seen in Voorhoeve's disease (osteopathia striata).

Diseases of bone and joints

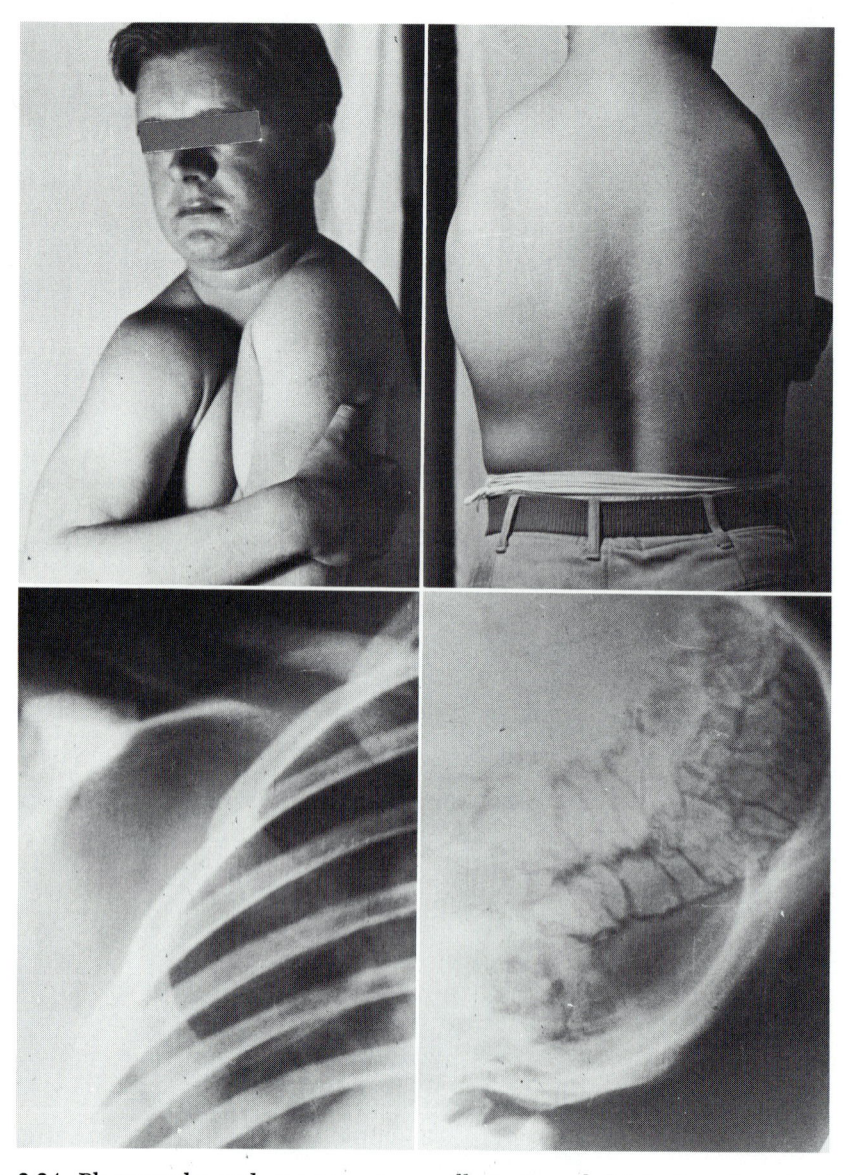

Fig. 2-24. Photographs and roentgenograms illustrating skeletal alterations in cleidocranial dysostosis. Note the defective clavicles and the anomalous ossification of the calvarium.

polysaccharide storage disease[56-61] exhibiting a number of variations, in which the affected skeletal and visceral tissues are stuffed with abnormal polysaccharides, which are also excreted in the urine in one form or another. As might be expected, this deranged metabolism and storage seriously interferes with the development and function of affected structures.

In a valuable review by McKusick and his associates,[43] as many as five similar clinical states (MPS I to V) are described, each of which is a primary,

Systemic anomalies of skeletal development

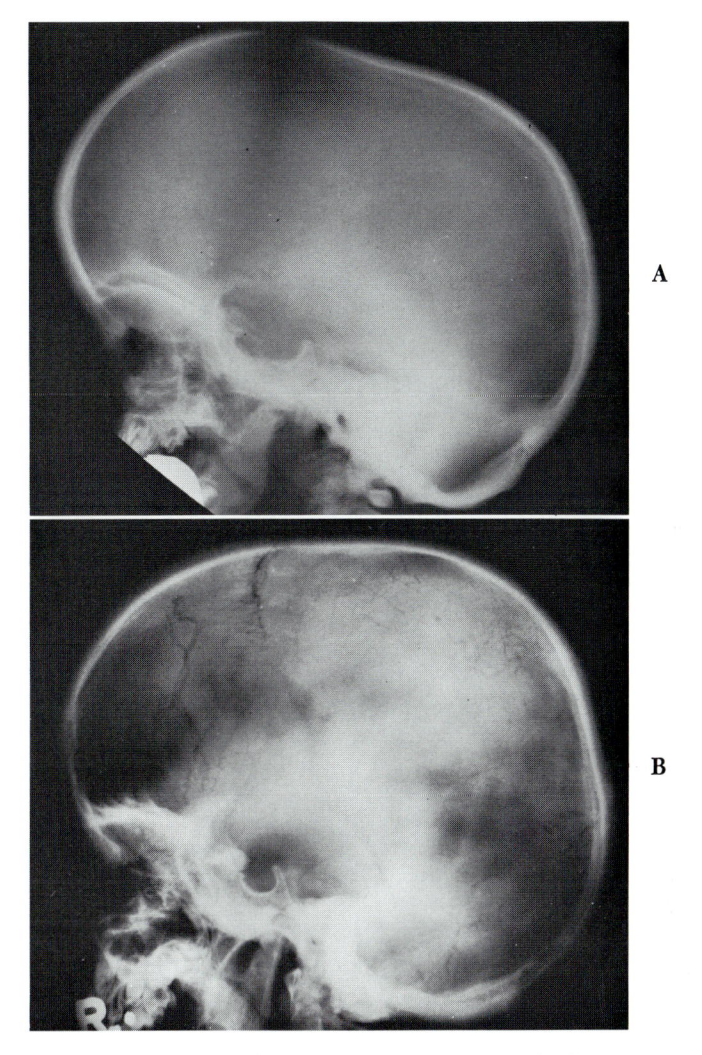

Fig. 2-25. **A,** The skull of a young child with gargoylism. **B,** Skull changes in gargoylism of another child at age 10.

gene-determined disorder of mucopolysaccharide metabolism. According to this concept, MPS I is the prototype mucopolysaccharidosis, inherited as an autosomal recessive trait, which leads to severe malformations and early death. MPS II, a milder sex-linked variety, represents clinical gargoylism (Hunter's syndrome). MPS III (Sanfilipo syndrome), another variant featuring heparitinuria, is characterized by severe mental retardation of late onset, which dominates the clinical picture. MPS IV represents the Morquio, or Morquio-Brailsford, syndrome, in which there are visceral as well as skeletal manifestations and in which keratosulfate is excreted in the urine in large amounts. MPS V (Scheie's syndrome) is still another recently described variant of Hurler's syndrome, with distinctive clinical and biochemical features, in which excessive amounts of chondroitin sulfate

Diseases of bone and joints

are excreted in the urine. Among its major clinical manifestations are stiff joints, claw hands, hirsutism, retinitis pigmentosa, carpal tunnel syndrome, and significant aortic valvular disease. At last report, a sixth subtype (MPS VI) has also been delineated, with more to come, in all probability.

Clinically, the fully developed disorder is characterized by stunting of stature (dwarfism), some shortening of the limbs (micromelia), heavy grotesque facies (large head, eyes set wide apart, bridge of the nose depressed, and, occasionally, hydrocephalus), corneal opacity, deafness, mental deficiency, marked dorsolumbar kyphosis, and distension of the abdomen from hepatosplenomegaly. Other features that may be noted are limited motion in the joints, umbilical hernia, hirsutism, and clawed hands.

The roentgenographic reflections of the skeletal alterations have been sufficiently well documented[62,63] to permit their ready recognition (Figs. 2-25 and 2-26).

For detailed information in regard to the pathologic changes, the reader may have recourse to the valuable paper by Lindsay and his associates[58] reporting their findings in some eight autopsied cases, supplemented by additional biopsy material. They described striking gross and microscopic alterations attributable to abnormal storage in almost all tissues of the body, including those of the central nervous system, the cardiovascular, reticuloendothelial, and endocrine systems, as well as the skeletal system. Some of the most striking changes were observed in the mesodermal connective tissue cells, including fibroblasts, chondrocytes, and osteocytes. There has been a renewed surge of interest in the genetic mucopolysaccharidoses recently, and studies of the ultrastructure of skin fibroblasts[64] and of cartilage cells[65] have opened up new avenues of investigation.

MELORHEOSTOSIS *(Léri type of osteopetrosis; osteosi eburnizzante monomelica*[66]*)*

Melorheostosis is a comparatively rare skeletal anomaly usually confined to a single limb bud, though it is sometimes more extensive. The affected bones show irregular linear, streaky, or flowing hyperostosis on their external surfaces (reminiscent of the flow of melted candle wax).[66-71] When an upper extremity is affected, the bones of the contiguous shoulder girdle may also be involved; similarly, with involvement of a lower limb, the ipsilateral iliac bone may likewise be transformed. Gradually increasing pain, often associated with stiffness and deformity of the affected region, is the usual clinical manifestation. Léri and Joanny[69] are generally credited with the first clinical report of this remarkable condition. Subsequently many other relevant papers appeared, both in the United States and abroad. The total number of cases in the literature as of 1963 was tallied at 131.[71] In 80% of these only a single limb was affected; in the remainder there was involvement of more than one limb and of other bones, particularly the skull, vertebrae, and ribs.

The onset of the condition in childhood, its slow evolution, and its monomelic

Systemic anomalies of skeletal development

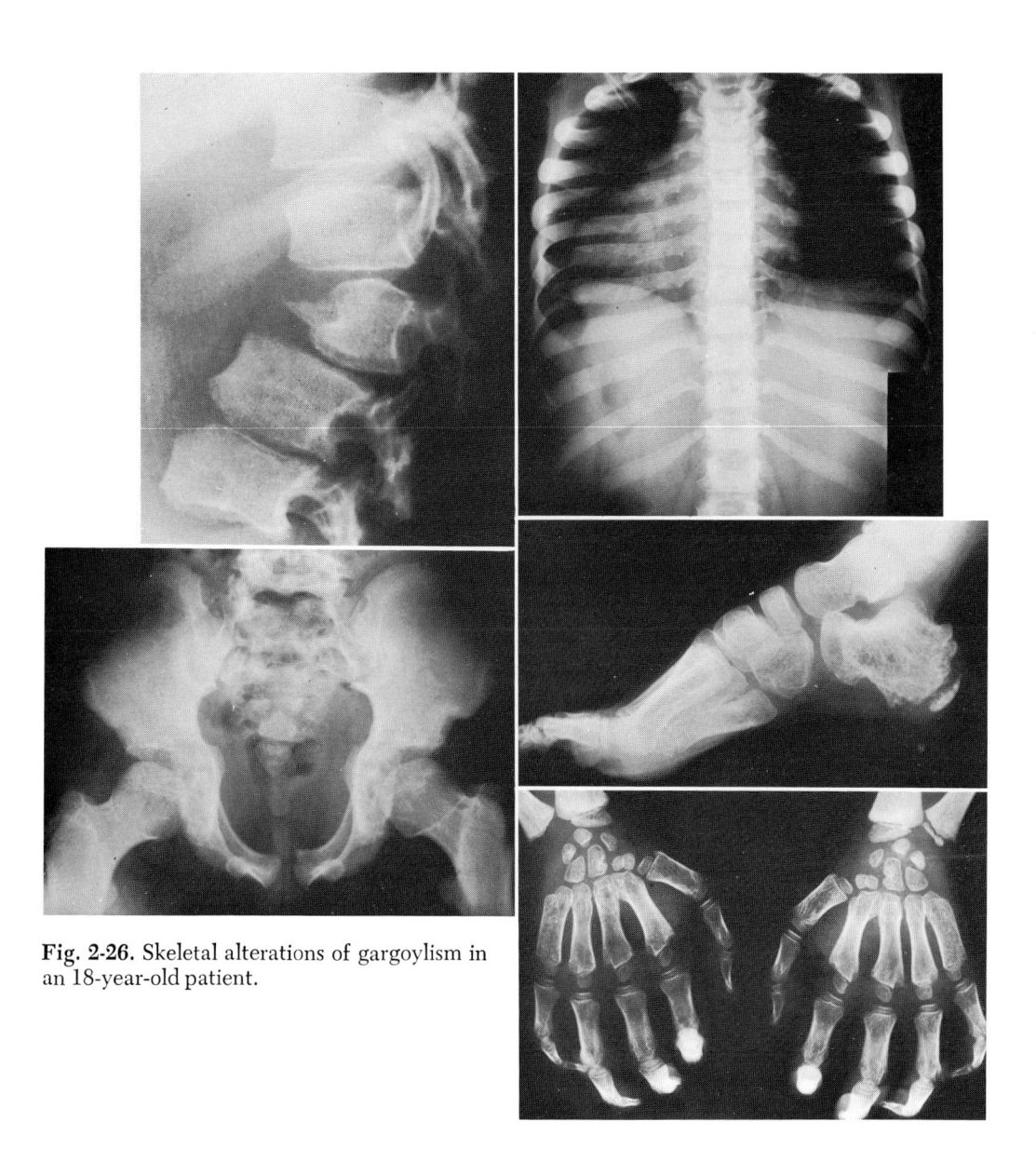

Fig. 2-26. Skeletal alterations of gargoylism in an 18-year-old patient.

Diseases of bone and joints

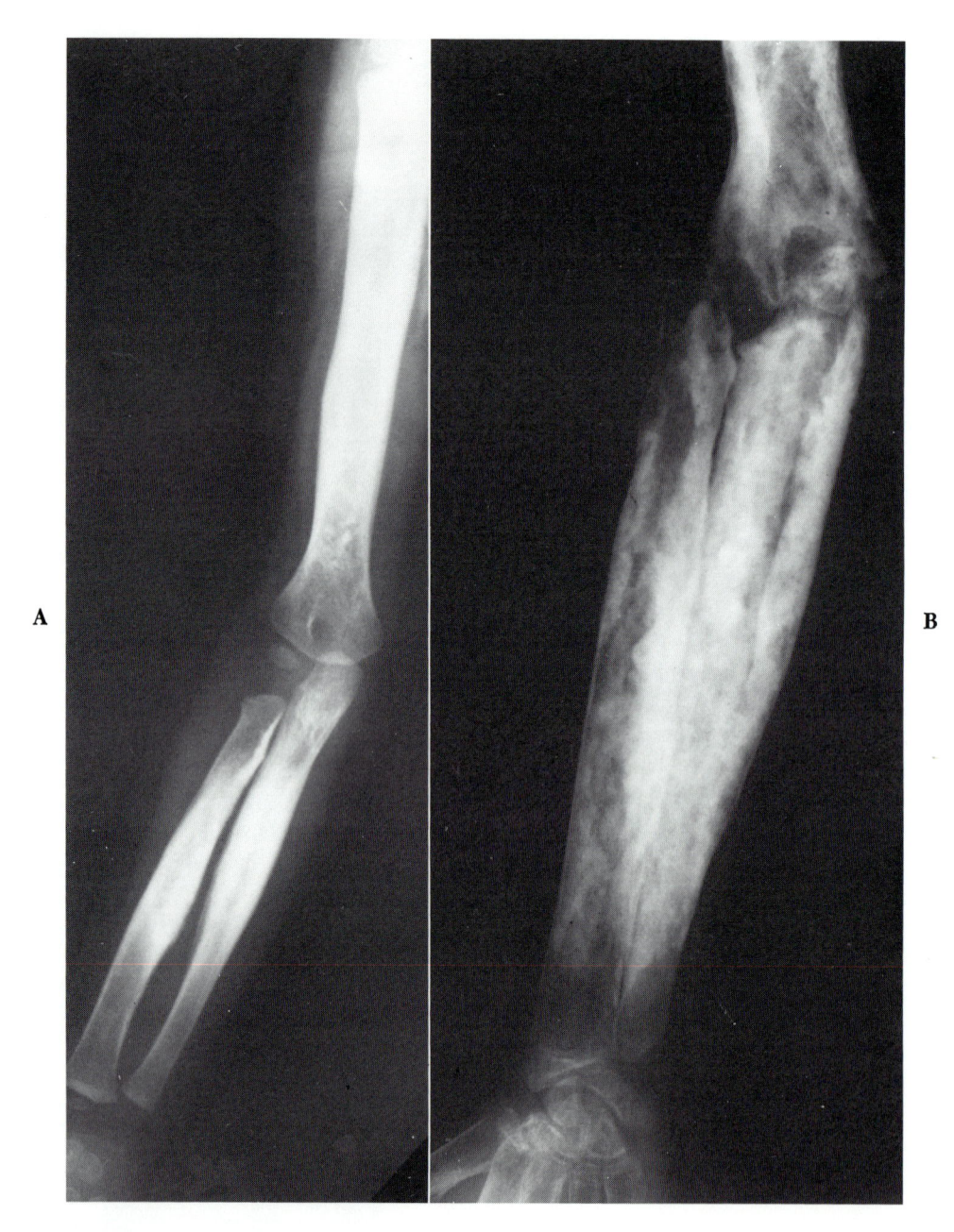

Fig. 2-27. A, Roentgenogram showing the changes of progressive diaphyseal dysplasia (Engelmann's disease) in the humerus and forearm bones. Note the widening and sclerosis of the shafts of the limb bones. **B,** Long-term followup showing the appearance of the same bones 16 years later. (Courtesy of Dr. M. E. Mottram,[78] San Francisco.)

or unilateral localization strongly suggest that it represents a congenital developmental anomaly. The limited number of biopsy specimens examined have confirmed the presence of marked abnormal condensation or sclerosis of the affected bone. New bone formation is predominantly periosteal in origin and only in part endosteal. There may also be paraarticular bone deposits in advanced cases that may be responsible for pain and limitation of motion.

PROGRESSIVE DIAPHYSEAL DYSPLASIA
(Engelmann's disease; osteopathia hyperostotica [sclerotisans] multiplex infantilis; hereditary multiple diaphyseal sclerosis)

Progressive diaphyseal dysplasia is another uncommon skeletal developmental anomaly whose manifestations have been clarified in comparatively recent years. The name currently favored to designate the disorder is that introduced by Neuhauser and his associates[72] in 1948, although earlier cases reports[73-74] date back to the 1920's. The pertinent literature was surveyed in 1956 by Griffiths,[75] who accepted some twenty-two cases as instances in point. Additional observations of interest were published in 1958 by Mikity and Jacobson[76] (who followed a patient for fully 22 years) and in 1964 by Clausen and Loop.[77]

The disorder is characterized roentgenographically by symmetrical sclerosis and fusiform widening of the shafts of the long bones, and often by thickening of the skull, especially at its base. Other bones (ribs, scapulae, pelvis, clavicles, hands, and feet) are infrequently involved. The condition manifests itself in childhood and may lead to physical underdevelopment, pains in the extremities, abnormal waddling gait, occasional deformities, fatigability, and weakness. The available reports indicate a tendency to progression of varying extent in childhood, but not necessarily in adult life. Presumably, some gene defect is responsible for this peculiar anomaly, as Griffiths[75] has suggested, although its pattern of hereditary transmission has not as yet been fully elucidated.[77]

Biopsies of affected limb bones in an appreciable number of instances[75-78] have indicated that the strikingly thickened bone results from endosteal and subperiosteal new bone deposition; this encroaches upon the marrow cavity, as one might expect from the roentgenograms (Fig. 2-27, A and B). Apart from its abnormal density, the structure of the new bone does not appear particularly unusual. For detailed study of these pathologic changes one may refer to the paper by Cohen and States,[79] who had occasion to examine a subject at autopsy.

MONOMELIC MEDULLARY OSTEOSCLEROSIS

Monomelic medullary osteosclerosis is still another comparatively rare developmental anomaly in which the bones of a single lower limb bud come to show a peculiar internal or medullary sclerosis—something like melorheostosis turned outside-in. The condition was described by Horwitz[80] in 1941, and Sotelo-Ortiz[81] in 1954 also reported a case in an 11-year-old girl who manifested unequal leg length and valgus deformity requiring surgical correction (Fig. 2-28).

Diseases of bone and joints

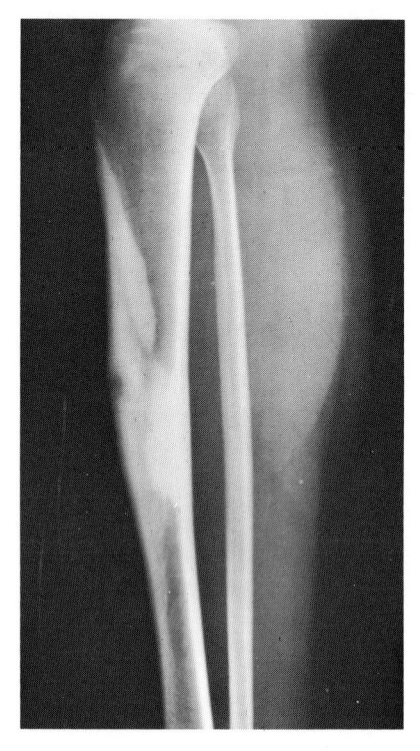

Fig. 2-28. Roentgenogram of a tibia showing peculiar medullary osteosclerosis, from the case reported by Sotelo-Ortiz.[81]

It is quite possible, as Sotelo-Ortiz pointed out, that additional instances have been recorded or compiled under the head of melorheostosis because their distinctive character was not recognized.

Histologically, as Horwitz indicated,[80] there is replacement of the normal spongiosa by densely sclerotic bone of unusual architecture, made up of compact, irregular segments of immature and adult bone arranged in a bizarre pattern.

OTHER ANOMALIES

In addition to the well-defined systemic anomalies of skeletal development already considered, there are a number of rarely observed disorders about which too little is known at present to serve as a basis for comprehensive discussion. Among these are *metaphyseal dysostosis* (Jansen[82]), which leads to a rare form of dwarfism; *familial metaphyseal dysplasia* (Bakwin and Krida[83]), which results in symmetrical enlargement of one or both ends of the shafts of the long bones; *dysplasia epiphysealis multiplex* (Fairbank[1]), characterized by mottled density and irregularity of affected epiphyses, dwarfism, and stubby digits; and *dysplasia epiphysealis punctata* (Fairbank[1] and Frank and Denny[84]), manifested in stippled or speckled epiphyses. For the limited information available in regard to these and some other rare anomalies, the reader is referred again to the valuable atlas of Sir Thomas Fairbank.

REFERENCES

1. Fairbank, H. A. T.: An atlas of general affections of the skeleton, Edinburgh, 1951, E. & S. Livingstone Ltd.
2. Lichtenstein, L.: Polyostotic fibrous dysplasia, Arch. Surg. 36:874, 1938.
3. Schlumberger, H. G.: Fibrous dysplasia of single bones (monostotic fibrous dysplasia), Mil. Surg. 99:504, 1946.
4. McCune, D. J., and Bruch, H.: Osteodystrophia fibrosa; report of case in which condition was combined with precocious puberty, pathologic pigmentation of skin and hyperthyroidism, Am. J. Dis. Child. 52:734, 1936; ibid. 54:806, 1937.
5. Albright, F., Butler, A. M., Hampton, A. O., and Smith, P.: Syndrome characterized by osteitis fibrosa disseminata, areas of pigmentation and endocrine dysfunction, with precocious puberty in females; report of 5 cases, N. Engl. J. Med. 216:272, 1937.
6. Albright, F., Scoville, W. B., and Sulkowitch, H. W.: Syndrome characterized by osteitis fibrosa disseminata, areas of pigmentation, and gonadal dysfunction, Endocrinology 22:411, 1938.
7. Lichtenstein, L., and Jaffe, H. L.: Fibrous dysplasia of bone: a condition affecting one, several or many bones, the graver cases of which may present abnormal pigmentation of the skin, premature sexual development, hyperthyroidism or still other extra-skeletal abnormalities, Arch. Pathol. 33:777, 1942.
8. Falconer, M. A., Cope, C. L., and Robb-Smith, A.: Fibrous dysplasia of bone with endocrine disorders and cutaneous pigmentation (Albright's disease), Q. J. Med. 11:121, 1942.
9. Jaffe, H. L.: Fibrous dysplasia of bone, a disease entity and specifically not an expression of neurofibromatosis, J. Mount Sinai Hosp. 12:364, 1945.
10. Jaffe, H. L.: Fibrous dysplasia of bone, Bull. N. Y. Acad. Med. 22:588, 1946.
11. Benjamin, D. R., and McRoberts, J. W.: Polyostotic fibrous dysplasia associated with Cushing syndrome: case report with autopsy findings, Arch. Pathol. 96:175, 1973.
12. Changus, G. W.: Osteoblastic hyperplasia of bone: a histochemical appraisal of fibrous dysplasia of bone, Cancer 10:1157, 1957.
13. Perkinson, N. B., and Higinbotham, N. L.: Osteogenic sarcoma arising in polyostotic fibrous dysplasia: report of a case, Cancer 8:396, 1955.
14. Coley, B. L., and Stewart, F. W.: Bone sarcoma in polyostotic fibrous dysplasia, Ann. Surg. 121:872, 1945.
15. Schwartz, D. T., and Alpert, M.: The malignant transformation of fibrous dysplasia, Am. J. Med. Sci. 247:350, 1964.
16. Ollier, L.: Lyon Méd. 88:484, 1898.
17. Stocks, P., and Barrington, A.: Hereditary disorders of bone development, University of London, Francis Galton Laboratory for National Eugenics, Memoir 22, 1925.
18. Keith, A.: J. Anat. 54:101, 1920.
19. Jaffe, H. L.: Hereditary multiple exostosis, Arch. Pathol. 36:335, 1943.
20. Müller, E.: Beitr. Path. Anat. 57:232, 1913.
21. Bethge, J. F. J.: Hereditäre multiple Exostosen und ihre pathogenetische Deutung, Arch. Orthop. Unfallchir. 54:667-696, 1963. (Contains extensive bibliography.)
22. Lichtenstein, L.: Bone tumors, ed. 4, St. Louis, 1972, The C. V. Mosby Co.
23. Carleton, A., Elkington, J. St. C., Greenfield, J. G., and Robb-Smith, A. H. T.: Maffucci's syndrome (dyschondroplasia with haemangiomata), Q. J. Med. 35:203, 1942.
24. Hunter, D., and Wiles, P.: Dyschondroplasia (Ollier's disease), with report of a case, Br. J. Surg. 22:507, 1935.
25. Albers-Schönberg, H.: Münchener Med. Wschr. 51:365, 1904.
26. Karshner, R. G.: Am. J. Roentgenol. Radium Ther. Nucl. Med. 16:405, 1926.
27. McKusick, V. A.: Hereditary disorders of connective tissue, Bull. N. Y. Acad. Med. 35:143-156, 1959.
28. Chowers, I., Czaczkes, J. W., Ehrenfeld, E. N., and Landau, S.: Familial aminoaciduria in osteogenesis imperfecta, J.A.M.A. 181:771, 1962.
29. Follis, R. H., Jr.: Osteogenesis imperfecta congenita: a connective tissue diathesis, J. Pediatr. 41:713, 1952.

30. Follis, R. H., Jr.: Maldevelopment of the corium in the osteogenesis imperfecta syndrome, Bull. Johns Hopkins Hosp. 93:225, 1953.
31. Hreno, A., and Haust, M. D.: Osteogenesis imperfecta congenita, J. Pediatr. 62:908, 1963.
32. Stern, C.: Principles of human genetics, San Francisco, 1949, W. H. Freeman & Co., Publishers.
33. Caffey, J.: In Brennemann's practice of pediatrics, vol. 4, Hagerstown, Md., 1957, W. F. Prior, pp. 1-22.
34. Hecktoen, L.: Anatomical study of short-limbed dwarf, with special reference to osteogenesis imperfecta and chondrodystrophia foetalis, Am. J. Med. Sci. 125:751, 1903.
35. Hughes Jones, E. W. A.: Studies in achondroplasia, J. Anat. 66:565, 1932.
36. Kaufmann, E.: Die Chondrodystrophia hyperplastica, Beitr. Path. Anat. 13:32, 1893.
37. Morquio, L.: Sur une forme de dystrophie osseuse familiale, Arch. Méd. Enf. 32:139, 1929.
38. Brailsford, J. F.: Chondro-osteodystrophy: roentgenographic and clinical features of child with dislocation of vertebrae, Am. J. Surg. 7:404, 1929.
39. Einhorn, N. H., Moore, J. R., and Rowntree, L. G.: Osteochondrodystrophia deformans (Morquio's disease): observations at autopsy in 1 case, Am. J. Dis. Child. 72:536, 1946.
40. Jacobsen, A. W.: Hereditary osteochondrodystrophia deformans: family with twenty members affected in five generations, J.A.M.A. 113:121, 1939.
41. Pohl, J. F.: Chondro-osteodystrophy (Morquio's disease), J. Bone Joint Surg. 12:187, 1939.
42. Robins, M. M., Stevens, H. F., and Linker, A.: Morquio's disease: an abnormality of mucopolysaccharide metabolism, J. Pediatr. 62:881, 1963.
43. McKusick, V. A., and others: The genetic mucopolysaccharidoses, Medicine 44:445, 1965.
44. Albers-Schönberg, H.: Eine Seltene, bisher nicht bekannte Struktur-anomalie des Skelettes, Fortschr. Roentgenstr. 23:174, 1915.
45. Newcomet, W. S.: Spotted bones, Am. J. Roentgenol. Radium Ther. Nucl. Med. 22:460, 1929.
46. Schmorl, G.: Anatomische Befunde bei Einen Falle von Osteopoikilie, Fortsch. Roentgenstr. 44:1, 1931.
47. Voorhoeve, N.: L'image radiologique non encore décrite d'une anomalie du squelette, Acta Radiol. 3:407, 1924.
48. Bethge, J. F. J., and Ridderbush, K. E.: Uber die osteopoikilie und das neue Krankeitsbild Hyperostose bei osteopoikilie, Ergebn. d. Chir. u. Orthop. 49:138-182, 1967. (Contains extensive bibliography.)
49. Marie, P., and Sainton, P.: Observation d'hydrocéphalie héréditaire (père e fils) par via de développement du crane et du cerveau, Bull. Soc. Méd. Hôp. Paris 14:706, 1897; ibid. 15:436, 1898.
50. Fitzwilliams, D. C. L.: Lancet, 2,1466, 1910.
51. Fitchet, S. M.: Cleidocranial dysostosis, hereditary and familial, J. Bone Joint Surg. 11:838, 1929.
52. Soule, A. B. Jr.: Mutational dysostosis (cleidocranial dysostosis), J. Bone Joint Surg. 28:81, 1946.
53. Engle, D.: Dysostosis multiplex; Pfaundler-Hurler syndrome—report of 2 cases, Arch. Dis. Child. 14:217, 1939.
54. Harvey, R. M.: Hurler-Pfaundler syndrome (gargoylism), Am. J. Roentgenol. Radium Ther. Nucl. Med. 48:732, 1942.
55. Hunter, C.: A rare disease in two brothers, Proc. R. Soc. Med. 10:104-116, 1917.
56. Klenk, E.: The pathological chemistry of the developing brain. In Waelsch, H., editor: Biochemistry of the developing nervous system, New York, 1955, Academic Press, Inc., pp. 397-410.
57. Kobayashi, N.: Acid mucopolysaccharide granules in the glomerular epithelium in gargolylism, Am. J. Pathol. 35:591, 1959.
58. Lindsay, S., Reilly, W. A., Gotham, T. J., and Skahen, R.: Gargoylism. II. Study of pathologic lesions and clinical review of 12 cases, Am. J. Dis. Child. 76:239, 1948.
59. Meyer, K., Grumbach, M. M., Linker, A., and Hoffman, P.: Excretion of sulfated mucopolysaccharides in gargoylism (Hurler's syndrome), Proc. Soc. Exp. Biol. Med. 97:275-279, 1958.
60. Meyer, K., and Hoffman, P. Hurler's syndrome, Arthritis Rheum. 4:552, 1961.
61. Tuthill, C. R.: Juvenile amaurotic idiocy; marked adventitial growth associated with skeletal malformation and tuberculomas, Arch. Neurol. 32:198, 1934.
62. Ellis, R. W. B., Sheldon, W., and Capon, N. B.: Gargolylism (chrondro-osteo-dys-

trophy, corneal opacities, hepatosplenomegaly, and mental deficiency), Q. J. Med. 5:119-139, 1936.
63. Hurler, G.: Über einen Typ Multiplex Abartungen, vorwiegend am Skelettsystem, Z. Kinderheilh. 24:220, 1920.
64. Belcher, R. W.: Ultrastructure of the skin in the genetic mucopolysaccharidoses, Arch. Pathol. 44:511, 1972.
65. Silberberg, R., Rimoin, D. L., Rosenthal, R. E., and Hasler, M. B.: Ultrastructure of cartilage in the Hurler and Sanfilippo syndromes, Arch. Pathol. 94:500, 1972.
66. Putti, V.: L'osteosi eburnizzante monomelica, Chir. Organi Mov. 11:335, 1927.
67. Franklin, E. L., and Matheson, I.: Melorheostosis: report of case with review of literature, Br. J. Radiol. 15:185, 1942.
68. Kraft, E.: Melorheostosis Léri; flowing hyperostosis of single extremity, report of 2 cases, J.A.M.A. 98:705, 1932.
69. Léri, A., and Joanny, S.: Une affection non décrite des os: hyperostose "en coulée" sur toute le longeur d'un membre ou "melorhéostose," Bull. Soc. Méd. Hôp. Paris 46:1141-1145, 1922.
70. Lewin, P., and MacLeod, S. B.: Osteosclerosis with distribution suggesting that of ulnar nerve, unclassified bone condition, J. Bone Joint Surg. 7:968, 1925.
71. Morris, J. M., Samilson, R. L., and Corley, C. L.: Melorheostosis: review of the literature and report of an interesting case with a nineteen-year follow-up, J. Bone Joint Surg. 45-A:1191, 1963. (Contains extensive bibliography.)
72. Neuhauser, E. B. D., Schwachman, H., Wittenborg, M., and Cohen, J.: Progressive diaphyseal dysplasia, Radiology 51: 11-22, 1948.
73. Camurati, M.: Di un raro caso di osteite simmetrica ereditaria degli arti inferori, Chir. Organi Mov. 6:662-665, 1922.
74. Engelmann, G.: Ein Fall von Osteopathia hyperostotica (sclerotisans) multiplex infantilis, Fortschr. Roentgenstr. 39:1101-1106, 1929.
75. Griffiths, D. W.: Engelmann's disease, J. Bone Joint Surg. 38-B:312-326, 1956.
76. Mikity, V. G., and Jacobson, G.: Progressive diaphyseal dysplasia (Engelmann's disease: report of a case with twenty-two years follow-up, J. Bone Joint Surg. 40-A:312-326, 1958.
77. Clausen, D. K., and Loop, J. W.: Progressive diaphyseal dysplasia (Engelmann's disease), J. Bone Joint Surg. 46-A:143, 1964.
78. Mottram, M. E., and Hill, H. H.: Diaphyseal dysplasia: report of a case, Am. J. Roentgenol. Radium Ther. Nucl. Med. 95:162, 1965.
79. Cohen, J., and States, J. D.: Progressive diaphyseal dysplasia: report of a case with autopsy findings, Lab. Invest. 5: 492-508, 1956.
80. Horwitz, T.: Monomelic medullary osteosclerosis of unknown etiology, Radiology 36:343, 1941.
81. Sotelo-Ortiz, F.: Monomelic medullary osteosclerosis; case report, Bull, Hosp. Joint Dis. 15:95, 1954.
82. Jansen, M.: Über atypische Chondrodystrophie (Achondroplasie) und über eine noch nicht beschrieben angeborene Wachstumsstörung des Knochensystems: Metaphysäre Dysostosis, Z. Orthop. Chir. 61:253, 1934.
83. Bakwin, H., and Krida, A.: Familial metaphysial dysplasia, Am. J. Dis. Child. 53:1521, 1937.
84. Frank, W. W., and Denny, M. B.: Dysplasia epiphysealis punctata, J. Bone Joint Surg. 36-B:118, 1954.

chapter 3

Infections of bone

PYOGENIC OSTEOMYELITIS

The widespread use of antibiotics has drastically altered the incidence and course of infection of bone by pyogenic organisms to the point where the pertinent articles of the 1920's and 1930's are now largely of historic interest.[1,2] One no longer has to stand by helplessly in the case of a child with acute hematogenous osteomyelitis[3,4] while pus formed by *Staphylococcus aureus* or hemolytic streptococci spreads from the richly vascular metaphysis of a long bone up the medullary cavity and through the cortex to the periosteum. By the same token, today one seldom sees specimens of massive sequestrum resulting from thrombosis of nutrient vessels or of involucrum (a tube of cortical new bone deposited around a necrotic shaft as a core; Fig. 3-1). Also, the spread of infection to neighboring joints (pyarthrosis) with impairment of articular function, if not ankylosis, is no longer as serious a problem as it once was.[5] In many instances, the infection may be aborted, or at least significantly modified by adequate antibiotic therapy.

To be sure, chronic bone abscess is still with us (Fig. 3-2), as is chronic osteomyelitis complicating compound fractures or orthopedic surgical procedures (a vexatious problem at times in hospital practice). Furthermore, antibiotic therapy has not altogether obviated the necessity for surgical drainage in cases of chronic osteomyelitis with small sequestra, pockets of residual infection, or persistent sinus tracts, for reasons to be indicated.

The pathologic reaction to infection in bone does not differ essentially from that in other tissues, although it is modified by the mineralized structure of bone in ways that can create special problems in successful treatment. As infected bone undergoes vascular and osteoclastic resorption, it is replaced by fibrous connective tisue. If the loss of bone is extensive, this can create a problem in reconstruction as well as in effective drainage. Also, as the periosteum is irritated, it lays down new cortical bone that can become quite dense (Fig. 3-3); this, too, may impede the evacuation of pus and sequestra. In these circumstances it is more difficult to attain adequate concentration of the antibiotic at the site

Infections of bone

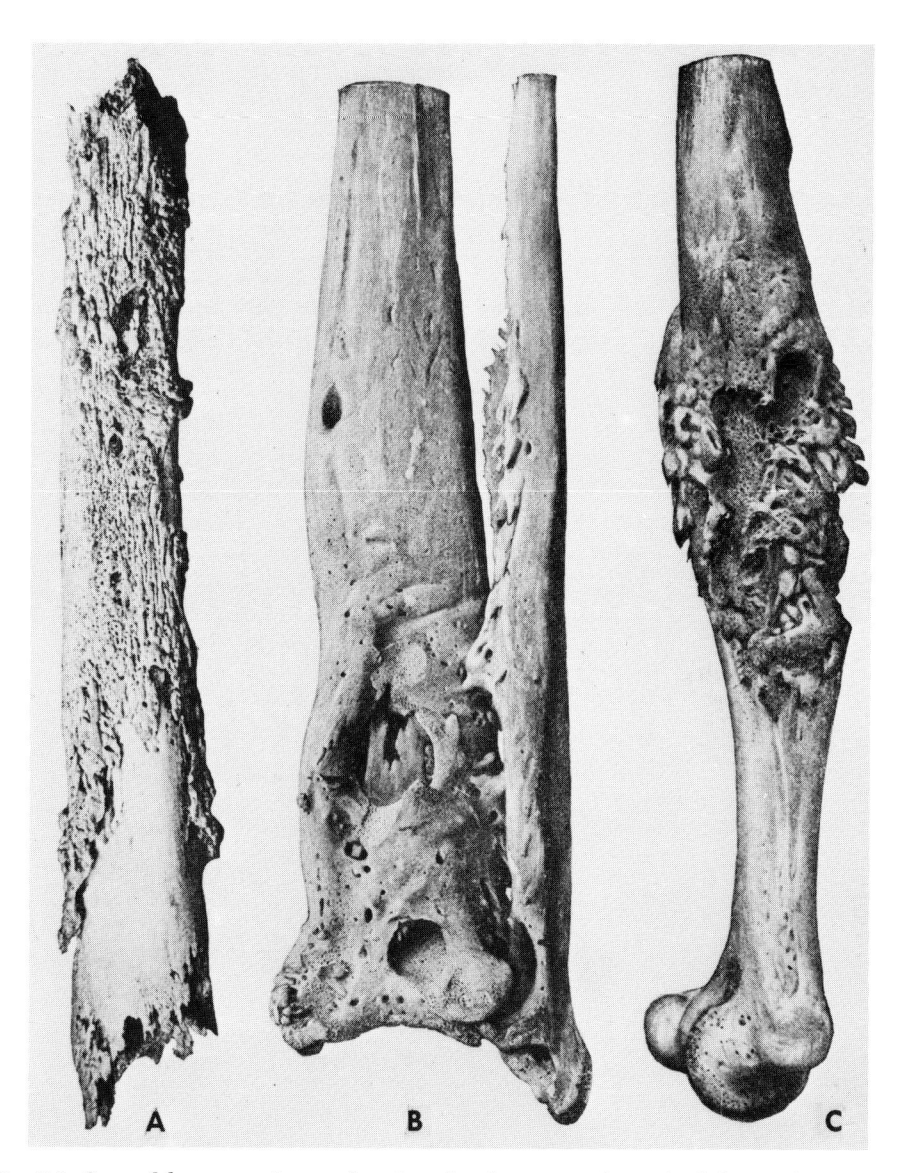

Fig. 3-1. Several bone specimens showing the changes in large limb bones from severe chronic osteomyelitis, as seen in the preantibiotic era. **A**, Large sequestrum in a tibia. **B**, Sequestrum in distal tibia with involucrum, and periosteal osteophytes on the contiguous fibula. **C**, Infection of the shaft of a femur with irregular periosteal new bone reaction. (From MacCallum, W. G.: A text-book of pathology, ed. 3, Philadelphia, 1924, W. B. Saunders Co.)

Diseases of bone and joints

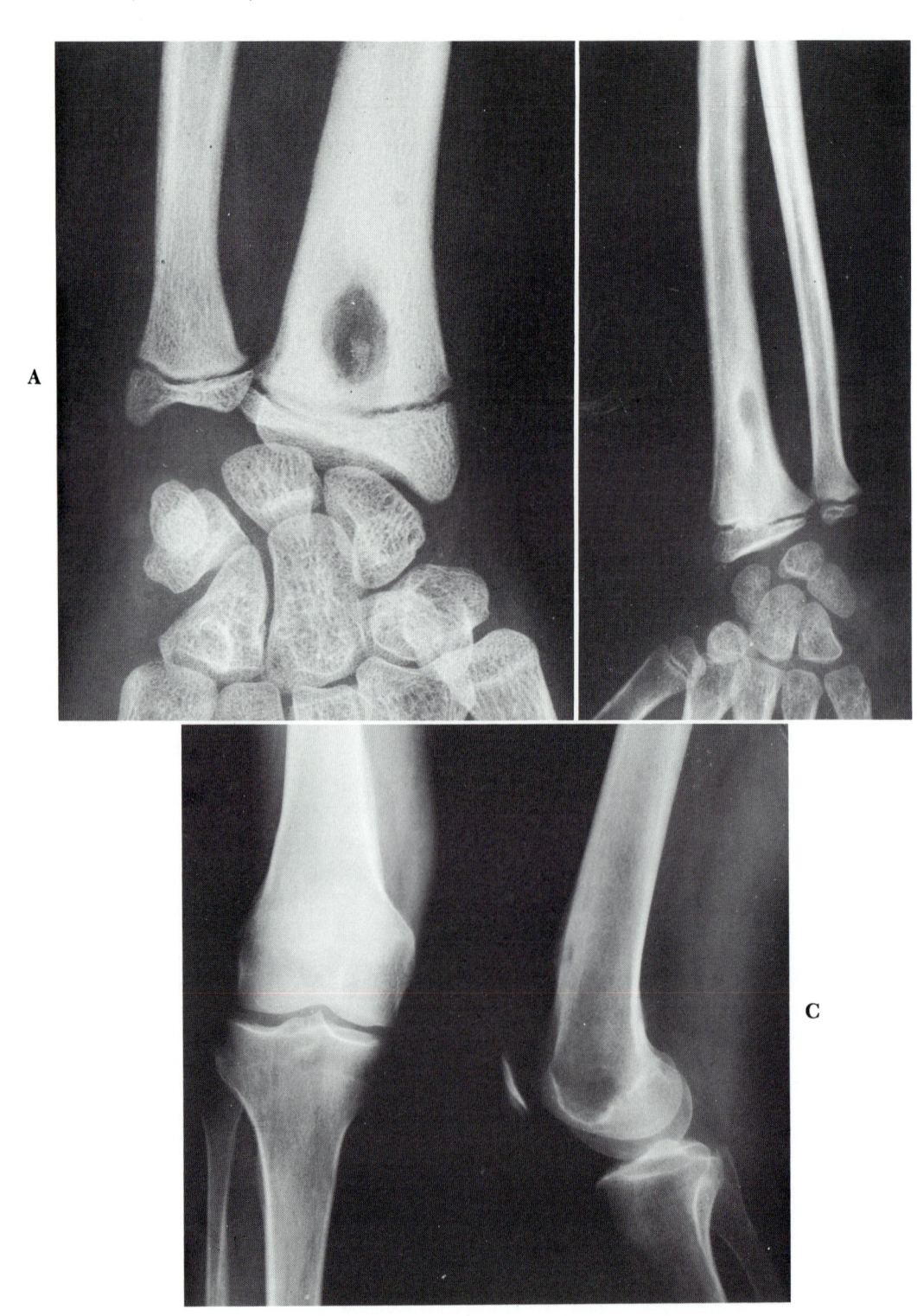

Fig. 3-2. For legend see opposite page.

Infections of bone

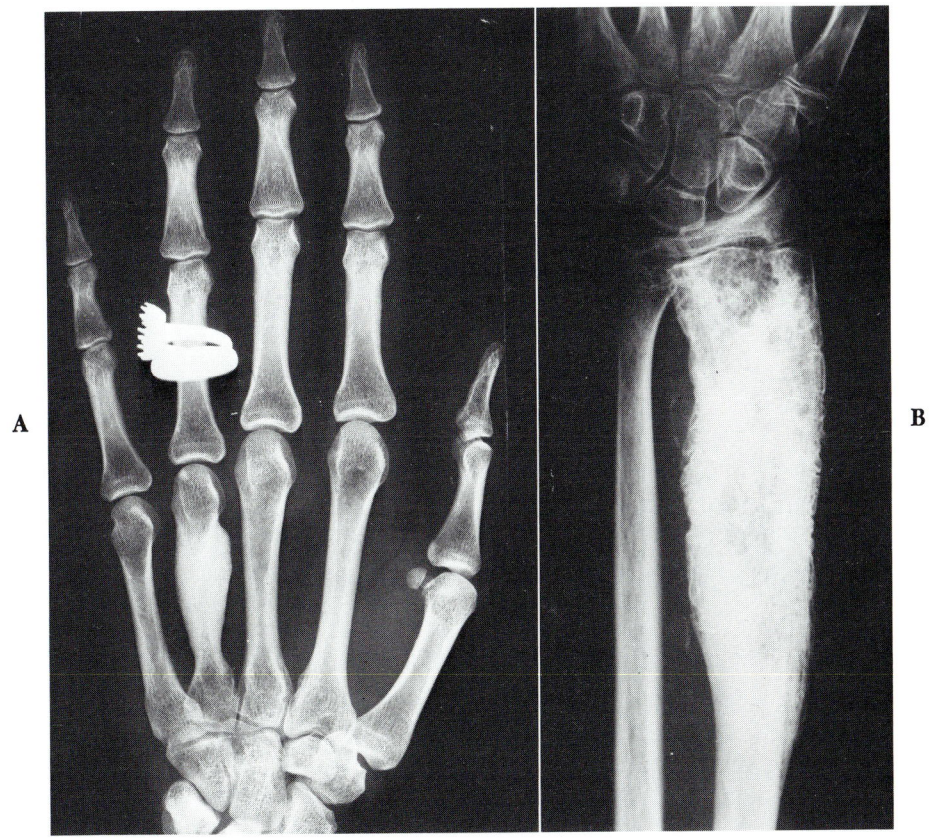

Continued.

Fig. 3-3. **A,** Roentgenogram showing a lesion of sclerosing osteomyelitis in the shaft of a metacarpal bone of an adult. Lesions such as this are sometimes referred to as the Garré type of osteomyelitis. **B,** Another unusual instance of sclerosing osteomyelitis in the distal metaphysis of a radius, which simulated osteogenic sarcoma. **C,** Roentgenogram of a sternum and attached ribs (autopsy specimen) showing marked radiopacity of the manubrium, reflecting the presence microscopically of a low-grade sclerosing osteomyelitis of long standing. This patient had a sternal marrow biopsy performed 20 years previously, and presumably the site became infected.

Fig. 3-2. **A,** Roentgenogram of a chronic bone abscess in the distal metaphysis of a radius. **B,** Another chronic bone abscess in the distal radius of an 8-year-old girl with a 2-year history. The metaphyseal location and the ovoid outline of the abscess, with slight sclerosis around it, are quite characteristic. **C,** Cortical bone abscess in the distal femur of an adult. The possibility of a small osteoid-osteoma was also considered clinically. This is a not uncommon problem in differential diagnosis prior to surgery.

Diseases of bone and joints

C

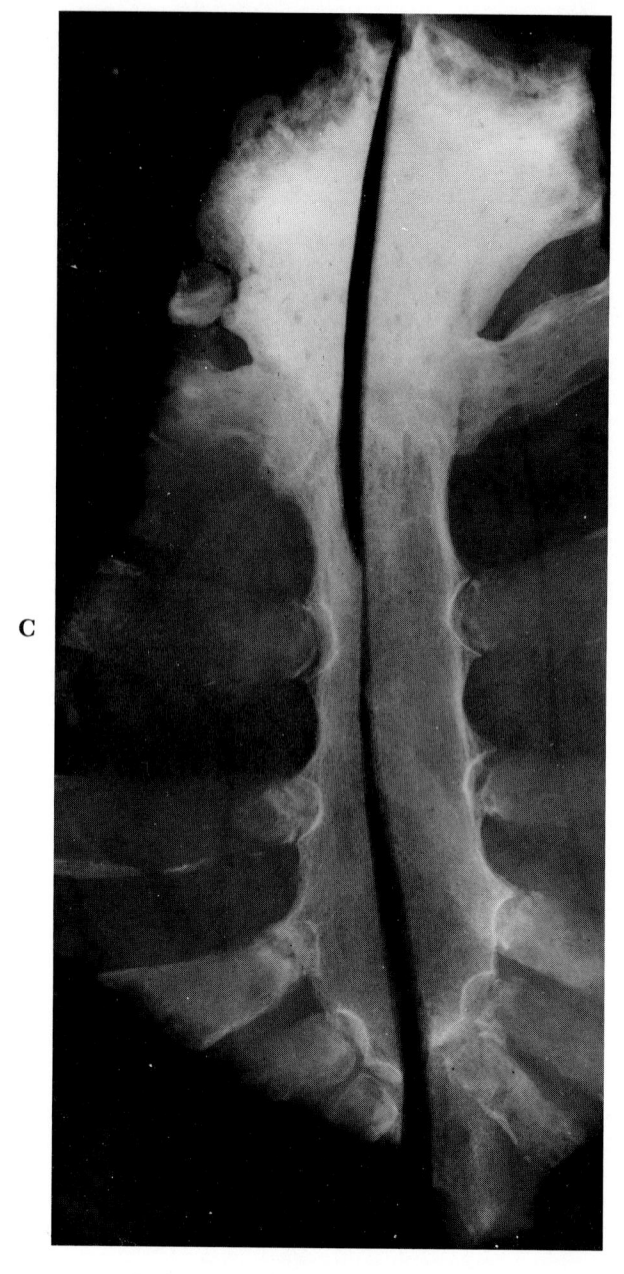

Fig. 3-3, cont'd. For legend see p. 55.

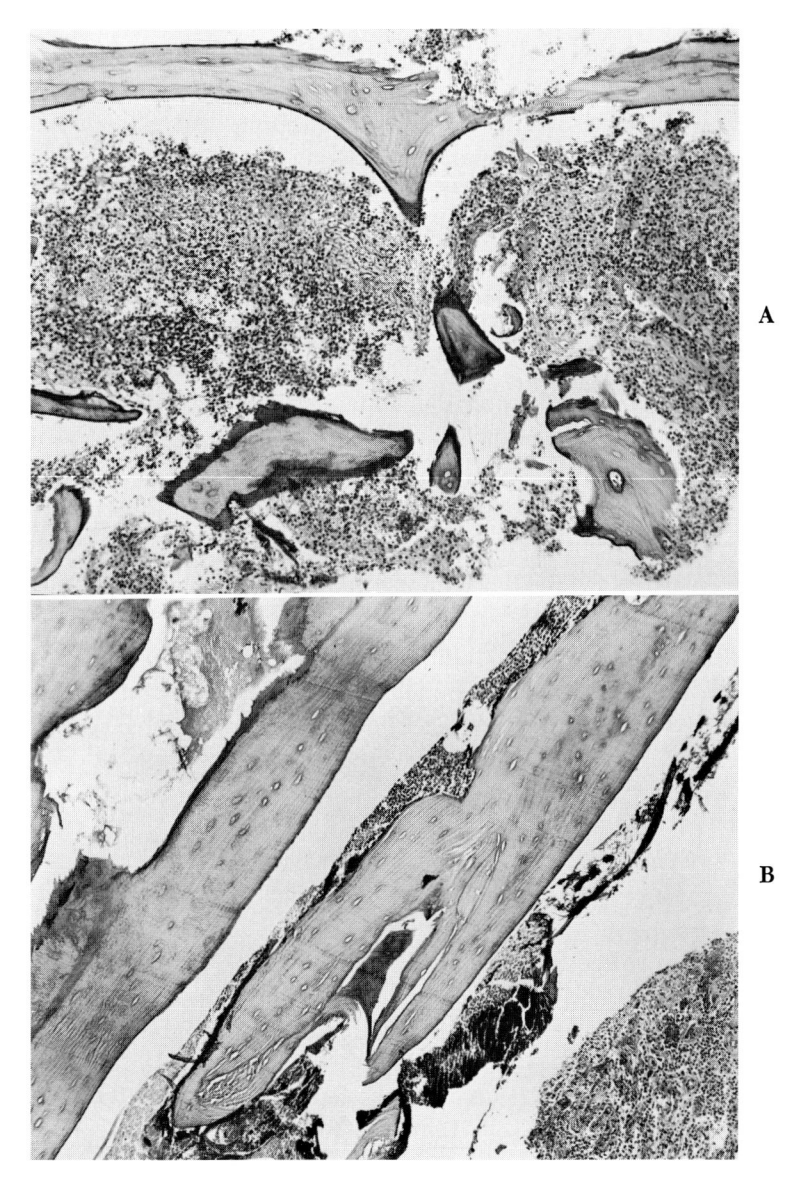

Fig. 3-4. **A,** Low-power photomicrograph of a focus of acute osteomyelitis showing necrosis of bone and the presence of pus in the marrow spaces. The inflammatory cells were virtually all polymorphonuclear leukocytes. **B,** Infected sequestrum showing dead bone and adherent pus and infected granulation tissue. Note that the osteocytes within the lacunae have entirely disappeared.

of infection. Altogether, one can readily perceive why time-honored surgical procedures such as saucerization, removal of sequestra, and excision of sinus tracts must still be employed with some frequency to supplement the limited beneficial effect of antibiotic therapy, quite apart from the factor of bacterial resistance, through mutation, to specific antibiotic agents.

In *acute osteomyelitis* (as seen in a bone of a toe in a diabetic patient, for example), there are two cardinal histologic features: (1) extensive necrosis of bone, evidenced by loss of osteocytes in lacunae, and (2) the presence of numerous pus cells (polymorphonuclear leukocytes) in the marrow spaces (Fig. 3-4, *A*). Similarly, in sections of an infected sequestrum one also finds dead bone and adherent pus or infected granulation tissue (Fig. 3-4, *B*).

If one examines sections of infected cortical bone in a case of *chronic osteomyelitis*, removed in the course of saucerization of a limb bone, for example, one notes at once that there has been more or less extensive resorption of bone and (inevitably) fibrous replacement. If there has been an attempt at reconstruction, and there usually is, this is manifested in a layer of osteoblasts on the surface of the residual blocks of bone, which lay down slender strips of new bone (Fig. 3-5, *A*). Within the fibrous tissue, there are numerous chronic inflammatory cells, including lymphocytes, plasma cells, and mononuclear macrophages; polymorphonuclear leukocytes are in a minority. At times, these inflammatory cells may be so concentrated focally as to constitute a microabscess (Fig. 3-5, *B*).

In a *chronic bone abscess*, necrotic debris and bacterial colonies may become walled off by fibrous tissue and inflamed granulation tissue (Fig. 3-6, *A*). Such an abscess may persist for years if it is not eradicated surgically, although culture may be sterile. Some surgeons are prone to designate any bone abscess as "Brodie's abscess," although Brodie in his old paper,* written long before Roentgen's work, actually described some five cases in point, *all in the tibia,* in which the manifestations of localized suppuration were ameliorated by drilling and evacuation of pus.

Because of their unusual effects, specific mention should be made of osteomyelitis caused by certain bacteria other than the common pyogenic pathogens. *Salmonella* infection may be complicated occasionally by bone abscess (Fig. 3-6, *B*) or by osteomyelitis in multiple foci, particularly in children and curiously in patients with sickle cell anemia. Unusual manifestations of osteomyelitis may also be caused by *Proteus* and by *Klebsiella pneumoniae*.

In *brucellosis*, which is endemic to the Midwest, in hogs and cattle and in humans who contract the infection from them, skeletal complications are well known. It has been estimated by Spink[6] that about 10% of all patients with chronic brucellosis have bone or joint lesions in the course of the disease. Within this group of brucella osteomyelitis, in fully 75% of patients the vertebral column is involved, mainly at the lower thoracic and upper lumbar levels. The

---

*Available in reprints of the Sydenham Society.

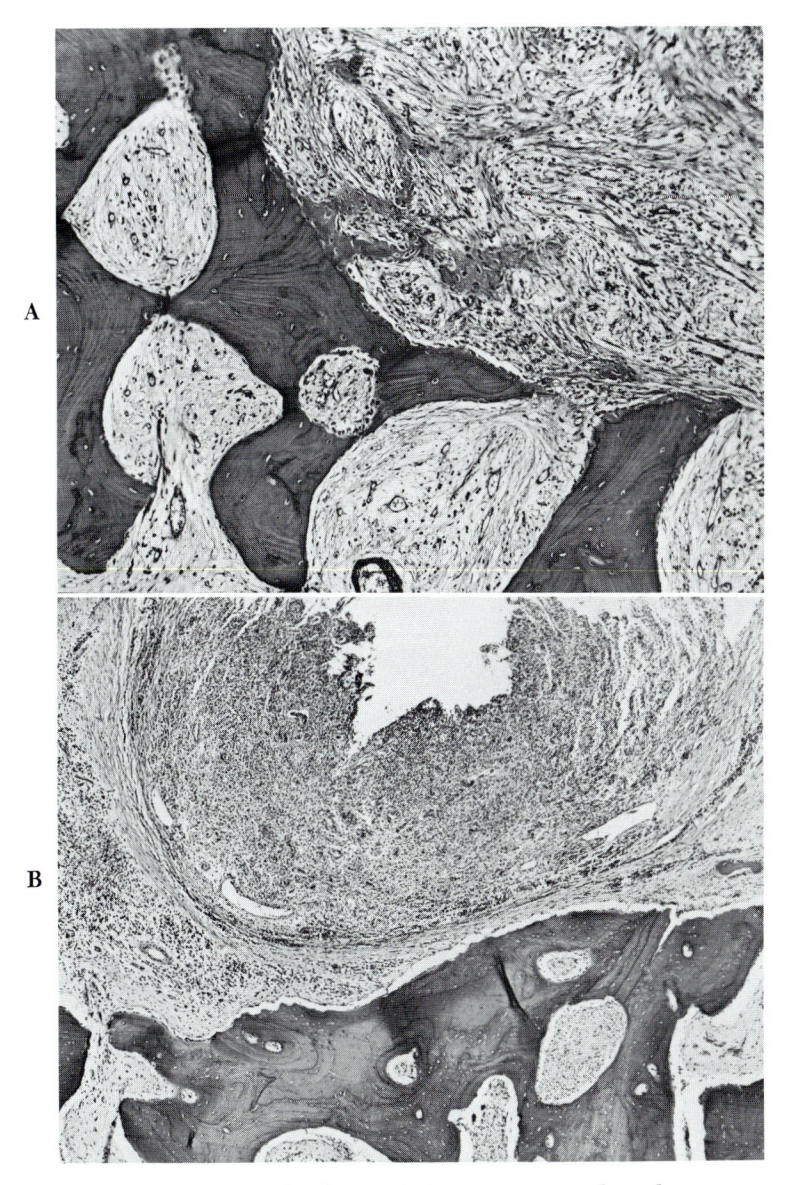

Fig. 3-5. A, Photomicrograph of a focus of chronic osteomyelitis showing resorption of bone and replacement by fibrous tissue and inflamed granulation tissue. There is also an attempt at new bone formation. **B,** Photomicrograph of another instance of chronic osteomyelitis with a microabscess lined by chronically inflamed granulation tissue.

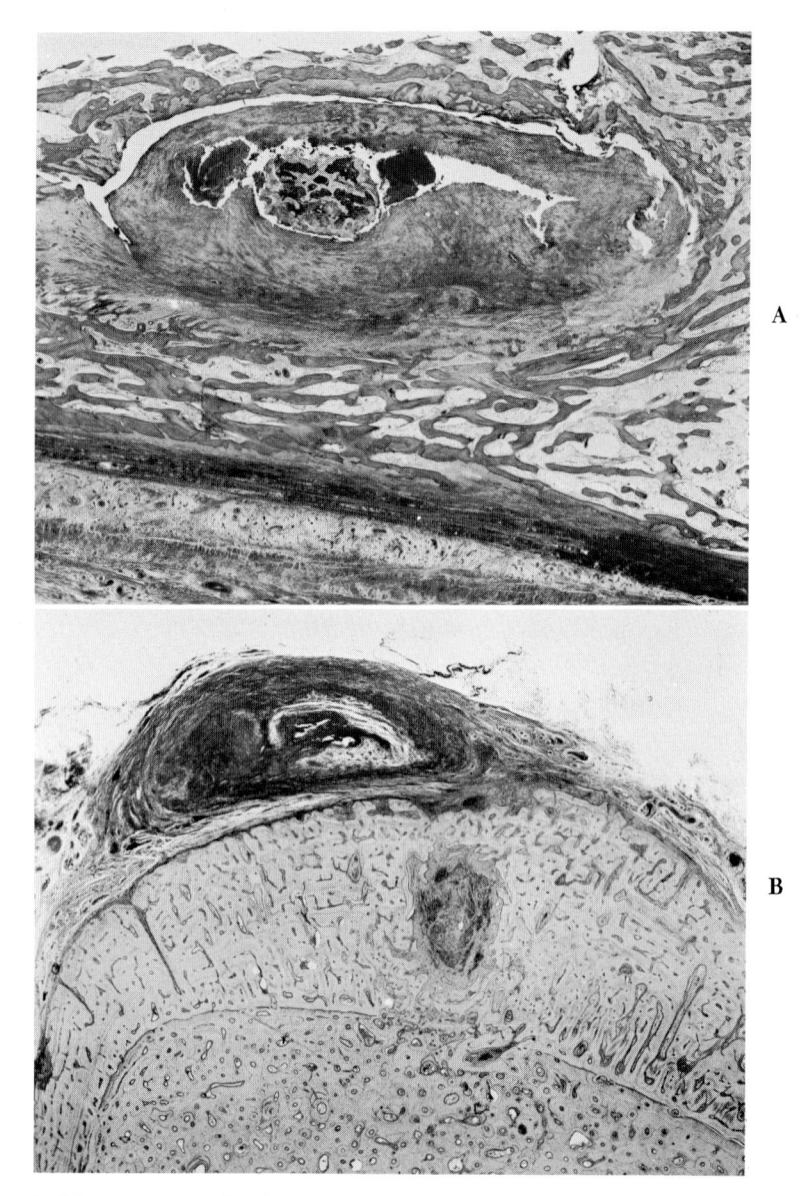

Fig. 3-6. **A**, Photomicrograph of a cortical chronic bone abscess of several years' standing. Although bacterial colonies were still discernible within this walled-off abscess at higher magnification, cultures were sterile. **B**, Periosteal abscess *(Salmonella)* overlying a layer of dense cortical new bone. The tract of infected granulation tissue within the thickened cortex was continuous at another level with the abscess on its surface. (This patient was found to have a sharply rising titer on Widal test, indicative of typhoid fever.)

spondylitis is chronic and at first may be mistaken for that of tuberculosis. It is likely to affect two adjacent vertebrae and the intervening disc, which is destroyed and replaced by granulomatous tissue. At times, a sizable paravertebral inflammatory mass develops and leads to abundant osteophytic reactive bone.

Less frequent manifestations of skeletal brucellosis are osteomyelitis of long bones, leading to chronic bone abscess (with *B. suis* particularly), and also chronic suppurative arthritis of large joints, especially the hip.

The tissue reaction to *Brucella* is peculiar and warrants brief comment. In occasional chronic lesions, one may find epitheloid cell follicles, not unlike sarcoid granulomas, but in the main they resemble chronic suppurative (pyogenic) osteomyelitis. Necrosis and abscess formation is limited, however, and there is abundant reparative fibrous tissue and bone regeneration (Lowbeer).[7]

The antibiotic agents currently favored are the tetracycline derivatives and streptomycin used in combination, but these are not always as effective as they might be.

Attention should also be directed here to two possible sequelae of persistent chronic osteomyelitis of long standing, which are familiar to clinicians and pathologists alike: (1) amyloidosis, developing at times in patients with neglected or unsuccessfully treated infection, and (2) the appearance of malignant tumor in old sinus tracts, which may necessitate amputation. This is usually squamous cell carcinoma[8] but, on rare occasions, it may be fibrosarcoma.[9] It seems altogether probable that these complications will occur with diminishing frequency in the future.

SKELETAL TUBERCULOSIS

Tuberculosis of bone and joints is always secondary to some other, previously established focus of tuberculous infection elsewhere in the body, commonly in the lungs. Skeletal tuberculosis takes three major forms: arthritis, spondylitis, and osteomyelitis of the shafts of long bones, although these are not the only ones.

Tuberculous arthritis (Fig. 3-7, *A*) is discussed further on in Chapter 15, and to avoid repetition, it will not be considered at this point.

As for tuberculous spondylitis (Pott's disease), it is commonly the vertebral bodies that are affected, and frequently a whole segment of the vertebral column is involved. The thoracic vertebrae are most often attacked, then the lumbar, and occasionally the cervical (Fig. 3-7, *F*). Progressive destruction of the bone leads to collapse of the vertebral body, and since two or more adjacent bodies are often affected, a severe angular kyphosis (hunchback) typically results. The intervertebral discs are more resistant than the bone, but they, too, become distorted and eventually disappear. At the site of angulation, there is usually a focus of active tuberculosis close to the dura, but the latter resists spread of infection, so that the meninges and the spinal cord are seldom infected by direct extension. When a cold abscess develops in these circumstances,

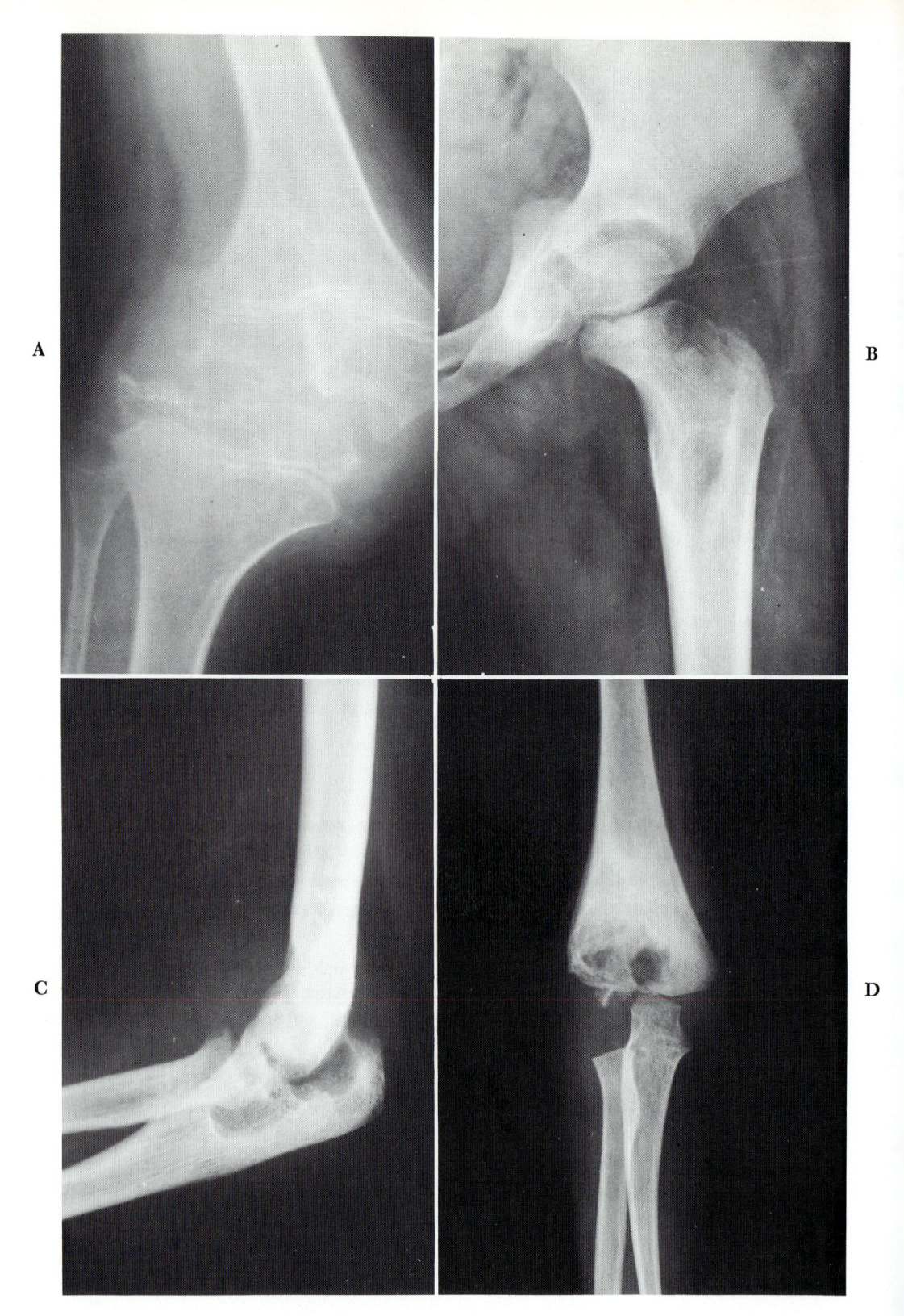

Fig. 3-7. For legend see opposite page.

62

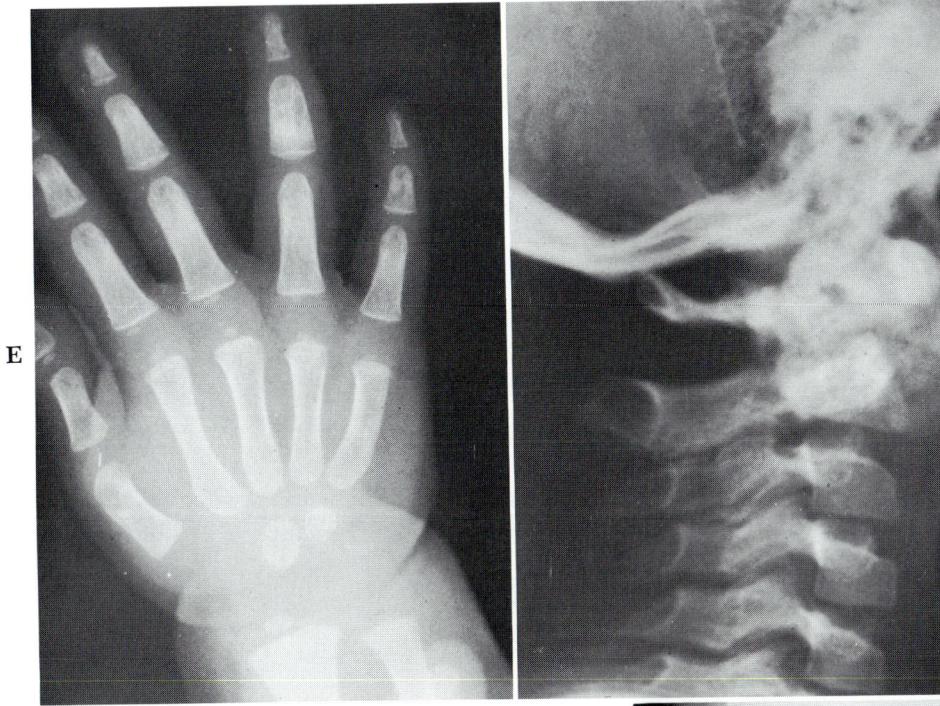

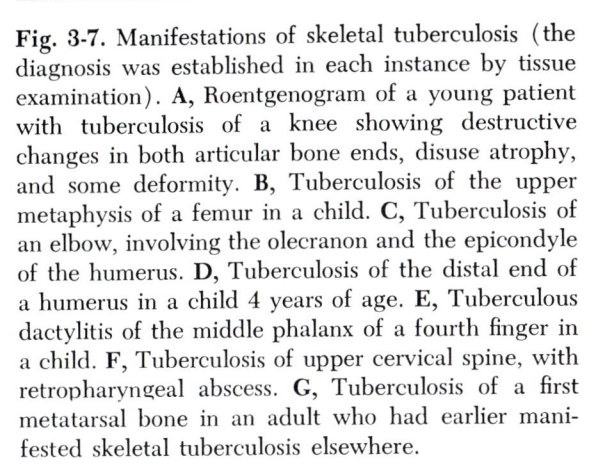

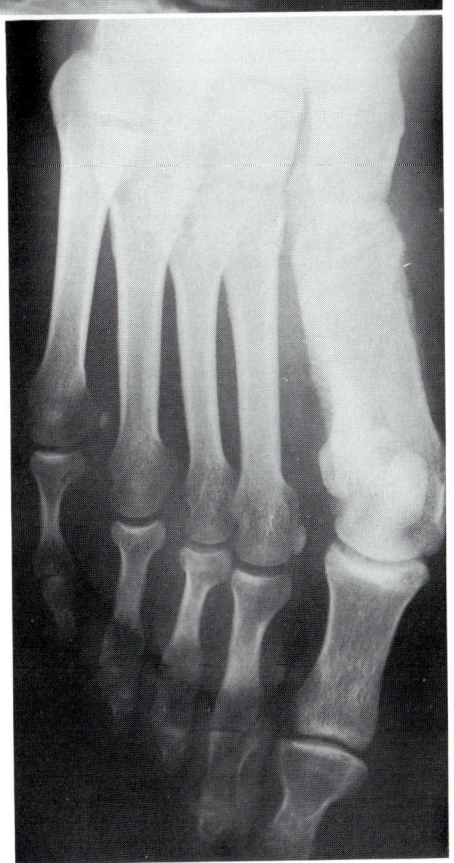

Fig. 3-7. Manifestations of skeletal tuberculosis (the diagnosis was established in each instance by tissue examination). **A,** Roentgenogram of a young patient with tuberculosis of a knee showing destructive changes in both articular bone ends, disuse atrophy, and some deformity. **B,** Tuberculosis of the upper metaphysis of a femur in a child. **C,** Tuberculosis of an elbow, involving the olecranon and the epicondyle of the humerus. **D,** Tuberculosis of the distal end of a humerus in a child 4 years of age. **E,** Tuberculous dactylitis of the middle phalanx of a fourth finger in a child. **F,** Tuberculosis of upper cervical spine, with retropharyngeal abscess. **G,** Tuberculosis of a first metatarsal bone in an adult who had earlier manifested skeletal tuberculosis elsewhere.

Diseases of bone and joints

it contains necrotic (caseous) debris, a few leukocytes, and usually some tubercle bacilli.

Tuberculosis of long bones, other than in association with tuberculous arthritis, is distinctly unusual. Like pyogenic osteomyelitis, it tends to localize at the metaphysis, and a chronic tuberculous abscess in that site may interfere with growth at the adjacent plate. Occasionally, one may observe tuberculosis of the tubular bones of the hand and foot, and examples of this are illustrated radiographically in Fig. 3-7, *E* and *G*.

The advent of effective chemotherapy has had as great an impact on the incidence and course of bone and joint tuberculosis as it has on pyogenic osteomyelitis. Specifically, the widespread use of streptomycin and nicotinic acid hydrazides, especially iproniazid, as well as other agents, has brought about a dramatic change, to the point that whole specialty hospitals formerly in great demand have gone out of business. Pott's disease with gibbus,[10-12] caries sicca (shoulder), and spina ventosa (tuberculous dactylitis) are just names to many younger medical men who see these conditions infrequently, if at all. For that matter, I now get most of my teaching material from Mexico, where skeletal tuberculosis is still prevalent (Fig. 3-7). For historic perspective, the reader may have profitable recourse to the authoritative account by Bosworth,[13] which has reference to conditions in the United States. However, skeletal tuberculosis is still a serious problem in some other parts of the world, and, in particular, Hodgson in Hong Kong has made many valuable clinical contributions.

To be sure, chemotherapy is not invariably successful and the need for selected surgical procedures—particularly spine fusion for the stabilization of tuberculous spondylitis and arthrodesis of badly damaged weight-bearing joints—has not been entirely eliminated. But the surgeon can now do what he has to under specific antibiotic cover, without being fearful of local spread of infection, persistent sinus formation, or miliary dissemination.

The pathologic reaction to tuberculosis in skeletal structures is not essentially different from that in soft tissues. Productive (tubercle formation) and exudative aspects occur in varying proportion, depending largely on the severity of the infection and the degree of acquired hypersensitivity of the patient. It may be remarked, however, that tubercles in bone are not likely to resemble the textbook picture, since they generally lack a mantle of lymphocytes and, frequently, Langhans' giant cells as well.

A few instances of serious bone infection simulating tuberculosis, caused by antibiotic resistant chromogenic acid-fast organisms (differing from *Myobacterium tuberculosis* culturally and in other respects), have been cited by Aegerter and Kirkpatrick.[14] These authors also called attention to several cases of osteomyelitis caused by acid-fast organisms that provoked a tissue reaction resembling that of tuberculosis or leprosy, but that, because of their branching tendency on culture, were classified as *Nocardia*.

With further reference to infection by *Nocardia*, I have had occasion to examine an amputated Madura foot[15] presenting numerous abscesses both in

Infections of bone

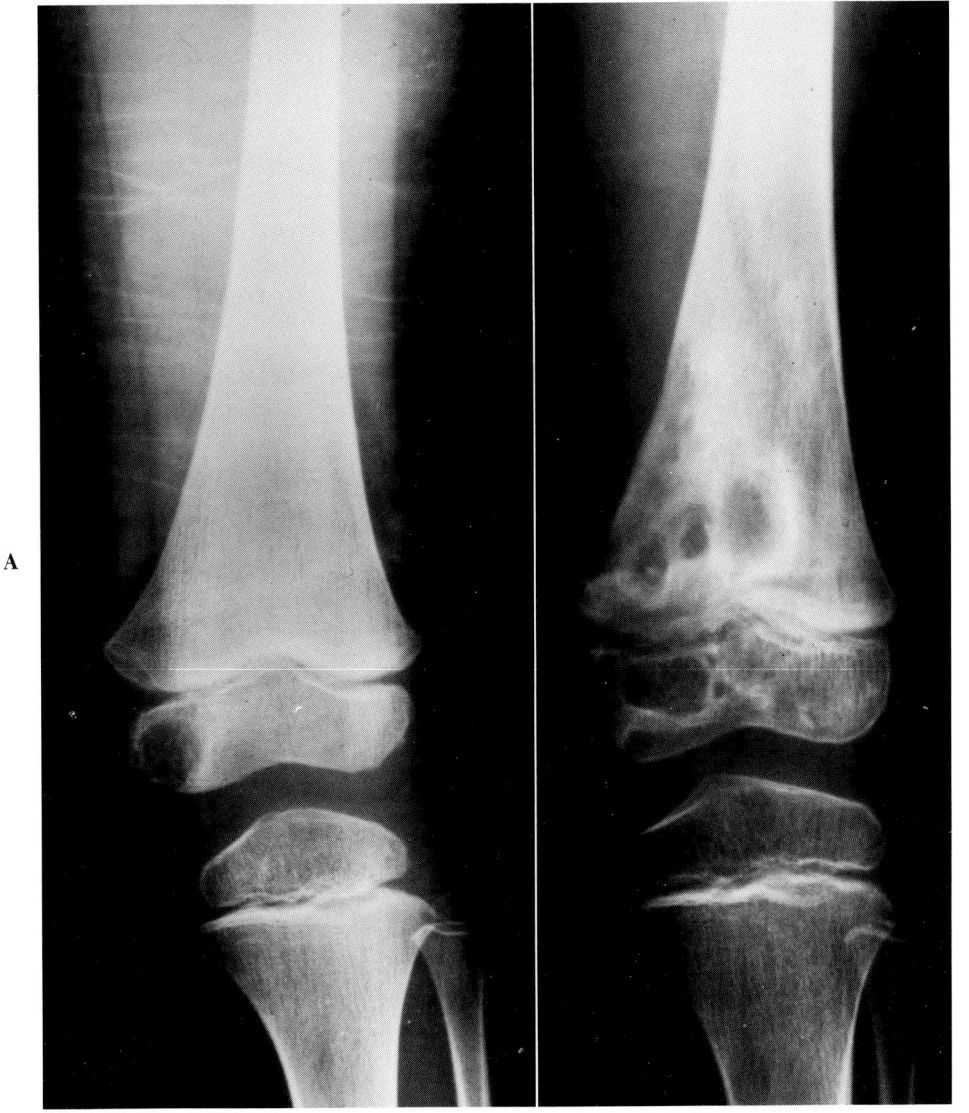

Fig. 3-8. **A,** Roentgenogram showing a lucent defect reflecting early tuberculous infection in the distal femoral epiphysis. **B,** Spread of the tuberculous infection 2 years later, involving more of the epiphysis and also the adjacent metaphysis.

the bones and in the soft parts. In the vicinity of the abscesses there were branching colonies with clubs at their periphery, which morphologically resembled ray fungi but which were identified on culture as *Nocardia*.

Many species of filamentous fungi have been described as causative organisms of *maduromycosis* (Madura foot, or mycetoma). The infection is contracted, as a rule, through the soles of bare feet, and most of the organisms isolated from the lesions are related to soil fungi. The disease runs an extremely chronic

Diseases of bone and joints

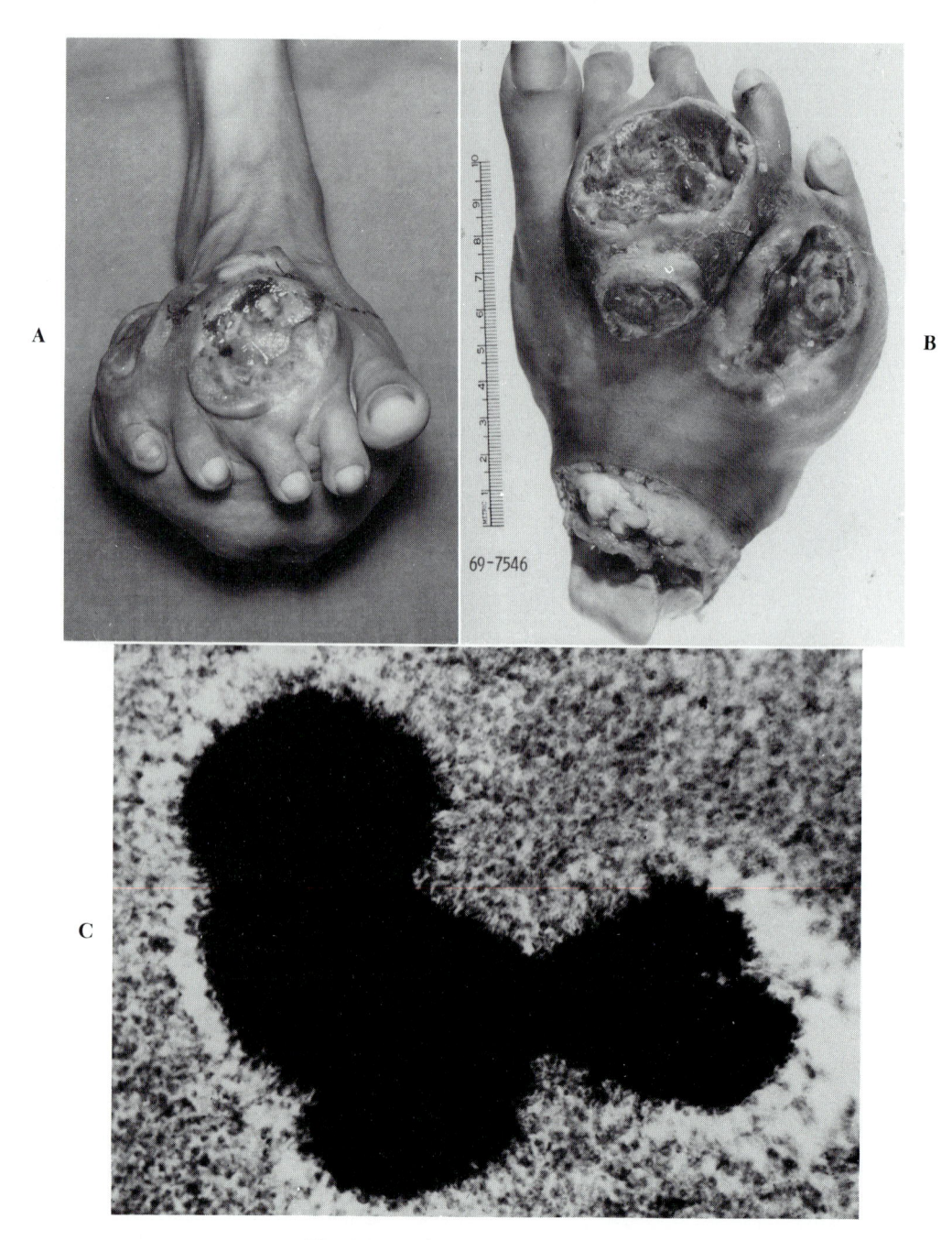

Fig. 3-9. For legend see opposite page.

Infections of bone

course, with slow but inexorable destruction of both the osseous and soft tissues. The end result is likely to be a grossly deformed, club-shaped, almost boneless foot whose surface is a mass of discharging sinuses (Fig. 3-9). The histologic picture is essentially that of chronic suppuration, with abscess formation and extensive necrosis of bone, as noted.

SKELETAL CHANGES IN LEPROSY

Leprosy, an ancient disease caused by *Mycobacterium leprae,* is not unknown in the United States.[16-18] There are endemic foci in Louisiana, for example; when I was at Charity Hospital in New Orleans, there were always a number of patients with leprosy there, as well as an appreciable number under treatment in the leprosarium at Carville.

This section will deal briefly with the skeletal alterations that may ensue in leprosy, especially in patients whose clinical manifestations have not been modified by prolonged sulfone therapy.

The most significant changes in the bones are associated with leprous neuritis or perineuritis (neural or anesthetic form). In this common expression of the disease, the scarring and cordlike thickening of nerve bundles lead to loss of sensation, striking trophic changes in the extremities, and eventual mutilation of the hands and feet, with clawlike contractures or hideous stumps that may develop penetrating ulcers (see Fig. 9-3).[19] It appears that secondary infection is a contributing factor in this process. In the cutaneous form of leprosy, there may be secondary destruction of the cartilage of the nose and even of the bones of the face. Finally, there is also a kind of leprous osteomyelitis as part of advanced systemic dissemination, with lepromatous lesions analogous to those of the skin, but this is much less significant than the sequelae of neural involvement. These foci in the bones may be small and widely dispersed, producing cystlike rarefactions radiographically. Other comparatively unusual bone changes in leprosy are those of sclerosing periostitis and osteomyelitis from complicating pyogenic infection.

Fig. 3-9. **A,** Peculiar mycetoma, present for 6 years, involving the foot of a 12-year-old Central American boy. Note the massive enlargement of the foot and the large ulcers on the dorsum and plantar surface. **B,** Photograph of the amputated foot some months later. The muscles showed marked atrophy, and the bones were all osteoporotic, as one might expect. The infected tissue mass was soft, pasty, and orange-yellow in color. Although no fungal organisms were isolated on culture, the clinical history and course of disease, as well as the appearance of the lesion, strongly suggested so-called Madura foot. **C,** Photomicrograph (high magnification) showing a fungal colony in another lesion of Madura foot. The clubs at the periphery suggested a ray fungus, although cultural identification was that of Nocardia. Elsewhere there were numerous abscesses, both in the bones and soft tissues of the foot.

Diseases of bone and joints

The pathologic reaction to *Mycobacterium leprae*[20] may take one of two forms. The first is the lepromatous lesion, featuring focal or more diffuse collections of histiocytes or foamy macrophages (lepra cells), and sometimes giant cells as well. Acid-fast bacilli are found not only in these cells but also in large numbers in endothelial cells of the granulation tissue. The second pathologic reaction is tuberculids, that is, tubercle-like or sarcoid-like follicles of epithelioid cells, in which organisms are rarely observed. These are found particularly in the chronic maculoanesthetic cases.

SKELETAL INVOLVEMENT IN GRANULOMA INGUINALE

Granuloma inguinale, long held to be a venereal disease affecting young adults of both sexes, especially blacks, is quite familiar to physicians who have worked in the southern part of the United States. The condition characteristically involves the genital region (including the cervix in women), the inguinal region, or both. Only infrequently does it affect extragenital sites as well. The infection is apparently caused by Donovan bodies, which appear as intracellular inclusions and which are best demonstrated by Giemsa or Wright's stain. Dissemination, presumably hematogenous, does occur occasionally, so that a few instances of skeletal involvement have been reported.[21-23] In one such instance,[21] for example, there was osteomyelitis of the spine that destroyed the fourth lumbar vertebra and part of the fifth. Giemsa stain of a needle aspiration biopsy showed intracellular Donovan bodies in large number. It is noteworthy that the condition was successfully treated by chloramphenicol and subsequent spine fusion.

SKELETAL MANIFESTATIONS OF SYPHILIS

Although the control of syphilis, a common venereal disease, is still a serious public health problem, the availability of penicillin has dramatically reduced the incidence of its skeletal complications. Specifically, the use of penicillin in prenatal clinics has made the osseous manifestations of congenital lues far less common than they used to be, while gummatous syphilis in the adult is now seldom observed in hospital practice. For detailed accounts of the former skeletal ravages of syphilis one must have recourse to old texts and articles[17,24-27] or, by analogy, to current descriptions of the effects of *yaws* (a related, penicillin-sensitive, spirochetal infection), as seen in Africa and the South Pacific, for example. The superbly illustrated monograph of Hackett[28] on the bone lesions of yaws in Uganda is particularly recommended.

In *congenital lues,* the skeletal lesions appear during the fifth month of intrauterine life and are fully demonstrated at birth.

The best known and most consistent manifestation of untreated or inadequately treated *congenital syphilis* is osteochondritis of the upper and lower limb bones, which often leads to epiphyseal separation (Fig. 3-10, A). The spirochetes flourish in the richly vascular growth zones, and their noxious effect and the resulting inflammatory exudate disrupt the process of endochondral ossifica-

Infections of bone

tion (Fig. 3-10, *B*). Irregularity and widening of the affected zone are reflected roentgenographically, and a yellow line is grossly discernible.

Periostitis or osteoperiostitis affecting the shaft of the long bones, especially those of the leg, forearm, and hand, is another relatively frequent manifestation in infancy and is found occasionally in older children. The granulation tissue within or beneath the periosteum is likewise rich in spirochetes, and may provoke extensive deposition of new bone on the original cortex. Gummas may form in affected bones (as they may elsewhere), particularly in long bones or the skull, and the gummatous nodes can undergo softening and suppuration with sinus formation.

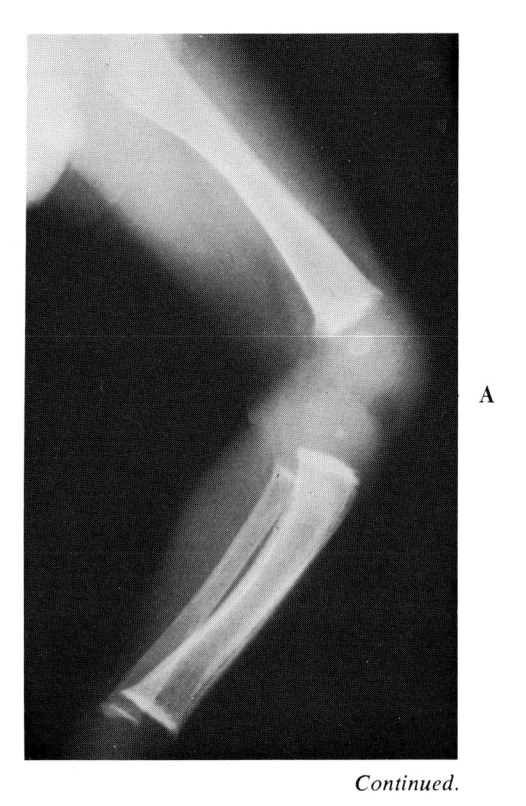

Continued.

Fig. 3-10. **A**, Roentgenogram showing the changes of osteochondritis in congenital syphilis. **B**, Photomicrograph showing luetic osteochondritis of the distal femur in a dead neonate examined at autopsy. (The mother had received only partial, inadequate treatment in prenatal clinic.) Note disruption of endochondral ossification at the plate. Special stain showed spirochetes in abundance within the inflammatory exudate. **C**, Photomicrograph of a partially necrotic, destructive skeletal focus (one of many) in a South Pacific native with yaws. The area of necrosis is bordered by inflamed granulation tissue containing occasional histiocytic nodes. This picture is quite analogous to that of gummatous syphilis. **D**, Roentgenogram illustrating a lesion of acquired syphilis in a tibia of an adult. This skeletal manifestation was once much more common than it is at present.

Diseases of bone and joints

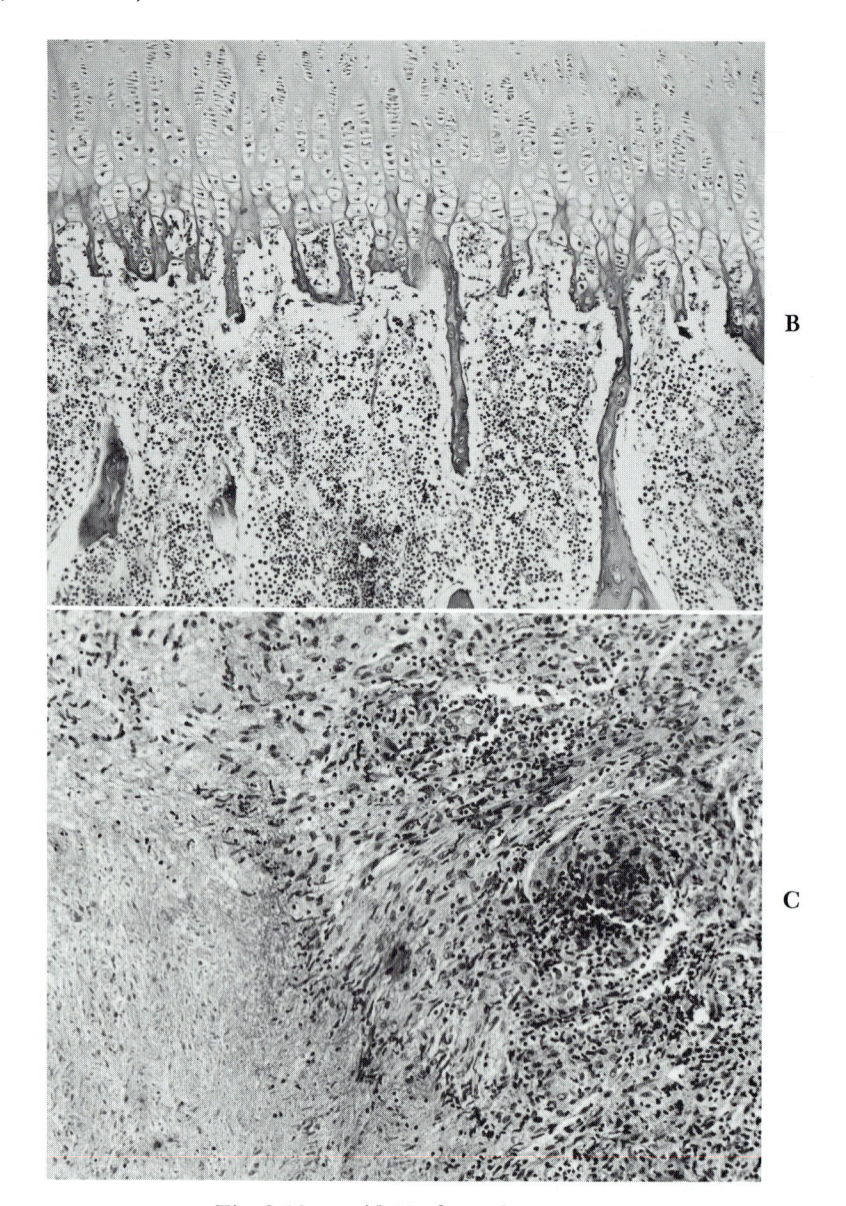

Fig. 3-10, cont'd. For legend see p. 69.

Severe untreated infection results in death of the fetus or neonate. Those who survive may go on to show such familiar late manifestations as interstitial keratitis; deformed teeth, particularly the upper central incisors of the second set (Hutchinson's teeth); leukoderma; nerve deafness; juvenile taboparesis; saddle nose (from destruction of the septum and turbinates); saber shin (from osteoperiostitis of the tibia); dactylitis, with spindle-shaped enlargement[24-28]; and occasionally chronic synovitis, especially of knee joints (Clutton's joints).[29]

The skeletal lesions of *acquired syphilis* usually appear as an early manifes-

Infections of bone

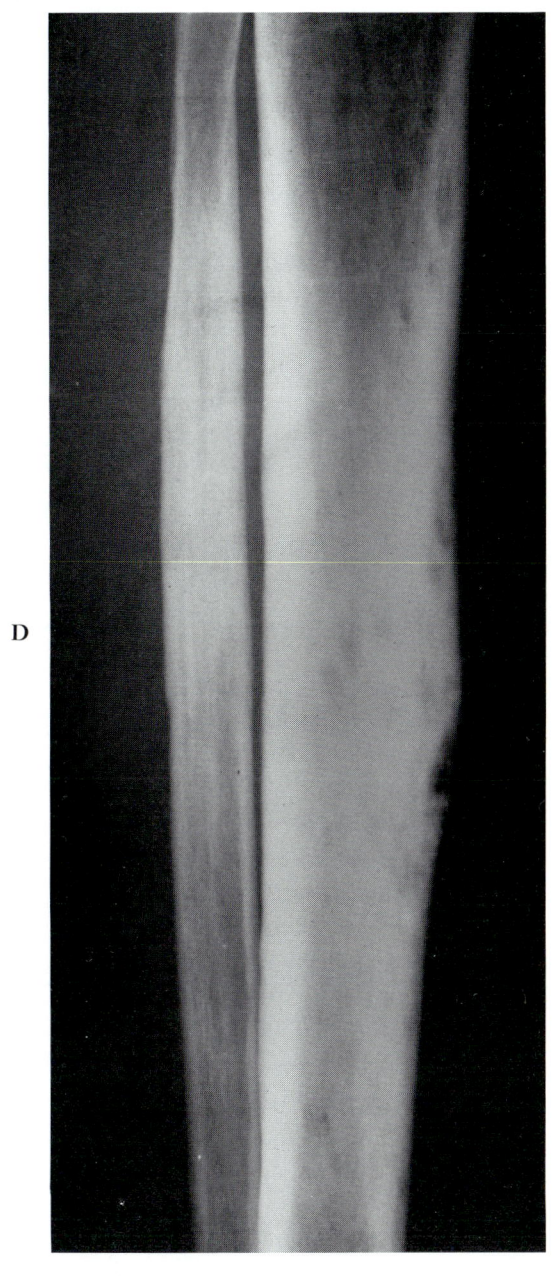

D

Fig. 3-10, cont'd. For legend see p. 69.

Diseases of bone and joints

tation of the tertiary stage, some 2 to 5 years after (untreated) infection. The bones most often involved are the tibia (Fig. 3-10, *D*), the bones of the nose and palate, and the skull. The bone changes include periostitis, resulting in irregularly dense osseous thickening, notably of the tibia, where it may produce the saber shin. Less frequently, nongummatous syphilis takes the form of osteomyelitis, featuring foci of granulation tissue and reactive new bone within the medullary cavity. The formation of gummas, leading to perforation of the skull, palate, or vomer, once familiar manifestations of tertiary syphilis, are now seldom observed, as noted, and for good examples one must have recourse to old museum specimens. In the vertebral column, gummatous necrosis may result in collapse of vertebral bodies and kyphosis, but this, too, is a rarity (see spondylitis syphylitica in the old German literature).[30]

Specific joint involvement (synovitis of large joints, especially the knee, with effusion) once seen as an occasional manifestation has also become a rarity, although damage to articular cartilage may result from involvement of contiguous bone ends. On the other hand, more or less extensive destruction of weight-bearing joints secondary to tabes (Charcot's joint), especially in the lower extremity and the vertebral column, is still a formidable clinical problem. This will be discussed in the section on neurotrophic disorders of joints (see Chapter 9).

BONE INVOLVEMENT IN FUNGAL INFECTIONS— COCCIDIOMYCOSIS

Of all the fungal infections that may give rise to osseous lesions, coccidiomycosis is by far the most common, at least in the Central Valley of California, in southwestern United States, and in the adjacent arid states of northern Mexico (fungi do not respect geographic boundaries). By comparison, skeletal lesions in other pathogenic mycoses—such as actinomycosis, blastomycosis, histoplasmosis, cryptococcosis, and sporotrichosis—are unusual, if not rare.

Although coccidiomycosis is primarily and predominantly a self-limited pulmonary disease, as Forbus and Bestebreurtje[31] and others have pointed out, the bones (and occasionally the joints as well) are among the more common sites of infection resulting from hematogenous dissemination of *Coccidioides immitis*.[32-34] One or more osseous sites may be affected. There is a curious predilection for bony prominences such as the radial styloid, tibial tubercle, malleoli of the ankle, olecranon, acromion, and sternoclavicular area, although the skull, vertebral column, ribs, and sternum, as well as other bones, may also be involved on occasion. Infection at any of these sites may be complicated by suppuration and persistent sinus formation. There is a widely held belief that skeletal involvement in dissemination is inevitably serious, but there are undoubtedly cases in which the clinical course is chronic and protracted over a period of many years (Fig. 3-11, *A*). No altogether satisfactory chemotherapeutic agent has as yet been discovered for coccidiomycosis, although a number have been given clinical trial over the years, and the search continues.

Infections of bone

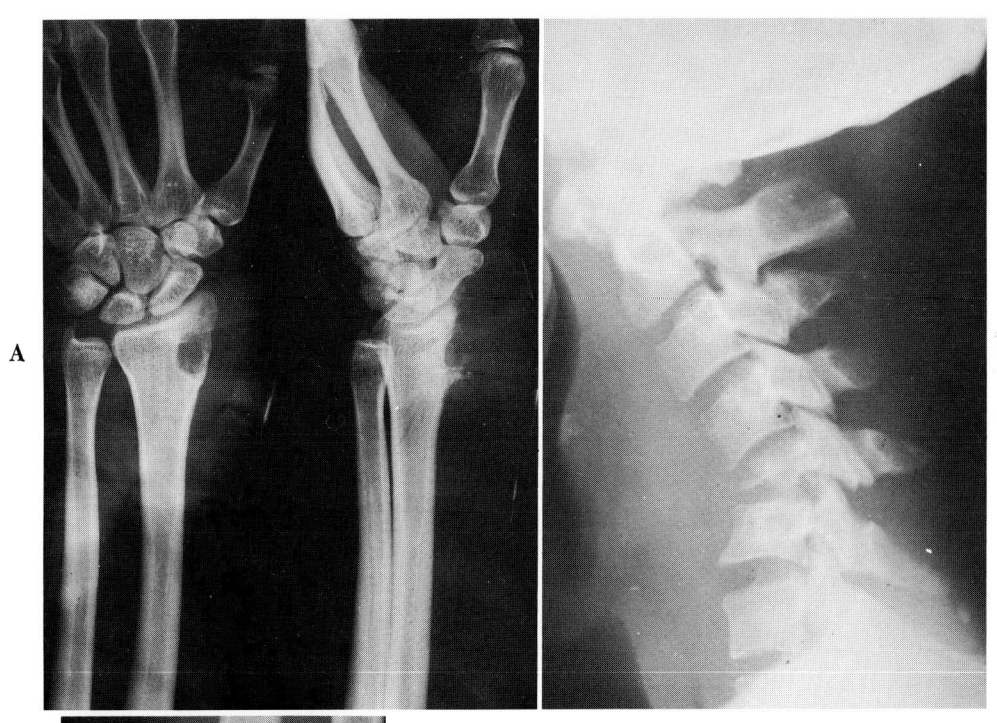

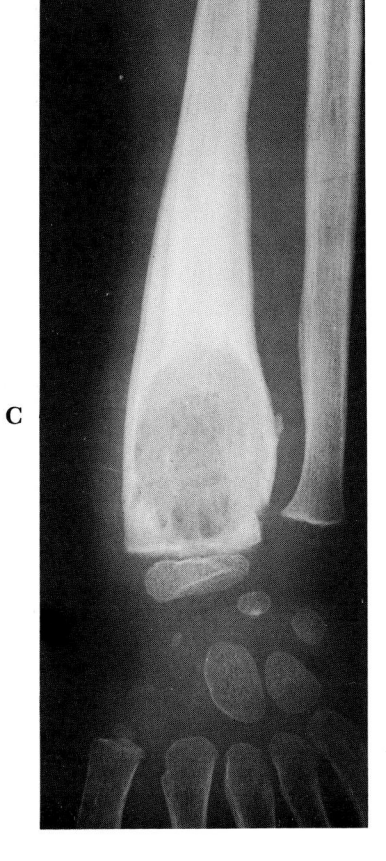

Fig. 3-11. **A,** Roentgenograms showing a lesion of coccidiomycosis in the distal radius and adjacent soft parts (sinus formation). The patient was a Filipino man who had had exacerbations from time to time over a period of almost 10 years. **B,** Coccidiomycosis causing collapse of a cervical vertebra (in a young black adult). Diagnosis was established by needle aspiration (see Fig. 3-12). **C,** Roentgenogram of a destructive focus in the distal metaphysis of a radius of a child. Before tissue examination it was thought to be a focus of eosinophilic granuloma, but subsequently proved to be a lesion of coccidiomycosis.

Diseases of bone and joints

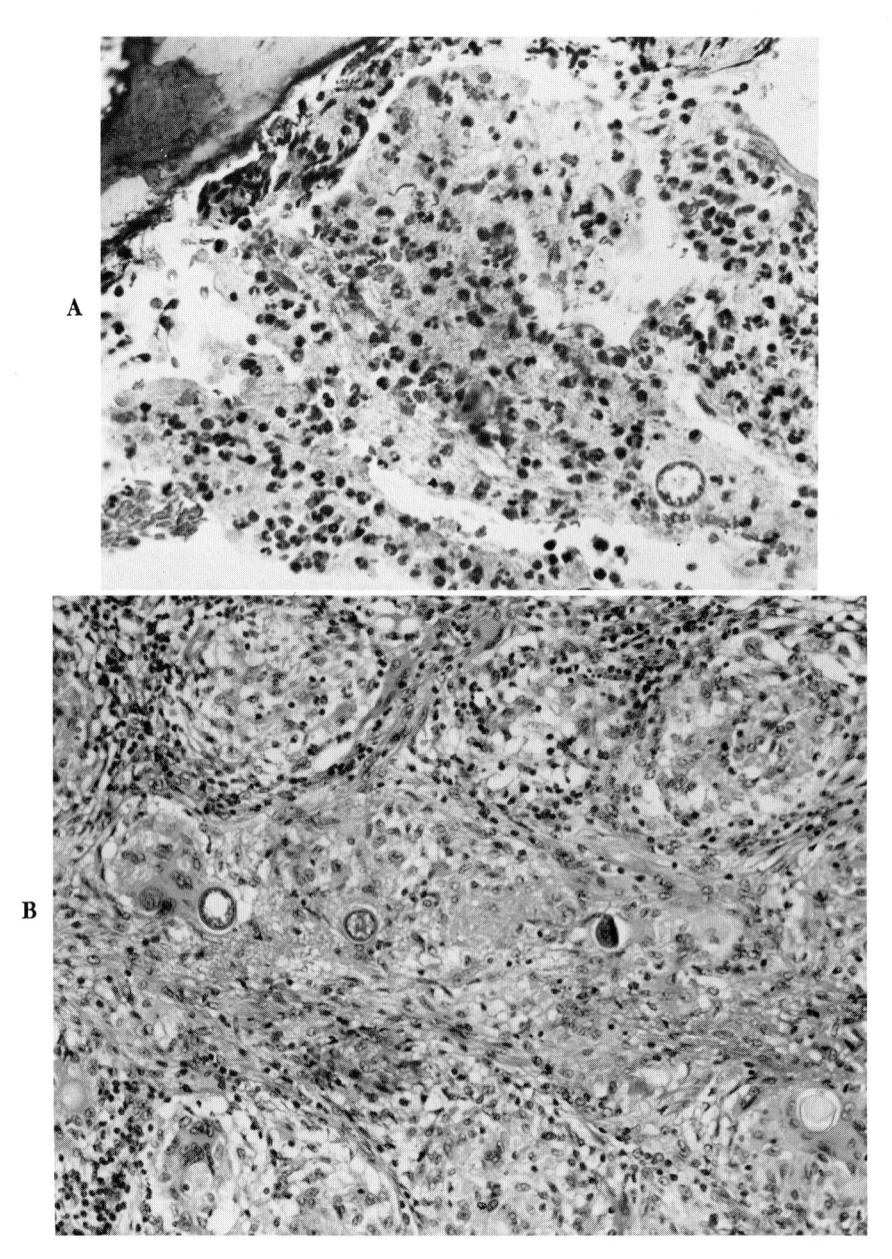

Fig. 3-12. **A,** Photomicrograph of a needle aspiration biopsy of the lesion shown in Fig. 3-11, **B.** The response in this instance was acute inflammation, but the presence of scattered spherules of *Coccidioides immitis,* (lower right) established the diagnosis. **B,** Photomicrograph showing proliferative tuberclelike reaction in a lesion of coccidiomycosis of a knee joint. Were it not for the finding of spherules of *Coccidioides immitis* (some still contain spores, others are empty), this lesion might have been called tuberculous. Many of the spherules were contained within giant cells. Elsewhere in this section, there was necrosis and leucocytic reaction. (×165.)

The pathologic response to *Coccidioides immitis* has both suppurative and granulomatous aspects, and frequently the two are combined (Fig. 3-12). When healing occurs in lesions that have gone beyond early resolution, it is usually a result of scarring and hyalinization (as may occur in tuberculosis). In predominantly granulomatous lesions, the mimicry of the tuberculous reaction may be remarkable; it is only by meticulous search for the spherules of *Coccidioides immitis* (often found within giant cells) that the problem in differentiation can be readily resolved.

Unusual expressions of mycotic osteomyelitis. In *actinomycosis*, involvement of bones (as well as of joints and paraskeletal connective tissues) usually results from direct extension and burrowing of neighboring soft tissue lesions. Specifically, the infection may spread from the mouth to the mandible (analogous to lumpy jaw of cattle); from the lungs to the ribs and even vertebrae; from the ileocecal region to the lumbar spine, sacrum, or iliac bone; or from the skin, burrowing into deeper tissue, including fascia, bones, and joints.[35-38]

That the ray fungus may cause infection in man has been known since 1879.[39] A good account of its pathologic manifestations may be found in MacCallum.[17] In essence, the tissue reaction, wherever it may be, is characterized by destruction and liquefaction, with abscess and sinus formation. The branched organisms grow in tangled mycelia (strahlenpilz), and colonies found in pus may appear as yellow "sulfur" granules. In tissue sections, one may have to make an extended search through many levels to find a single ray fungus, which suffices for a firm diagnosis.

Although osteomyelitis caused by the fungus *Blastomyces dermatitidis* was described as early as 1894 by Gilchrist, this manifestation is infrequent in man.[40-41] Infection of bone may develop by deep extension of cutaneous lesions (for example, on an extremity) or, more often, from hematogenous dissemination with systemic involvement. In the latter circumstance, destructive lesions may develop in the vertebral column, in limb bones, or elsewhere. Such lesions have been described radiographically as simulating skeletal tuberculosis rather than pyogenic osteomyelitis.

Diagnosis is established by the finding in pus or in tissue specimens of doubly refractile blastomyces, which tend to be engulfed by foreign body giant cells. The tissue reaction to this fungus is essentially suppurative with pseudotubercle formation. With reference to therapy, aromatic diamidines have been found effective against systemic blastomycosis (and possibly other systemic fungus infections).[42]

Sporotrichosis, caused by a filamentous spore-forming fungus *(Sporotrichium),* produces bone or joint lesions only rarely in man.[43,44] As in some other fungal infections, osteomyelitis is described as developing either by direct extension from cutaneous lesions or by hematogenous spread. In the latter event, the skeletal lesions may be multiple,[45] affecting the skull, ribs, long bones, and phalanges (simulating the dactylitis of syphilis or tuberculosis).

Cryptococcosis (torulosis) and *histoplasmosis,* while relatively common fungal infections,[46] only occasionally produce clinically detectable bone lesions.[47-50] However, infection of the knee joint (pyarthrosis) has been reported in both conditions.[51] Interestingly enough, in each instance the condition was thought to be tuberculous arthritis until the causative organisms were identified.

In a review of some 200 cases of cryptococcosis, Collins[52] found 17 patients with bone involvement. The lesions are said to be osteolytic and characteristically very slow to evolve. As in coccidiomycosis, the lesions are prone to develop in bony prominences.

In a recent comprehensive article by Williams, Lawson, and Lucas[53] on histoplasmosis, with particular reference to *Histoplasma duboisii* prevalent in Nigeria, there is much clinical and pathologic information of value. While the skull is the most common site for an isolated lesion, hematogenous dissemination and even lymphatic spread often ensue, with involvement of one or more bones, as well as other sites. The bones commonly involved are vertebrae, femora, humeri, ribs, sternum, tibiae, skull, and carpal bones. In the vertebral column in particular, histoplasma infection is characterized by liquefaction necrosis of several bodies, with resulting collapse, paravertebral abcess, kyphosis, and sometimes spinal cord compression and paraplegia.

LESIONS OF BONE CAUSED BY PARASITIC DISEASE

Of all the numerous diseases in man caused by animal parasites, only one is relevant here, that caused by the cestode worm *Taenia echinococcus,* for which man may be the intermediate host (the mature form is a parasite of the intestine of the dog). The disease is most common in sheep raising areas;[54] it is seen only occasionally in the United States. The parasitic eggs are transmitted to the human digestive tract, and the wandering of the embryos can take them to any organ of the body, where they develop as huge cysts (or hydatids) with daughter cysts and scolices contained by chitinous walls. As is well known, the liver is the chief site of the disease. Localization in bone and the development of significant disease there are said to occur in no more than 1% of the cases of infestation with recognized clinical disease.

As a rule, only a single bone is affected by echinococcosis. Its site, of course, is fortuitous,[54-57] although involvement of the vertebral column, especially of the thoracic spine, appears to be relatively frequent.[11] The pelvis and the large limb bones may also be affected. The disease may remain localized, or it may slowly extend to involve the entire bone. Radiographically such lesions are described as cystic and multilocular, with little or no expansion of the cortex and no periosteal new bone reaction. Pathologic fracture may occur, with some hazard of spread.

The only effective treatment is complete surgical excision, although this may not always be feasible.

BONE CHANGES IN VIRAL INFECTIONS

The finding of osseous lesions in *smallpox* is an old observation.[58-60] In children, growth arrest and premature fusion of epiphyses have been described. It appears also that in adults, as well as in children, nonsuppurative osteomyelitis (designated "osteomyelitis variolosa" in older literature[61,62]) may be a sequel of smallpox, as may also arthritis of the elbow and other joints, ending in ankylosis and deformity. That these skeletal complications are not rare is evidenced by the fact that Bose[63] reported as many as twelve cases from Calcutta, where smallpox is still prevalent. He could not be certain whether the osteoarticular lesions resulted from the viral infection per se or whether some of them may have reflected secondary pyogenic infection in debilitated young patients.

In *rubella* (German measles), bone changes in the newborn held to be specific and virtually diagnostic have been reported by Singleton and his associates at Texas Children's Hospital in Houston. These infants were born of mothers who had had rubella during the first trimester of pregnancy (contracted during the course of an epidemic); they showed, in addition to the usual defects of cataracts and cardiac anomalies, thrombocytopenic purpura, a large anterior fontanelle, and, on roentgenographic survey, poorly defined irregular growth plates and altered trabecular patterns in the metaphyses of long bones, especially of the distal femora and proximal tibiae.

Aegerter and Kirkpatrick[14] have briefly cited an instance in which "multiple areas of bone destruction" appeared in a patient with severe *vaccinia* (the patient eventually recovered).

Osteolytic lesions have also been described as complications in occasional patients with *cat-scratch fever*,[64] although their precise nature was not clearly stated. Bone and joint infections of pyogenic nature have also been noted as unusual complications of *chickenpox*.[65]

INFANTILE CORTICAL HYPEROSTOSIS
(Caffey's disease)

Infantile cortical hyperostosis, first delineated by Caffey and Silverman[66] in 1945, affects young infants, particularly between 2 and 6 months of age. It is characterized pathologically by a peculiar inflammatory osteoperiostitis found most often in the long limb bones, mandible, clavicles, ribs, and scapulae. Occasionally other bones may be affected as well. The condition is by no means uncommon and is being recognized with increasing frequency in pediatric practice[67-70] (Fig. 3-13, *A*, *B*, and *C*).

Clinically, infantile cortical hyperostosis is commonly ushered in by fever, irritability, and tender indurated swellings at sites where bone lesions appear. During the acute phase, anemia, leukocytosis, elevated sedimentation rate, and pleural thickening and exudate may also be present. The condition is usually self-limited, although I have had an unusual opportunity to examine the bones in an autopsied baby who had developed thrombocytopenia and fatal cerebral hemorrhage (Fig. 3-13, *D* and *E*). There may be periods of remission and exacerbation, but, as a rule, the manifestations subside after some weeks or months, and the affected bones undergo gradual reconstruction that is said to be substantially complete by 3 years of age.[71] Only rarely, apparently, do bowing deformities persist beyond early childhood.[70]

Diseases of bone and joints

Radiographically, in the active phase of the disease the affected bones characteristically show more or less prominent periosteal new bone apposition (Fig. 3-13). This bone apposition may be lamellated and extensive and may lead to clublike thickening and deformity of the long limb bones (hyperostoses). These changes, although distinctive, may initially suggest scurvy, luetic osteoperiostitis, or severe trauma. As indicated, the cortical thickening gradually diminishes and tends to disappear after several months.

The essential pathologic lesion in affected bones, at least in the active stage of the disease, is a peculiar inflammatory osteoperiostitis (Fig. 3-13, *D* and *E*). As noted in Fig. 3-13, *D,* a photomicrograph of a cross section of a thickened affected bone (one of many examined at autopsy), there is partial resorption of the original cortex and, layered over it, concentric tiers of cortical new bone, the trabeculae of which are oriented, for the most part, at right angles to the attenuated original cortex. Fig. 3-13, *E,* at higher magnification, shows the nature of the granulation tissue within the thickened cortex. In addition to numerous fibroblasts, there are large histiocytes and an inflammatory exudate featuring small mononuclear cells and only an occasional polymorphonuclear leukocyte. In the matter of interpretation, as I see it, this type of reaction is quite consistent with the concept of a viral infection.

Caffey[66] suggested that infantile cortical hyperostosis might well be an infection, possibly viral in nature. This working hypothesis would indeed explain

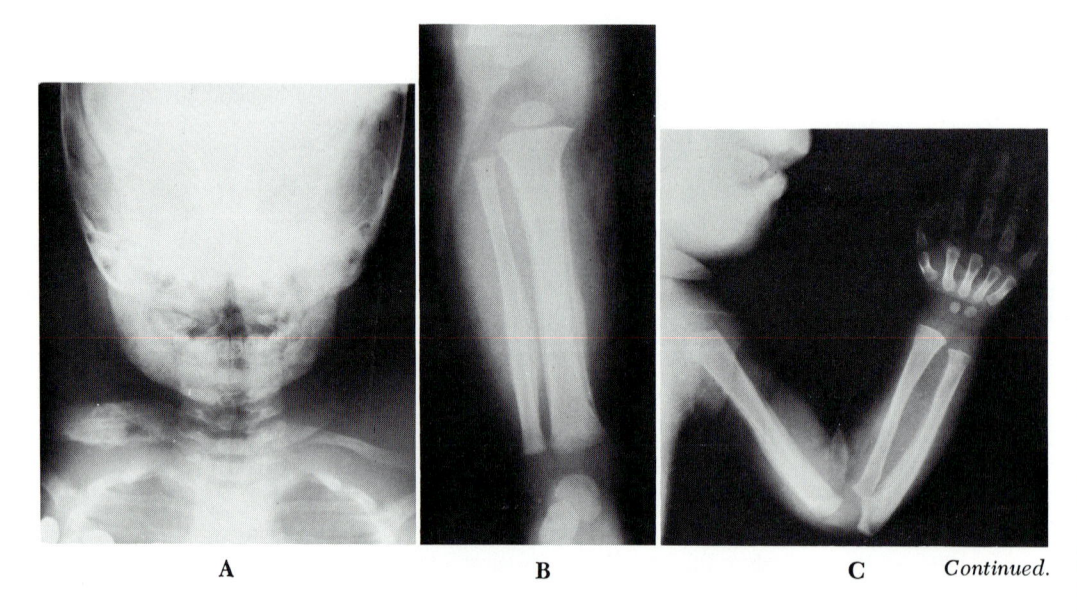

A B C *Continued.*

Fig. 3-13. **A,** Roentgenogram of a baby with infantile cortical hyperostoses showing involvement of the mandible bilaterally and a clavicle. The long limb bones were not examined. **B,** Periosteal new bone apposition on the tibia and fibula of another infant with Caffey's disease. **C,** Comparable changes in the humerus and ulna. Note also the enlargement of the lower jaw.

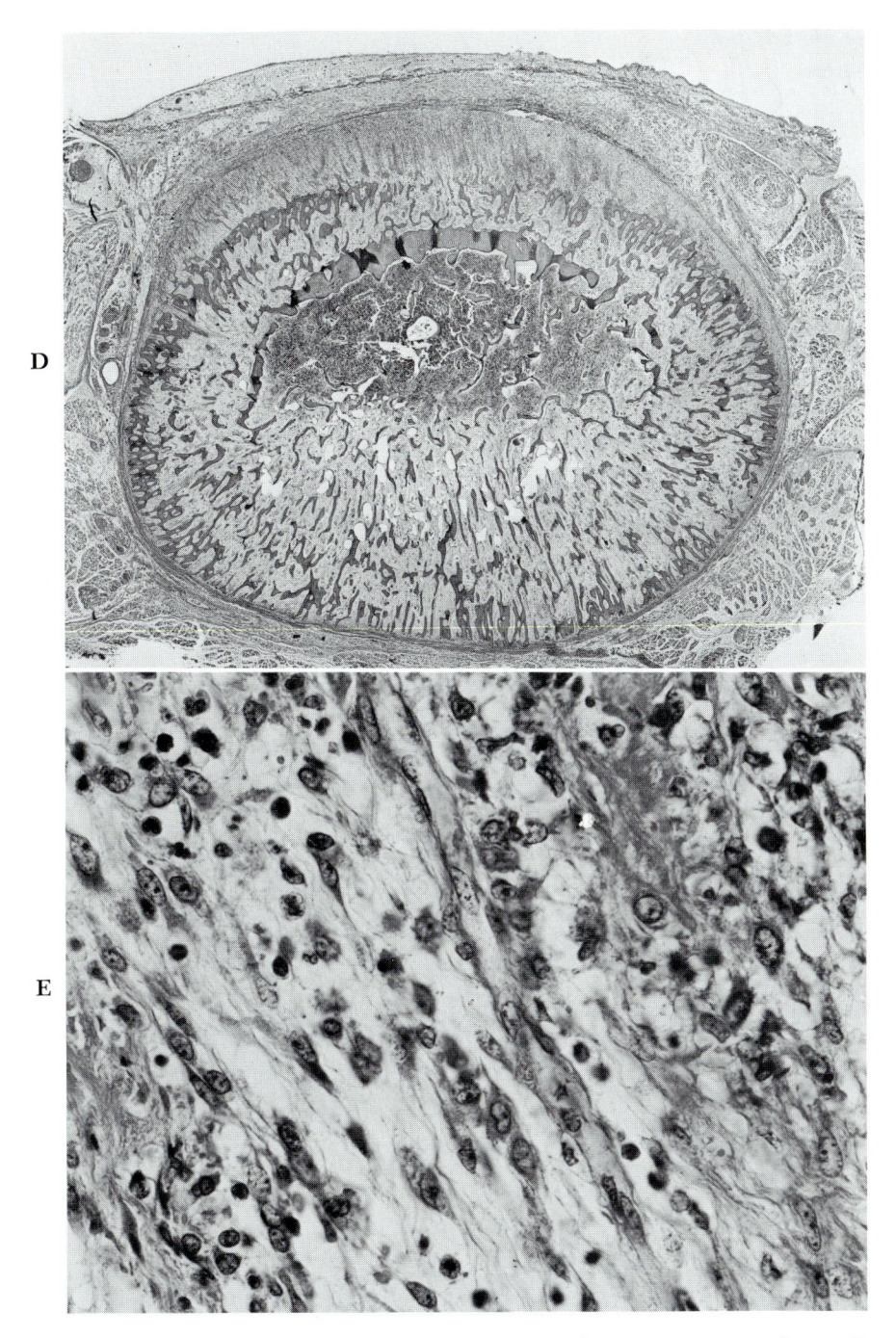

Fig. 3-13, cont'd. **D**, Low-power photomicrograph of a cross section of an affected bone in infantile cortical hyperostosis showing a peculiar inflammatory osteoperiostitis. **E**, Photomicrograph at higher magnification showing the character of the granulation tissue within the thickened cortex of the bone illustrated in **D**.

many of the clinical features of this disease, particularly the fever, leukocytosis, elevated sedimentation rate, and pleurisy with mononuclear exudate, as well as the peculiar inflammatory osteoperiostitis observed pathologically in the affected bones. It has also been suggested that there may be a hereditary or familial factor, based on occasional reports of incidence in two or three members of a family and, more importantly, on an account of eleven cases in a single family over a 14-year period.[67,70] While the latter observation is noteworthy, the familial incidence cited may reflect opportunity for contagion rather than a hereditary congenital disorder. It is conceivable also that adults can harbor a virus for a long time (as with herpes simplex) and transmit it to susceptible infants in the kindred. Altogether, it appears to me that one should reserve judgment concerning this problem of etiology, pending further study.

REFERENCES

1. Wilensky, A. O.: Osteomyelitis, New York, 1934, The Macmillan Co.
2. Wilson, J. C., and McKeever, F. M.: Hematogenous acute osteomyelitis in children, J. Bone Joint Surg. 18:323, 1936.
3. Shandling, B.: Acute hematogenous osteomyelitis; a review of 300 cases treated during 1952-1959, S. Afr. Med. J. 34: 520, 1960.
4. Trueta, J.: The three types of acute hematogenous osteomyelitis, J. Bone Joint Surg. 41-B:67, 1959.
5. Steindler, A.: Pyogenic arthritis: the musculoskeletal system: a symposium, New York, 1952, The Macmillan Co., pp. 287-312.
6. Spink, W. W.: The nature of brucellosis, Minneapolis, 1956, University of Minnesota Press.
7. Lowbeer, L.: Brucellotic osteomyelitis of the spinal column in man, Am. J. Pathol. 24:723, 1948.
8. Sedlin, E. D., and Fleming, J. L.: Epidermoid carcinoma arising in chronic osteomyelitic foci, J. Bone Joint Surg. 45-A:827-838, 1963.
9. Morris, J. M., and Lucas, D. B.: Fibrosarcoma within a sinus tract of chronic draining osteomyelitis, J. Bone Joint Surg. 46-A:853, 1964.
10. Carr, E. F.: Tuberculosis of the spine in children, Clin. Orthop., No. 1, p. 129.
11. Schmorl, G., and Junghanns, H.: Die Gesunde und die Kranke Wirbelsaüle in Roentgenbild und Klinik, ed. 4, Stuttgart, 1957, Georg Thieme Verlag.
12. Sanchis Olmos, V.: La tuberculosis del esqueleto, Barcelona, 1957, Editorial Ciéntifico Medica.
13. Bosworth, D. M.: Treatment of tuberculosis of bone and joint, Bull. N. Y. Acad. Med. 35:167-177, 1959.
14. Aegerter, E., and Kirkpatrick, J. A., Jr.: Orthopedic diseases, ed. 2, Philadelphia, 1963, W. B. Saunders Co., pp. 263-265.
15. Oyston, J. K.: Madura foot, a study of twenty cases, J. Bone Joint Surg. 43-B: 259, 1961.
16. Harbitz: Arch. Intern. Med. 6:147, 1910.
17. MacCallum, W. G.: A text-book of pathology, ed. 3, Philadelphia, 1924, W. B. Saunders Co.
18. Veterans Administration Technical Bulletin: Leprosy, TB 10-98, Washington, D. C., March 15, 1954. (For literature on treatment, particularly.)
19. Riordan, D. C.: The hand in leprosy. Part II. Orthopedic aspects of leprosy, J. Bone Joint Surg. 42-A:683.
20. Fife, G. L.: Leprosy from a histologic point of view, Arch. Pathol. 35:611, 1943.
21. Kalstone, B. M., Howell, J. A., Jr., and Cline, F. X., Jr.: Granuloma inguinale with hematogenous dissemination to the spine, J.A.M.A. 176:152, 1961.
22. Lyford, J. III, Scott, R. B., and Johnson, R. W., Jr.: Polyarticular arthritis and osteomyelitis due to granuloma inguinale, Am. J. Syph. 28:588, 1944.
23. Rajam, R. V., Rangiati, P. N., and Anguli, V. C.: Systemic donovaniasis, Br. J. Vener. Dis. 30:73, 1954.
24. Hodges, P. C., Phemister, D. E., and Brunschwig, A.: The roentgen-ray diagnosis of diseases of the bones and joints, New York, 1938, Thomas Nelson and Sons, pp. 37-48.

25. Holt, L. E., and Howland, J.: Diseases of infancy and childhood, ed. 9, New York, 1926, D. Appleton and Co., pp. 917-944.
26. Freund, E.: Über Knochensyphilis, Virch. Arch. Path. Anat. 288:146, 1933.
27. Pick, L.: Angeborene Knochensyphilis. In Henke and Lubarsch: Handbuch. der spec. Anatomie und Histologie, Berlin, 1929, Springer Verlag, p. 240.
28. Hackett, C. J.: Bone lesions of yaws in Uganda, Oxford, 1951, Blackwell Scientific Publications.
29. Argen, R. J., and Dixon, A. St. J.: Clutton's joints with keratitis and periostitis: a case report with histology of synovium, Arthritis Rheum. 6:341-348, 1963.
30. Schmorl, G., and Junghanns, H.: Die Gesunde und die Kranke Wirbelsäule in Rontgenbild und Klinik, ed. 4, Stuttgart, 1957, Georg Thieme Verlag, p. 126.
31. Forbus, W. D., and Bestebreurtje, A. M.: Coccidiomycosis: a study of 95 cases of the disseminated type with special reference to the pathogenesis of the disease, Mil. Surg. 99:653-719, 1946. (Well-documented references through 1945.)
32. Carter, R. A.: Infectious granulomas of bones and joints, with special reference to coccidioidal granuloma, Radiology 23:1-16, 1934.
33. McMaster, P. E., and Gilfillan, C. F.: Coccidioidal osteomyelitis, J.A.M.A. 112:1233-1237, 1939.
34. Schwartz, J., and Muth, J.: Coccidiomycosis: a review, Am. J. Med Sci. 221:89, 1951.
35. Parker, C. A.: Actinomycosis and blastomycosis of spine, J. Bone Joint Surg. 5:759, 1923.
36. Rhangos, W. C., and Chick, E. W.: Mycotic infections of bone, South. Med. J. 57:664-674, 1964.
37. Simpson, W. M., and McIntosh, C. A.: Actinomycosis of vertebrae (actinomycotic Pott's disease): report of 4 cases, Arch. Surg. 14:116, 1927.
38. Beitzke, H.: Aktinomykose der Knochen. In Handbuch. der spec. Anatomie und Histologie, vol. 9, part 2, Berlin, 1934, Springer Verlag.
39. Israel: Virch. Arch. 74:15, 1879; ibid. 78:421, 1879.
40. Colonna, P. A., and Gucker, T.: Blastomycosis of the skeletal system, J. Bone Joint Surg. 26:322, 1944.
41. Martin, D. S., and Smith, D. T.: Blastomycosis (review of literature), Am. Rev. Tuberc. 39:275, 488, 1938.
42. Editorial: Diamidine therapy of blastomycosis, J.A.M.A. 154:588, 1954.
43. Foerster, H. R., Sporotrichosis, Am. J. Med. Sci. 167:54, 1924.
44. Aetner, P. C., and Turner, R. R.: Sporotrichosis of bones and joints: review of the literature and report of six cases, Clin. Orthop. 68:138, 1970.
45. Reeves, R. J., and Pedersen, R.: Fungus infection of bone, Radiology 62:55, 1954.
46. Mitchel, L. A.: Torulosis, J.A.M.A. 106:450, 1936.
47. Allcock, E. A.: Torulosis, J. Bone Joint Surg. 43-B:71, 1961.
48. Allen, J. H.: Bone involvement with disseminated histoplasmosis, Am. J. Roentgen. 82:250, 1959.
49. Cox, L. B., Tolhurst, J. C.: Human torulosis: a clinical, pathological, and microbiological study, with a report of 13 cases, Melbourne, Australia, 1946, Melbourne University Press.
50. Klingberg, W. G.: Generalized histoplasmosis in infants and children: review of 10 cases with apparent recovery, J. Pediatr. 36:728, 1950.
51. Key, J. A., and Large, H. M.: Histoplasmosis of the knee, J. Bone Joint Surg. 24:28, 1942.
52. Collins, V. P.: Bone involvement in cryptoccosis (torulosis), Am. J. Roentgen. 63:102, 1950.
53. Williams, O. A., Lawson, E. A., and Lucas, A. O.: African histoplasmosis due to *Histoplasma duboisii*, Arch. Pathol. 92:305, 1971.
54. Dew, H. R.: Hydatid disease: its pathology, diagnosis, and treatment, Sydney, 1928, Australasian Medical Publishing Co. Ltd.
55. Coley, B. L.: Echinococcus disease of bone: report of 2 cases involving pelvic girdle, J. Bone Joint Surg. 14:577, 1932.
56. Howorth, M. B.: Echinococcus of bone (includes review of literature), J. Bone Joint Surg. 27:401, 1945.
57. Hsieh, C. K.: Echinococcus involvement of bone: report of case, Radiology 14:562, 1930.
58. Chiari, H.: Beitr. Path. Anat. 13:13, 1893.
59. Musgrave, W. E., and Sison, A. G.: Bone lesions of smallpox, Philippine J. Sci. 5:553, 1910; ibid. 8:67, 1913.
60. Cochran, W., Connolly, J. H., and

Thompson, I. D.: Bone involvement after vaccination against smallpox, Br. Med. J. **2**:285, 1963.
61. Brown, W. L., and Brown, C. P.: Osteomyelitis variolosa, J.A.M.A. **81**:1414, 1923.
62. Cockshott, P., and MacGregor, M.: Osteomyelitis variolosa, Q. J. Med. **27**: 369, 1958.
63. Bose, K. S.: Osteo-articular lesions in smallpox, J. Indian Med. Assoc. **31**:151, 1958.
64. Carithers, H. A., Carithers, C. M., and Edwards, R. O., Jr.: Cat-scratch disease: its natural history, J.A.M.A. **207**:312, 1969.
65. Buck, R. E.: Pyarthrosis of the hip complicating chickenpox, J.A.M.A. **206**:136, 1968.
66. Caffey, J., and Silverman, W. A.: Infantile cortical hyperostoses: preliminary report on a new syndrome, Am. J. Roentgen. **54**:1-16, 1945.
67. Editorial: Caffey's enigma, J.A.M.A. **175**: 495, 1961.
68. Sherman, M. S., and Hillyer, D. T.: Infantile cortical hyperostosis: review of literature and report of five cases, Am. J. Roentgen. **63**:212, 1950.
69. Smyth, F. S., Potter, A., and Silverman, W.: Periosteal reaction, fever and irritability in young infants: new syndrome, Am. J. Dis. Child. **71**:333-350, 1946.
70. Tampas, J. P., van Buskirk, F. W., Peterson, O. S., and Soule, A. B.: Infantile cortical hyperostosis, J.A.M.A. **175**:167, 1961.
71. Caffey, J.: On some late skeletal changes in chronic infantile cortical hyperostosis, Radiology **59**:651, 1952.

chapter 4

Skeletal changes in vitamin deficiencies and excesses

This chapter is concerned primarily with vitamin C deficiency (scurvy) and vitamin D deficiency (rickets and osteomalacia), and to a lesser extent with vitamin A deficiency. Vitamin B deficiencies in man are not accompanied by notable changes in the bones, although many skeletal aberrations and deformities attributable to various components of the vitamin B complex have been noted in experimental animals.[1] As for excessive administration, only the effects of vitamins A and D are relevant; inordinately large amounts of vitamin C (ascorbic acid) are apparently not harmful.

VITAMIN A DEFICIENCY

There is an optimal range of vitamin A dosage, just as there is for other dietary essentials, and deviations in either direction have been demonstrated to have deleterious effects. Vitamin A deficiency in infants was recognized[2] as early as 1933, but the condition is uncommon and only a limited number of case reports[3-6] have appeared since then. If the diet of the pregnant mother is extremely low in vitamin A, or if she is suffering from a malabsorption syndrome, the newborn infant may have low stores of vitamin A or even clinical vitamin A deficiency.[6,7]

The most consistent manifestation of such a deficiency is xerophthalmia (keratitis and scarring of the cornea, with impairment of vision) but many other signs have been noted,[8,9] among them mental and physical retardation, cornification of vaginal epithelium, refractory anemia, and some rather curious neurologic changes such as facial palsy, seventh cranial nerve injury, and hydrocephalus. The major effects are night blindness and epithelial changes affecting the skin and mucous membranes, featuring keratinization and squamous metaplasia. The skeletal alterations are not particularly noteworthy and relate to the general impairment of growth and development.[5] There may also be defective enamel

Diseases of bone and joints

and dentin formation in developing teeth. More specifically, one may observe squamous metaplasia of the enamel organ and whitening of the teeth.

VITAMIN A EXCESS OR POISONING
(hypervitaminosis A)

The harmful effects of hypervitaminosis A in infants and young children were described[10] in 1944. Subsequently, an appreciable number of similar reports appeared in the pediatric and radiologic literature.[11,12]

Hypervitaminosis A is characterized by anorexia, loss of weight, irritability, pruriginous rash, sparseness of hair, and hepatomegaly, as well as by swelling, pain, and tenderness over affected bones. The latter are usually long limb bones, although other bones such as the foot bones and calvarium may be involved. On roentgenographic examination, they show periosteal new bone apposition, the appearance of which is not unlike that of the milder expressions of infantile cortical hyperostosis (Fig. 4-1). Accompanying these changes, there is an increase in serum alkaline phosphatase activity.

The clinical histories of such babies and young children indicate, as a rule, entirely too much vitamin A in their diets, often supplemented by excessive amounts of vitamin A concentrate administered in error or through ignorance of its consequences. The suggestion has been advanced[12] that inability of the liver to store and handle the vitamin (hepatic dysfunction) is a contributing factor. Be that as it may, the toxic manifestations soon disappear when the con-

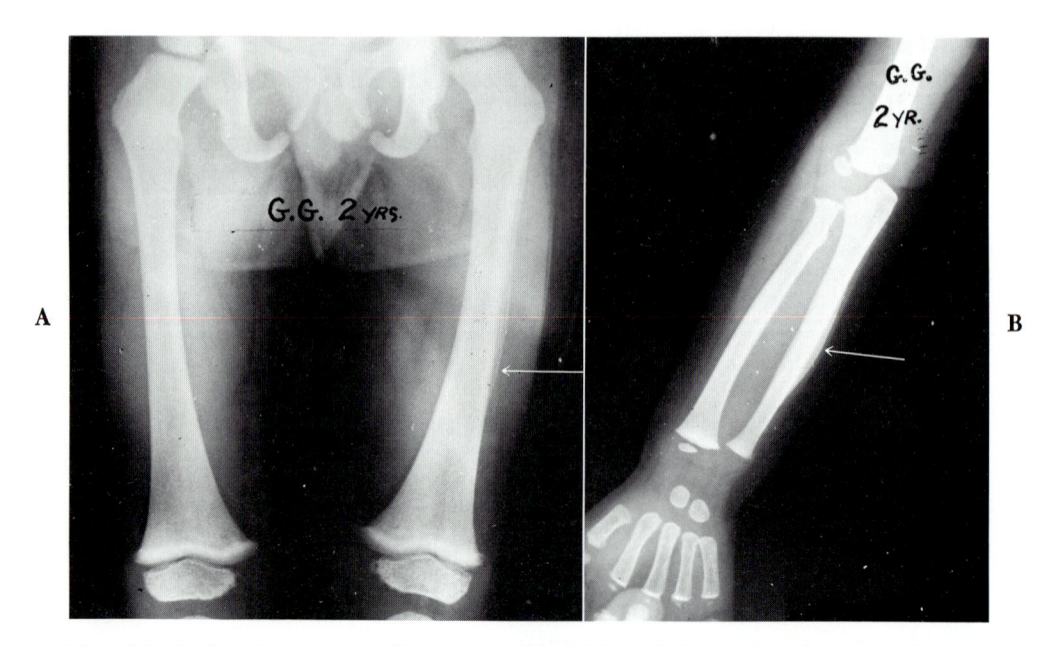

Fig. 4-1. **A**, Roentgenogram of a 2-year-old child with hypervitaminosis A, showing cortical thickening from periosteal new bone apposition *(arrows)* on the shaft of a femur. **B**, Comparable changes in the shaft of an ulna in the same patient.

dition is corrected, although the bone changes persist for some time, as one might expect.

There are some relevant experimental data that should be mentioned here. In the rat, excessive administration of vitamin A causes fragility and fractures of the bones. In dogs given an excess of the vitamin, the epiphyseal cartilage is greatly disturbed and premature ossifying union of the epiphysis results. In this connection, McElligott,[13] working with radioactive sulfate, has shown that excessive vitamin A interferes with the vitality of the chondrocytes and their synthesis of chondroitin sulfate. As Cohlan[14] has pointed out, the administration of excessive amounts of vitamin A to pregnant rats produces a diminished litter rate[15,16] and characteristic congenital malformations among the surviving young, commonly defective calvarium with extrusion of the brain, and, sporadically, other anomalies such as macroglossia, harelip, cleft palate, and gross defects in eye development. Another interesting observation[17] is that, in rabbits, cartilage can be dissolved by excess vitamin A; however, this effect can be prevented by the administration of cortisone.

VITAMIN C DEFICIENCY—SCURVY *(scorbutus; Möller-Barlow's disease; avitaminosis C)*

Because of its obvious and dramatic features, scurvy, especially in sailors and professional soldiers, has been known for a long time.[18] In fact, the word came into colloquial use as an adjective, in the sense of mean or contemptible (such as a scurvy trick). However, the delineation of this deficiency disease in precise clinical and pathologic terms proceeded at a pedestrian pace.

Although the curative effect of lemon (and lime) juice was discovered as early as 1753 by Lind,[18] it took more than a century thereafter for infantile scurvy to be clearly established as a clinical entity distinct from rickets and other disorders,[19] and another 25 years for scurvy to be produced experimentally in guinea pigs.[20] The elucidation of its pathologic changes came even later, while the classical chemical analysis and identification of vitamin C as ascorbic acid by Szent-Györgi dates back to 1928.

As is now well known, full-blown clinical scurvy is characterized by progressive secondary anemia, weakness, slight fever, swelling, bleeding and ulceration of the gums (with loosening of teeth), exquisite tenderness of the legs from painful hemorrhages about the joints and under the periosteum (particularly of long limb bones), and ecchymoses in the skin, muscles, and internal organs (kidney and bowel). The condition may be fatal if left untreated, since infections, especially pneumonia, may develop. On the other hand, rapid healing occurs following vitamin C administration, although it may be several months before there is complete restoration of the skeletal structures.

Scurvy is now unusual in adults except under war starvation conditions, but it may be seen occasionally in alcoholics, extreme diet faddists, or the very deprived. It is still observed in young children (usually from 6 to 15 months of age) who are fed boiled or condensed milk and no citrus juices. Subclinical

Diseases of bone and joints

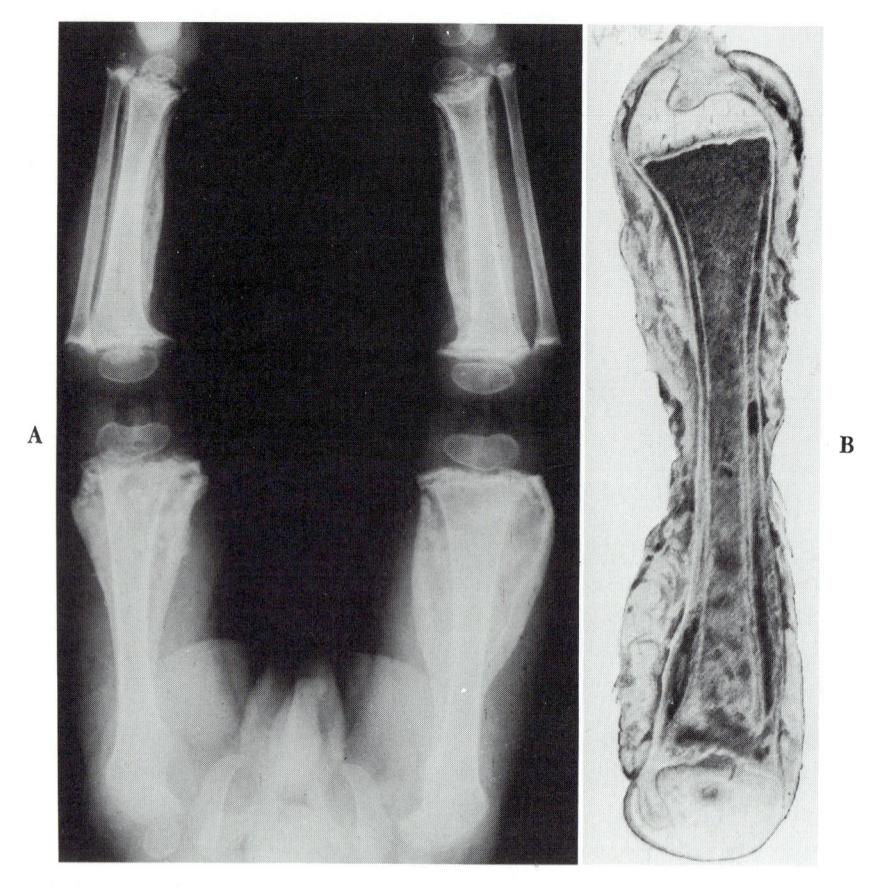

Fig. 4-2. **A**, Sagittal section of the femur of a young child who died of scurvy. Note the hemorrhages in the medullary cavity and under the raised periosteum. (From Mac-Callum, W. G.: A text-book of pathology, ed. 3, Philadelphia, 1924, W. B. Saunders Co.) **B**, Roentgenogram showing changes in the growth zones of both femora and tibiae in infantile scurvy, as well as striking periosteal new bone formation in consequence of subperiosteal hemorrhage.

vitamin C deficiency is believed to be not uncommon and is a possible cause of delayed healing of wounds and fractures.[21]

Pathologically, if one examines a long limb bone of a young scorbutic subject (Fig. 4-2, A), two unusual features are immediately apparent:

1. Hemorrhages may be found within the bone marrow (most conspicuous at the growing end of the bone) and also under the periosteum, which may be elevated over a large part of the shaft by the effusion of blood and which tends to form reactive new bone.[22,23] This is, of course, reflected roentgenographically, and the changes may be quite striking (Fig. 4-2, B).

2. The growth zone is broadened and irregular, reflecting stagnation or cessation of bone formation through endochondral ossification. More specifi-

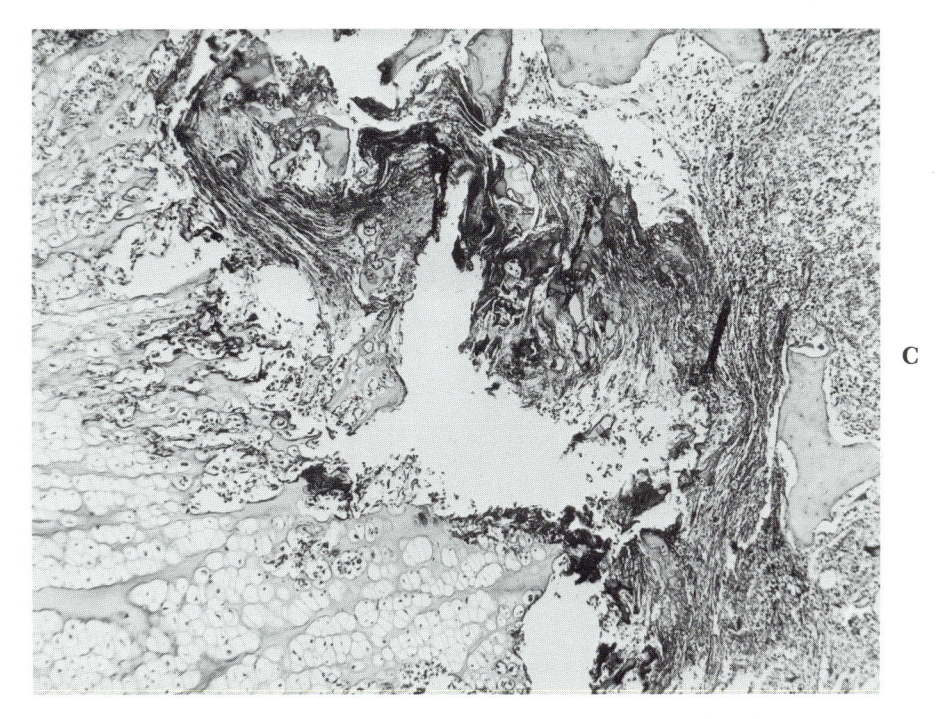

Fig. 4-2, cont'd. C, Photomicrograph of a growth plate in severe infantile scurvy showing disruption of endochondral ossification. The columns of calcified cartilage (on the left) are broken up and enmeshed in an irregular zone of necrosis and hemorrhage.

cally, there is lack of orderly invasion of calcified cartilage columns by osteoblastic vascular connective tissue, so that only sparse, scattered trabeculae of new bone are formed, or none at all.

In severe lesions there is complete disruption of this portion of the plate, with necrosis and hemorrhage (Fig. 4-2, C). Epiphyseal separation may occur and is often bilateral. This is observed most often in the lower femur, upper tibia, and upper humerus. There may also be costochondral separations.

Further, as a consequence of stagnation of new bone formation, whereas resorption proceeds normally (and is, in fact, accelerated by disuse or immobilization), there is a tendency to thinning of cortices and atrophy of the spongiosa, reflected roentgenographically in a washed-out appearance. As for the marrow, this in time loses its myeloid elements as well as its blood vessels and osteoblasts and is converted to an edematous fibrous tissue. It is remarkable that these profound changes are reversible, as noted, if vitamin C therapy is not too long delayed.

As to pathogenesis, an adequate concentration of vitamin C is required for the formation of collagen and ground substance,[24,25] which constitute the substrate of osteoid and bone. The widespread hemorrhages from capillaries, characteristic of scurvy, apparently result from a deficiency of the intercellular, basement membrane matrix materials in the capillary walls. In the teeth, dentin formation ceases and the odontoblasts revert to fibroblastlike cells. As Follis[26] has succinctly stated, the disorder in scurvy is a failure of fibroblasts, osteoblasts, and odontoblasts to promote the deposition of their respective fibrous proteins; namely, collagen, osteoid, and dentin.

VITAMIN D DEFICIENCY *(rickets and osteomalacia)*

The D vitamins are a group of biologically active sterols, which have profound effects on mineral, and especially calcium and phosphate, metabolism.[27] The three major antirachitic sterols of clinical importance are vitamin D_2 and dihydrotachysterol (from irradiated ergosterol), and vitamin D_3 (from potent fish liver oils). In the rat at least, administration of vitamin D promotes absorption of calcium from the gut and retention of phosphate, and also has a growth-stimulating effect. The major target organs are the gastrointestinal tract and bone, and quite possibly the kidney.

Rickets and osteomalacia are the diseases of infancy and adult life, respectively, that result from vitamin D deficiency. They are characterized by a lack of normal mineralization of bone and disordered calcium, magnesium, and phosphate metabolism, associated with abnormalities of growth and neuromuscular function.[27]

Rickets. At one time, rickets was probably, at least in northern cities, the disease from which infants most frequently suffered. In fact, among the poor in these cities it was an almost universal disease.[28]

Some 50 years ago it was recognized that ultraviolet light, potent fish liver oils, or both, could heal rickets.[29-32] As the administration of vitamin D in one form or another to babies became routine pediatric practice,[29-32] the incidence of rickets, at least in severe form, declined sharply, to the point that pathologic teaching material is now hard to come by. That is not to say that rickets may not still be encountered at times, particularly in its mild or subclinical expressions, or even in its advanced stage under unusual circumstances.[33]

Rickets is one of the so-called malacic diseases of bone. Its most striking feature is the presence of osteoid (limeless bone) throughout the skeleton. As a result of vitamin D deficiency the osteoid is not calcified and converted to bone. It has been cogently postulated that in the absence of adequate vitamin D there is faulty absorption of calcium from the gut (such intestinal disorders as idiopathic steatorrhea, celiac disease, or sprue may sometimes be a contributing factor); that the parathyroid homeostatic mechanism acts to maintain the serum calcium level by drawing calcium out of the skeleton; and that parathyroid hyperactivity concomitantly brings about the loss of phosphorus through the kidneys. Thus the serum phosphorus level is consistently low in rickets (as low as 1.0 mg./100 ml. in extreme cases), while the serum calcium level is likely to be in the low normal range. The stimulus to new bone formation by way of attempted reconstruction is reflected in significantly elevated alkaline phosphatase activity in the serum. The latter returns to normal only slowly and may remain somewhat increased even after clinical and roentgenographic evidence of healing is manifest.

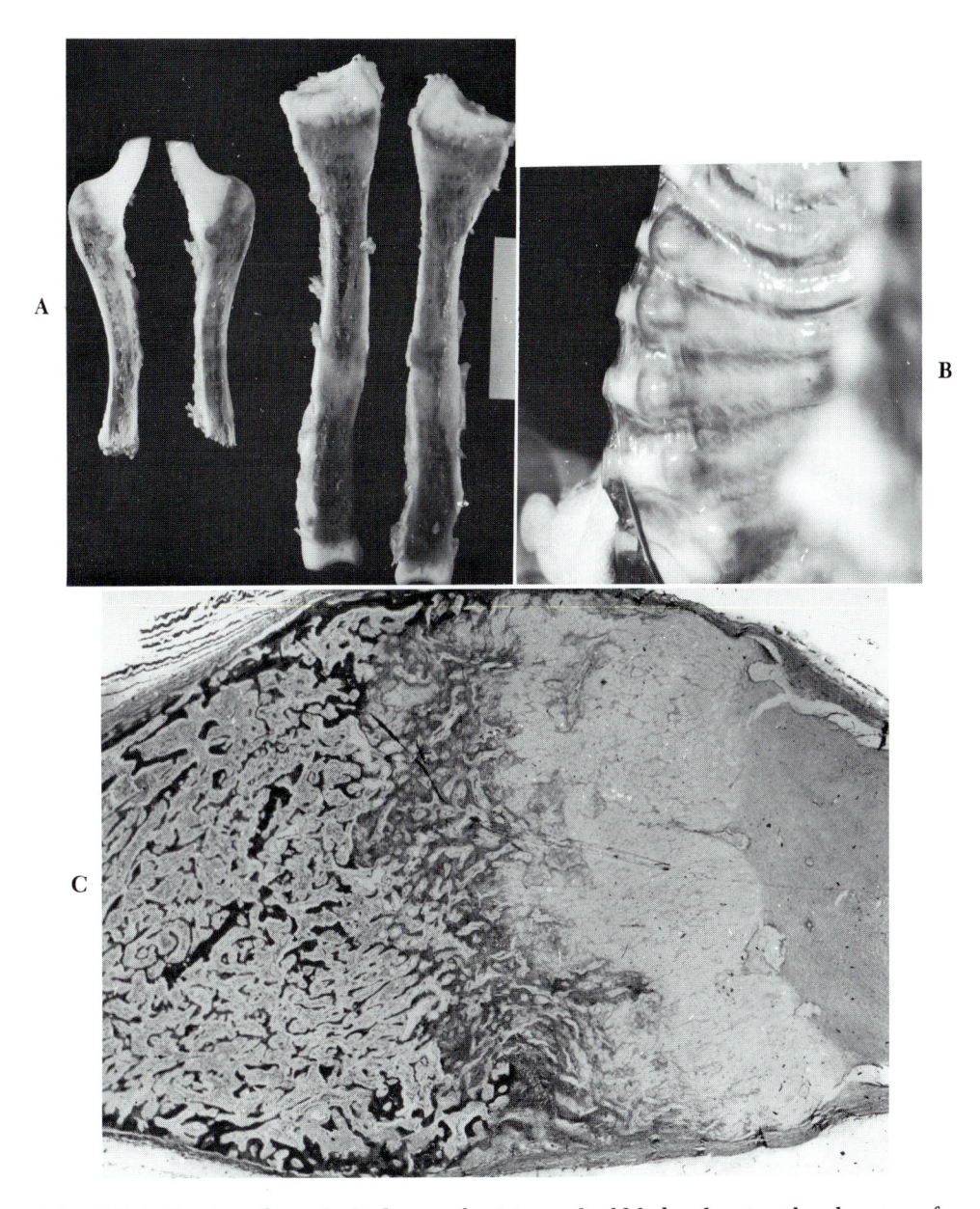

Skeletal changes in vitamin deficiencies and excesses

Fig. 4-3. **A,** Sections through the bones of a 14-month-old baby showing the changes of active rickets (the cause of death was bronchopneumonia). Note the irregular widening of the growth zones. **B,** Conspicuous enlargement of costochondral junctions in the same child. **C,** Photomicrograph of a section through a costochondral junction of a rib of a child with rickets (autopsy specimen). Note the widening of the preparatory zone of cartilage (to right of center), which is invaded by blood vessels. To the left is the irregularly widened growth zone, where osteoid is heaped up and not converted to bone, because of lack of available calcium and phosphate.

Diseases of bone and joints

When rickets is observed clinically, it begins usually at 6 to 18 months of age and last for several to many months, sometimes for years, with remissions and final healing. The active process ends, as a rule, by the time the child is 2 or 2½ years old in all but the severe or resistant cases. The disease has systemic effects and, at the height of its development, the old commonplace picture was that of a pale, sickly child restless at night and sweating about the head, with secondary anemia, lowered resistance to infection, lymphadenopathy (especially of tonsils, adenoids, and cervical nodes), protrusion of the abdomen (potbelly), splenomegaly (from hyperplasia), retarded dentition, poor development, flabbiness of musculature, and laxity of ligaments.

The most constant and characteristic lesions, however, are found in the skeleton. There is enlargement of epiphyses (especially at the wrists, knees, and ankles) and of costochondral junctions (beaded ribs or rachitic rosary) (Fig. 4-3, *B*). There may also be thoracic deformity, scoliosis, bending or greenstick fractures of long bones (particularly of the forearm bones and femora), deformed pelvis, bowing of femora and tibiae (knock knees), and coxa vara from general softening and thinning of the bones. There is also enlargement of the skull with prominent forehead (spongy thickenings over the frontal and parietal fossas) and thin occiput (craniotabes). The capacity for skeletal reconstruction in young children is so remarkable, fortunately, that most cases end with gradual restoration of normal consistency and structure of affected bones. If orthopedic corrective measures are neglected, however, the changes described may leave lasting deformities in adults, notably of the chest (with diminished vital capacity) and of the pelvis (with narrowed outlet, interfering with parturition in women), as well as flat feet, coxa vara, scoliosis, and the familiar bowlegs and knock knees.

The changes outlined are, of course, reflected roentgenographically and are of diagnostic importance, as are also the altered serum chemistry findings. In essence, the significant roentgenographic alterations relate to failure of centers of ossification in epiphyses to appear or to be clearly outlined (osteoid is not radiopaque); to demineralization of the skeleton (in variable degree and for the reason previously indicated); and, most importantly, to irregular broadening of epiphyseal cartilage plates and to "cupping" of the metaphyses (Figs. 4-4 and 4-5).

Pathologic examination of a rachitic long bone, sectioned through the epiphysis and shaft (Fig. 4-3, *A*), or of a rib through the costochondral junction (Fig. 4-3, *C*), shows widening of the preparatory zone of cartilage (which may be irregularly invaded by perichondral and marrow vessels), lack of calcification of this cartilage (except perhaps in occasional small foci), and an irregular piling up of osteoid at the growth plate for lack of calcification and conversion to bone. The cortical and spongy trabeculae in the adjacent metaphysis may also be covered by osteoid. In severe rickets, the marrow may become somewhat fibrous.

In this concise description, the salient characteristic features of the pathologic

Skeletal changes in vitamin deficiencies and excesses

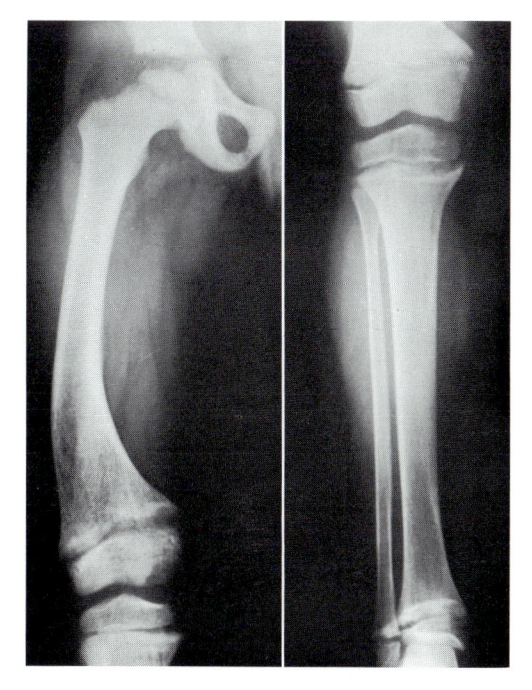

Fig. 4-4. Roentgenograms showing the changes of vitamin D–resistant rickets.

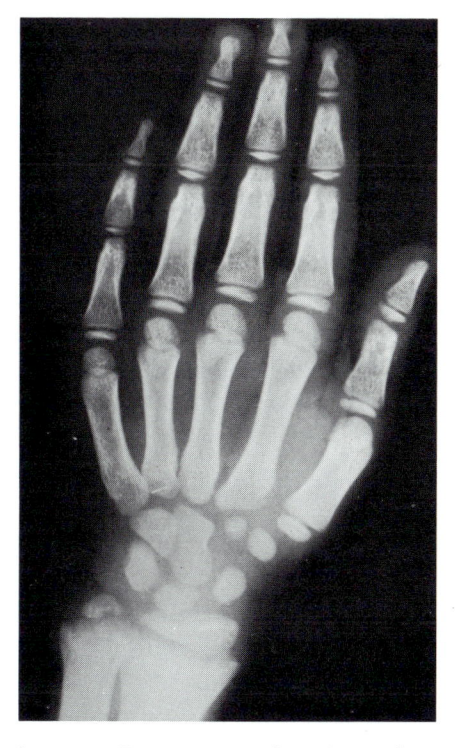

Fig. 4-5. Another case of vitamin D–resistant rickets. Note the irregular widening of the growth zones and metaphyseal "cupping" at the distal radius and ulna.

alterations have been stressed. For a meticulously detailed account of these changes in various sites, the reader may have recourse to the discussion by Jaffe.[34]

Late rickets (rickets tarda). There are undoubtedly instances (Schmorl[28] and M. B. Schmidt) of rickets occurring late in childhood (from about 6 to 15 years of age) and attributable to dietary insufficiency. This is unusual, however, except under war starvation conditions. Such cases respond readily to treatment (Holt and Howland). The deformities are seldom extreme and the skeletal changes are most marked in the lower extremities.

Vitamin D–resistant rickets (hypophosphatemic–vitamin D refractory rickets; de Toni-Debré-Fanconi syndrome). There are occasional instances of more or less severe clinical rickets (Figs. 4-4 and 4-5) that require very large if not massive doses of vitamin D for effective control. Dwarfing has been noted in such cases (de Toni). There also seems to be a history of familial incidence for this condition.

The prevailing view in regard to such cases is that the skeletal and other changes that develop are attributable to a defect in renal tubular reabsorption, whereby the kidneys leak phosphate, glucose, various amino acids, and possibly other metabolites.[35,36] Vitamin D–resistant rickets will be considered at greater length in Chapter 7, which deals with the skeletal changes in renal disease.

Renal rickets (renal osteodystrophy). "Renal rickets" is an old, somewhat confusing designation for the rachitic skeletal changes (in a growing child) that develop as a result of secondary hyperparathyroidism complicating chronic renal insufficiency of long standing (Fig. 4-6). This condition will also be discussed in Chapter 7.

Hypophosphatasia. Mention should be made of still another unusual condition, hypophosphatasia, first described by Rathbun[37] in 1948. In this disease skeletal changes resembling those of severe classical infantile rickets, or of osteomalacia in older patients, occur[38-40] for an entirely different reason. Failure to form bone by mineralization of osteoid at sites of endochondral ossification, and also to form adequate bone preformed in membrane in the calvarium, results not from lack of available bone-forming minerals (the serum calcium and phosphorus levels are actually at the upper limits of their normal range), but rather from failure of their utilization because of an inbred gene defect blocking the formation of the enzyme, phosphatase. Not only is there pronounced lowering of serum alkaline phosphatase activity, but there is also marked reduction of phosphatases in all tissues where they are ordinarily abundant. A survey of the literature on this disorder may be found in an informative article by Fraser.[38]

The disease is also characterized biochemically by the urinary excretion of phosphoethanolamine and of increased amounts of pyrophosphates, whereas the output of hydroxyproline is diminished.

The less severely affected patients surviving into adult life usually give a history of rickets followed by an asymptomatic interlude, and as adults they may develop pseudofractures, as seen in osteomalacia. In the matter of therapy,

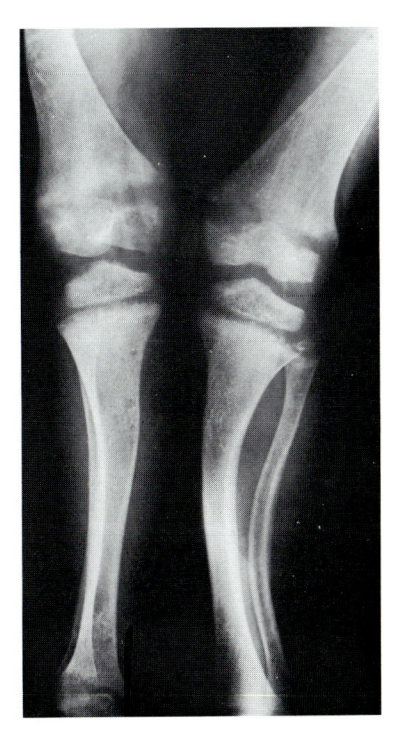

Skeletal changes in vitamin deficiencies and excesses

Fig. 4-6. Roentgenogram of the lower femora and tibiae of a child with secondary hyperparathyroidism associated with long-standing renal insufficiency—so-called renal rickets.

vitamin D has proved ineffective and may be hazardous in large doses because of the tendency to hypercalcemia and nephrocalcinosis, but ordinarily administered phosphate is said to be of value.[27]

Osteomalacia. Osteomalacia, which must be distinguished from osteoporosis (Chapter 8), is the counterpart of rickets in adults or in any patients beyond the growth period. Like rickets, osteomalacia is characterized by a tendency to demineralization of the skeleton and by lack of adequate calcification of osteoid and its conversion thereby to bone.[41-43] Osteomalacia results from deficient absorption of calcium, phosphorus, or both, from the gut, or from their excessive excretion in either the stool or urine. While dietary deficiency may be the primary factor, this is comparatively rare under present conditions, at least in the United States. By far the most common causes are intestinal malabsorption, for whatever reason, and certain renal disorders.

To be sure, severe osteomalacia of the type found in women in India and China[44] after repeated child-bearing and lactation, on rations often deficient in vitamin D and bone-forming minerals, can lead to extreme skeletal demineralization and fantastic deformities of the pelvis, spine, and lower limb bones. After all, if far more calcium is used than is available, the deficit can come only from the skeleton. While osteomalacic bones have little tendency to break, if they get soft enough they can, under stress, bend like a pretzel. In the United States

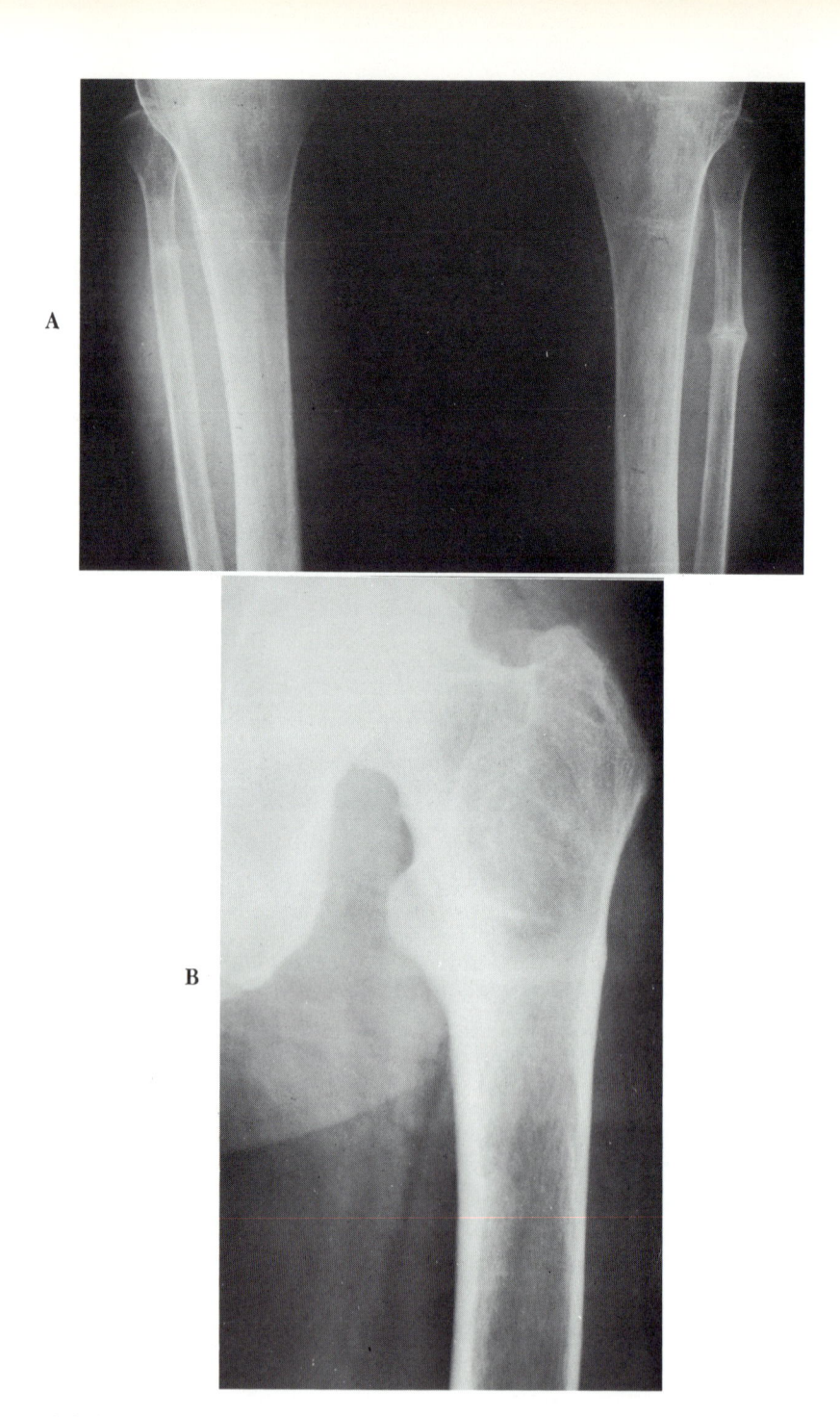

Fig. 4-7. **A,** Roentgenogram of an adult with osteomalacia. Note the uniform thinning of the cortices and the transverse pseudofractures in the upper tibiae and fibulae. **B,** The upper femur of the same patient, showing a transverse Looser, or "umbau," zone with pseudofracture just below the lesser trochanter. **C,** Photomicrograph (low magnification) of a bone of an adult with a renal tubular reabsorption defect (Fanconi syndrome) showing striking manifestations of osteomalacia. Note the broad osteoid seams, or borders, on the surface of the spongy trabeculae.

Skeletal changes in vitamin deficiencies and excesses

C

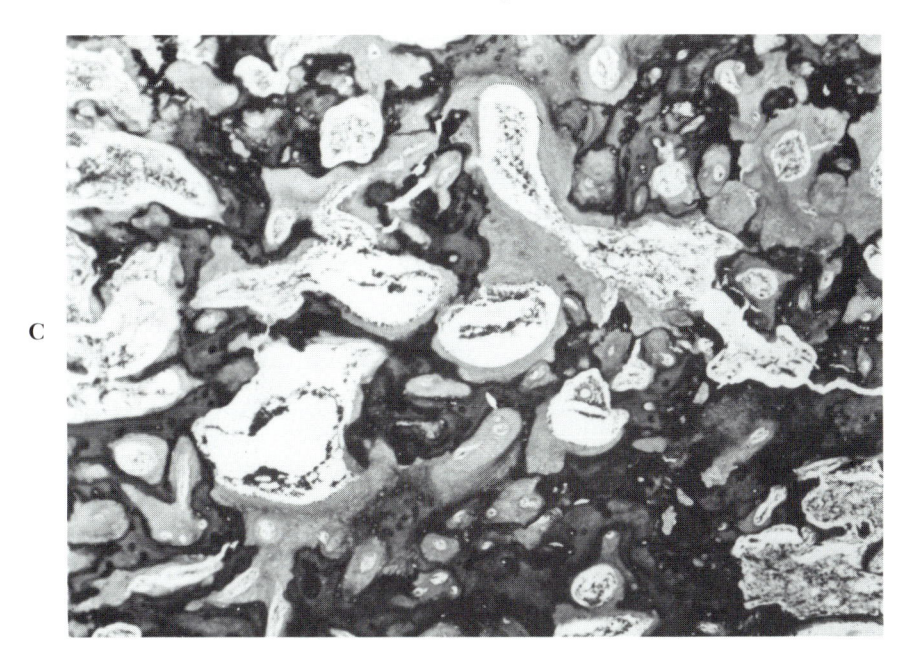

Fig. 4-7, cont'd. For legend see opposite page.

and in western Europe, one observes this only under extraordinary circumstances, such as war hunger or slow starvation, or in a few eccentric individuals on offbeat, vitamin-deficient diets. A notable example of hunger "osteopathy" or osteomalacia on a large scale was documented in Vienna during the lean years following World War I.[45] I have seen some of this abundant material at first hand from the pathologic collection of Professor Erdheim, and the preparations show exquisite osteomalacia.

Perhaps the most common cause of early or less severe forms of osteomalacia found in adults today (and this disease is by no means unusual) is intestinal malabsorption.[46] This may be associated with bypassing gastrointestinal operations, pancreatitis,[47] the steatorrhea of nontropical sprue,[48,49] or such intestinal disorders as regional enteritis or Whipple's disease. It would appear that the poor absorption of calcium and phosphorus in these circumstances is as important for the development of osteomalacia as the malabsorption of fat-soluble vitamin D, if not more so. According to Avioli and his coworkers,[50] intestinal malabsorption of calcium may be attributed to deficient activation of vitamin D_3 (to 25-OH-D).

The other common cause of osteomalacia is renal disease characterized by excessive urinary excretion of phosphate.[51] As previously noted, the congenital disorder of tubular transport of phosphate, glucose, and amino acids, described by Debré and de Toni,[52] as well as by Fanconi,[53] can lead to osteomalacia as well as rickets. It must be kept in mind, however, that hyperphosphaturia per se can also reflect parathyroid hyperplasia developing in response to hypocalcemia.

Whatever the cause of osteomalacia, appreciable thinning and rarefaction of bone cortices eventually ensue. Associated with this are generalized bone tenderness, bowing, compression of vertebral bodies, and, rather characteristically, Looser zones[54] ("umbauzonen," or bandlike radiolucent areas of osteoid remodeling) and painful symmetrical transverse fissure pseudofractures (so-called Milkman's syndrome).[55] The latter may be seen in the shafts of long limb bones (Fig. 4-7) and in such sites as the medial border of the scapula and the inferior ramus of the pubis.[56]

As for significant serum chemical changes, the calcium or the phosphorus level is on the low side; in advanced cases, both may be markedly reduced. The serum alkaline phosphatase activity is consistently elevated. Tubular reabsorption of phosphate is high early in the course of the disease, and low later on, when hypocalcemia has led to secondary hyperparathyroidism.

Biopsy of an affected bone or of the iliac crest in osteomalacia may present a complex picture in advanced cases, with their overlay of stress reaction and secondary hyperparathyroidism. The basic diagnostic feature, however, apart from thinning of cortical bone, is the finding of osteoid borders on the bone trabeculae. These are seen to best advantage after very slow decalcification (several weeks) in Müller's fluid. After the customary rapid decalcification with acid or a chelating agent, it may be difficult to distinguish the osteoid seams clearly from the contiguous bone. We have found it helpful to use acridine orange stain and ultraviolet light microscopy.

Osteomalacia can be cured, with restoration of skeletal function, by the administration of large doses of vitamin D, but therapy must be tailored to fit the individual patient. At times, as much as 1,000,000 units per day may be required. Care should be taken to prevent overdose with its hazards of hypercalcemia and nephrocalcinosis. It is self-evident also that an adequate source of calcium must be provided in the diet and that the deleterious effects of the underlying intestinal or renal disorder must be ameliorated if at all possible. With good clinical management and avoidance of vitamin D overdosage, pseudofractures become calcified and the bones become denser, although the bowing deformities persist and may require osteotomy for correction.[57] It is possible that the availability of 25-hydroxycholecalciferol (25-HCC), a more potent, active form of vitamin D, will make clinical management easier.

VITAMIN D EXCESS OR POISONING
(hypervitaminosis D)

As in the case of vitamin A, too much vitamin D can be harmful, if not dangerous. Hypervitaminosis D results from the administration of excessive or massive doses of vitamin D in one form or another, ostensibly with therapeutic intent. There was a spate of such cases some years ago[58-60] before the toxicity of excessive vitamin D was recognized. The substance was used (or commercially exploited) in the treatment of rheumatoid arthritis, as well as other conditions. In these circumstances, there is a significant increase in the serum calcium level,

Skeletal changes in vitamin deficiencies and excesses

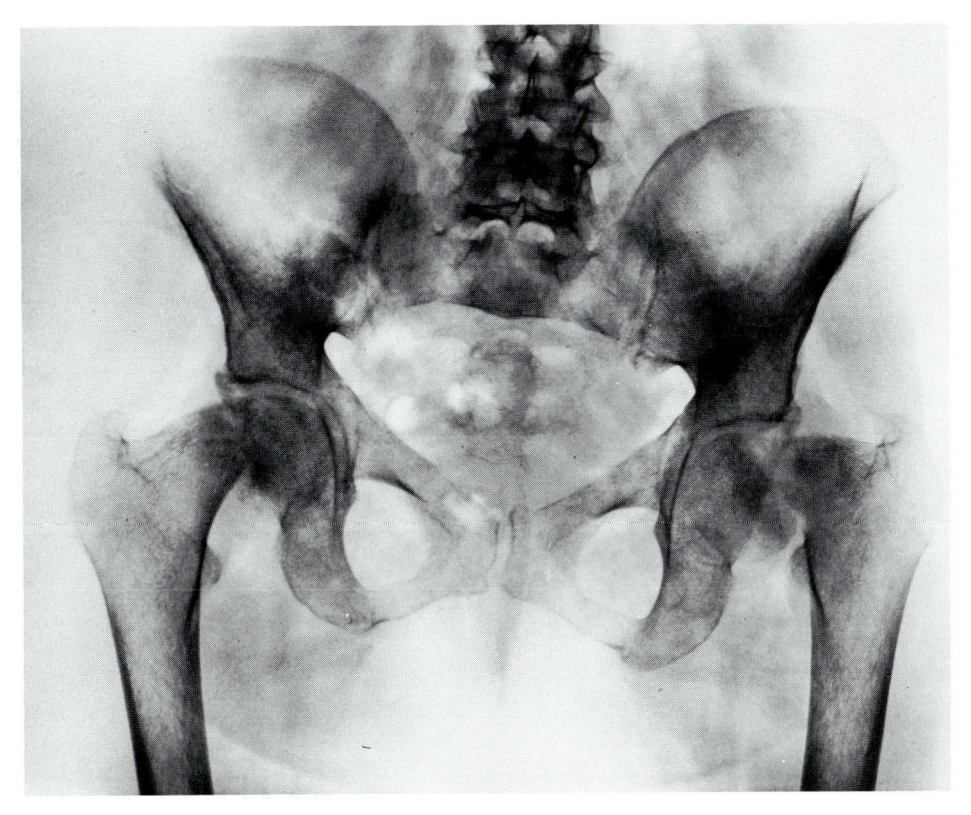

Fig. 4-8. Roentgenogram of another patient with osteomalacia showing multiple, spontaneous, symmetrical pseudofractures.

up to 16 mg. or more, presumably the result of increased absorption of calcium from the gut.

The two major manifestations of vitamin D poisoning are: (1) the usual untoward effects of marked hypercalcemia—polyuria, thirst, nausea, and lethargy, and (2) widespread calcific deposits, sometimes massive, in many sites throughout the body, both skeletal (joints) and visceral. Those in the kidneys (nephrocalcinosis) may be potentially serious. If the condition persists long enough, demineralization of the skeleton ensues, although the mechanism for this is not altogether clear. The obvious therapeutic measures are cessation of vitamin D administration, a low calcium diet, abundant fluid intake to flush out the kidneys, and the administration of corticoids to reduce hypercalcemia.[61]

REFERENCES

1. Putschar, W. G. J.: General pathology of the musculoskeletal system, Handbuch der Allgemeinen Pathologie, vol. 3, part 2, Berlin, 1960, Springer-Verlag, pp. 363-488 (see p. 419).
2. Blackfan, K. D., and Wolbach, S. B.: Vitamin A deficiency in infants: clinical and pathological study, J. Pediatr. 3:679, 1933.
3. Bass, M. H., and Caplan, J.: Vitamin A deficiency in infancy, J. Pediatr. 67:690, 1955.
4. Cornfeld, D., and Cooke, R. E.: Vitamin

97

A deficiency: case report, unusual manifestations in 5½ month old baby, Pediatrics **10**:33, 1952.
5. Wolbach, J. B.: Vitamin A deficiency and excess in relation to skeletal growth, J. Bone Joint Surg. **29**:171, 1947.
6. Wolf, I. J.: Vitamin A deficiency in an infant, J.A.M.A. **166**:1859, 1958.
7. Maxwell, J. P.: Vitamin deficiency in antenatal period: its effect on mother and infant, J. Obstet. Gynaecol. Br. Commonw. **39**:764, 1932.
8. Warkany, J., and Nelson, R. C.: The appearance of skeletal abnormalities in the offspring of rats reared on a deficient diet, Science **92**:383, 1940.
9. Wilson, J. G., and Barch, S.: Fetal death and maldevelopment resulting from maternal vitamin A deficiency in the rat, Proc. Soc. Exp. Biol. Med. **72**:687, 1949.
10. Josephs, H. W.: Hypervitaminosis A and carotinemia, Am. J. Dis. Child. **67**:33, 1944.
11. Caffey, J.: Chronic poisoning due to excess of vitamin A: description of clinical and roentgen manifestations in seven infants and young children, Pediatrics **5**:672, 1950.
12. Fried, C. T., and Grand, M. J.: Hypervitaminosis A, Am. J. Dis. Child. **79**:475, 1950.
13. McElligott, T. F.: Increased fixation of sulfate ($^{35}SO_4$) by chondrocytes in hypervitaminosis A, J. Pathol. Bact. **83**:347, 1962.
14. Cohlan, S. Q.: Excessive intake of vitamin A as a cause of congenital anomalies in the rat, Science **117**:535, 1953.
15. Moore, T., and Wang, Y. L.: Hypervitaminosis A, Biochem. J. **399**:222, 1945.
16. Rodahl, K.: Hypervitaminosis A, Norske Polarinstitut, Skrifter Nr. **95**:73, 1950.
17. Weissmann, G., Bell, E., and Thomas, L.: Prevention by hydrocortisone of changes in connective tissue induced by an excess of vitamin A, Am. J. Pathol. **42**:571, 1963.
18. Hess, A. F.: Scurvy, past and present, Philadelphia, 1920, J. B. Lippincott Co.
19. Barlow, T.: On cases described as acute rickets, Med. Clin. Trans. **66**:159, 1883.
20. Holt, H., and Frolich, T.: Ueber experimentallen Skorbut, Z. Hyg. Infektionskr. **72**:1, 1912.
21. Lauman, T. H., and Ingalls, T. H.: Vitamin C deficiency and wound healing, Ann. Surg. **105**:616, 1937.
22. MacCallum, W. G.: A text-book of pathology, ed. 3, Philadelphia, 1924. W. B. Saunders Co., pp. 927-929.
23. Follis, R. H., Jr.: Histochemical studies on cartilage and bone; ascorbic acid deficiency, Bull. Johns Hopkins Hosp. **89**:9, 1951.
24. Wolbach, S. B., and Howe, P. R.: Intercellular substance in experimental scorbutus, Arch. Path. Lab. Med. **1**:1, 1926.
25. Meiklejohn, A. P.: The physiology and biochemistry of ascorbic acid, Vitam. Horm. **11**:61, 1953.
26. Follis, R. H., Jr.: Histochemical studies on cartilage and bone. II. Ascorbic acid deficiency, Bull. Johns Hopkins Hosp. **89**:9, 1951.
27. Rasmussen, H.: The parathyroids. In Williams, R. H.: Textbook of endocrinology, ed. 4, Philadelphia, 1968, W. B. Saunders Co.
28. Schmorl, G.: Ergebn. Inn. Med. Kinderheilk. **4**:403, 1909.
29. Hess, A. F.: Rickets including osteomalacia and tetany, Philadelphia, 1929, Lea & Febiger.
30. Mellanby, E.: An experimental investigation on rickets, Lancet **1**:407, 1919.
31. Pappenheimer, A. M.: Anatomical changes accompanying healing experimental rat rickets under influence of cod liver oil or its active derivatives, J. Exp. Med. **36**:335, 1922.
32. Park, E. A.: Etiology of rickets, Physiol. Rev. **3**:106, 1923.
33. Richards, I. D. G., Sweet, E. M., and Arneil, G. C.: Infantile rickets persists in Glasgow, Lancet **1**:7546, 1968.
34. Jaffe, H. L.: Metabolic degenerative and inflammatory diseases of bone and joints, Philadelphia, 1972, Lea & Febiger.
35. Tapia, J., Stearns, G., and Ponseti, I. V.: Vitamin D resistant rickets: a long-term clinical study of 11 patients, J. Bone Joint Surg. **46-A**:935, 1964.
36. Winters, R. W., Graham, J. B., Williams, T. F., McFalls, V. W., and Burnett, C. H.: A genetic study of familial hypophosphatemia and vitamin D resistant rickets with a review of the literature, Medicine **37**:97, 1958.
37. Rathbun, J. C.: Hypophosphatasia: a new developmental anomaly, Am. J. Dis. Child. **75**:822, 1948.
38. Fraser, R.: Am. J. Med. **22**:730, 1957.
39. Bethune, J. E., and Dent, C. E.: Hypophosphatasia in the adult, Am. J. Med. **28**:615, 1960.

40. Kellsey, D. C.: Hypophosphatasia and congenital bowing of the long bones, J.A.M.A. **179**:187, 1962.
41. Albright, F., Burnett, C. H., Parson, W., Reifenstein, E. C., and Roos, A.: Osteomalacia and late rickets, Medicine **25**: 399, 1946.
42. Engle, R. L., and Wallis, L. A.: Am. J. Med. **22**:5-13, 1957.
43. McCrudden, F. M.: Studies in bone metabolism and osteomalacia, Arch. Intern. Med. **5**:596, 1910.
44. Maxwell, J. P.: Osteomalacia in China, China Med. J. **38**:349, 1924.
45. Dalyell, E. S., and Chick, H.: Hunger-osteomalacia in Vienna, 1920, Lancet **2**:842, 1921.
46. Picchi, J., Crane, J., Gordan, G. S., Sakai, H. Q., and Steinbach, H.: Parathyroid function in malabsorption osteomalacia, Clin. Res. Proc. **5**:67, 1957.
47. Plough, I. C., and Kyle, L. H.: Pancreatic insufficiency and hyperparathyroidism, Ann. Intern. Med. **47**:590, 1957.
48. Dent, C. E.: Hyperparathyroidism and steatorrhea, Br. Med. J. **2**:1546, 1956.
49. Fraser, R., and Nordin, B. E. C.: Hyperparathyroidism and steatorrhea, Br. Med. J. **2**:1363, 1956.
50. Avioli, L. V., and others: Metabolism of vitamin D_3-^{3}H in vitamin D–resistant rickets and familial hypophosphatemia, J. Clin. Invest. **46**:1907, 1967.
51. Dent, C. E.: Rickets and osteomalacia from renal tubule defects, J. Bone Joint Surg. **34-B**:266, 1952.
52. De Toni, G.: Renal rickets with phospho-gluco-amino renal diabetes (de Toni-Debré-Fanconi syndrome), Ann. Paediat. **187**:42, 1956.
53. Fanconi, G.: Der frühinfantile nephrotisch-glykosurische Zwergwuchs mit hypophosphatämischer Rachitis, Jahrbuch Kinderheilh. **147**:299, 1936.
54. Looser, E.: Über pathologische form von Infraktionen und Callusbildungen bei Rachitis und Osteomalacie und anderen Knochenerkrankungen, Zbl. Chir. **47**:1470, 1920.
55. Milkman, L. A.: Multiple spontaneous idiopathic symmetrical fractures, Am. J. Roentgen. **32**:622, 1934.
56. Steinbach, H. L., Kolb, F. O., and Gilfillan, R.: A mechanism of the production of pseudo-fractures in osteomalacia (Milkman's syndrome), Radiology **62**: 388, 1954.
57. Gordan, G. S.: Osteomalacia: diagnosis and treatment, Tex. Med. **59**:110, 1963.
58. Adams, F. D.: Reversible uremia with hypercalcemia due to vitamin D intoxication, N. Engl. J. Med. **244**:590, 1951.
59. Chaplin, H., Clark, L. D., and Ropes, M. W.: Vitamin D intoxication, Am. J. Med. Sci. **221**:369, 1951.
60. Christensen, W. R., Liebman, C., and Sosman, M. C.: Skeletal and periarticular manifestations of hypervitaminosis D, Am. J. Roentgen. **65**:27, 1951.
61. Verner, J., and others: Vitamin D intoxication and report of 2 cases treated with cortisone, Ann. Intern. Med. **48**:765, 1958.

chapter 5

Skeletal changes in endocrine disorders

In this highly active subspecialty of internal medicine and pediatrics, there are available a number of commendable monographs and otherwise a vast literature to which many gifted clinical investigators have contributed. Each new annual *Year Book of Endocrinology* directs attention to hundreds of relevant new observations. For me to attempt anything more than a thumbnail sketch of the skeletal changes found in the well-recognized disorders of the various endocrine glands resulting from hypo- or hyperfunction would be impractical as well as presumptuous.

PITUITARY GLAND

We are concerned here primarily with human growth hormone (HGH). In recent years, we have witnessed the purification and synthesis of this complex peptide hormone and its demonstrated effectiveness in the treatment of hypopituitary dwarfism, as well as the development of a specific HGH immunoassay. This has led to a rapid increase in our knowledge concerning the regulation of growth hormone secretion and has provided a specific test for the diagnosis of HGH deficiency and hypersecretion. As with the other pituitary hormones, the secretion of HGH appears to be regulated by a specific hypothalamic releasing factor. With the use of these new tools has come an increasing awareness of the complexity of the hypothalamic and pituitary abnormalities involved in the etiology of both acromegaly and pituitary dwarfism.[1]

Pituitary basophilism (basophil cell adenoma of the anterior lobe) was at one time thought by Cushing (1932) to be responsible for the clinical entity or syndrome that bears his name, although it is now recognized that this explanation is valid in relatively few instances. Even in these, the untoward effects may well be mediated through stimulation of excessive adrenal cortical activity. As indicated in Chapter 8, one of the major features of *Cushing's syndrome* is pronounced osteoporosis, manifested clinically in backache, round shoulders, and multiple fractures, especially of the ribs.

Skeletal changes in endocrine disorders

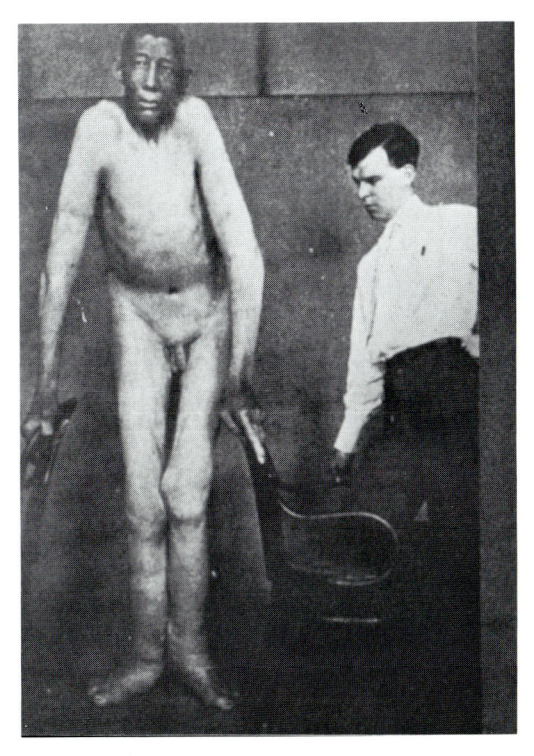

Fig. 5-1. Pituitary gigantism. Note feeble, eunuchoid appearance and hypotrichosis of patient, whose height was over 8 feet. (From Lisser, H., and Escamilla, R. F.: Atlas of clinical endocrinology, ed. 2, St. Louis, 1962, The C. V. Mosby Co.)

Hyperfunction of the eosinophil cells of the anterior lobe, resulting from either diffuse hyperplasia or adenoma, has a very striking effect on skeletal growth. The growth hormone that is produced in excess stimulates chondrogenesis and osteogenesis in skeletal tissues, even reawakening these processes in adult bones.[2] As Collins has emphasized, the anabolic properties of growth hormone reveal themselves nowhere better than in human gigantism, or acromegaly. Its excessive secretion promotes the continuing growth of all tissues, both mesenchymal and epithelial, somatic and visceral.

If the condition has its onset before puberty, *pituitary gigantism* results (Fig. 5-1). Persons with this condition are the 7- to 8-foot circus giants, whose exaggerated skeletal growth reflects inordinate stimulation of endochondral ossification or its reactivation. Other related manifestations are hypertrophy of the subcutaneous tissues and a tendency to periosteal new bone deposition, readily apparent on the jaw bones, for example. In such individuals, the early years of growth may be normal until the excess of growth hormone causes a spurt in general growth, which may then continue several years beyond the usual age for epiphyseal closure. If they survive long enough, the features of acromegaly may be superimposed on great stature.

If, as happens more often, the condition develops after the growth period,

Diseases of bone and joints

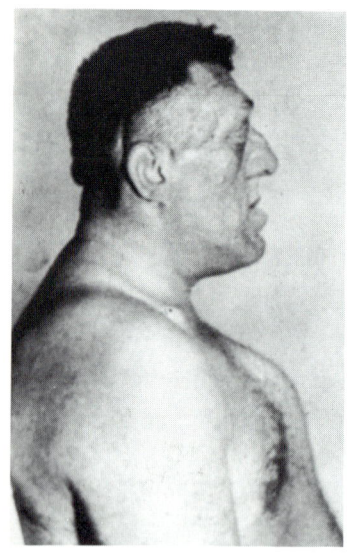

Fig. 5-2. **A,** Acromegalic patient showing protruding sternum, kyphosis, heavy coarse features, and prognathus. **B** and **C,** Comparison of acromegalic hand and foot with those of a normal adult male (on the right of each figure). (From Lisser, H., and Escamilla, R. F.: Atlas of clinical endocrinology, ed. 2, St. Louis, 1962, The C. V. Mosby Co.)

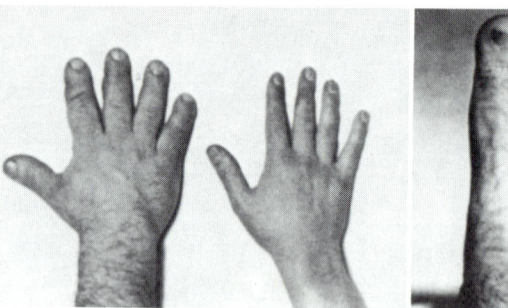

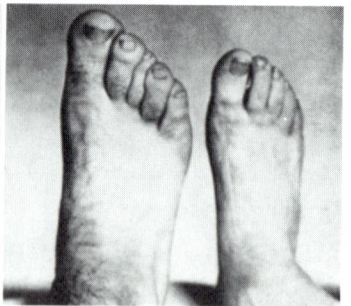

A   B   C

the condition of *acromegaly* (Fig. 5-2) is the result. This condition features the familiar thickset appearance, coarse face, narrow barrel chest with dorsal kyphosis (from reactivated growth at costochondral junctions), large joints, massive hands and feet with thickened digits, and conspicuous prognathism (lantern jaw).[3-9] Back pain, which is a common manifestation, may be the result of osteoporosis. The skull changes associated with prominent enlargement of the head are particularly noteworthy: balloonlike expansion of the sella turcica, great increase in the angle of the mandible with resulting malocclusion and separation of teeth, thickening of the calvarium, overdevelopment of the frontal sinuses and mastoids, and pronounced enlargement of the external occipital protuberance. Other parts of the skeleton, including the vertebral column, show comparable enlargement, particularly at sites of muscle attachment, while the spadelike hand bones show tufting of the terminal phalanges. There is also a high incidence of carpal tunnel compression.

In long-standing acromegaly, joint changes not unlike those of hypertrophic osteoarthritis eventually ensue, although their pathogenesis is somewhat different (so-called acromegalic arthritis or arthropathy). In general, articular symptoms are common in acromegaly, and vary from mild arthralgia to severe, crippling arthritis. Bony overgrowth leads to distortion of the articular plates, and fibrous thickening of joint capsules and ligaments may well be contributing factors.

Hypopituitarism, caused most often by tumors of the craniopharyngeal duct, or Rathke's pouch, results during childhood in the *Lorain type of dwarfism* (nanosomia pituitaria in the old terminology of Erdheim[10]), which is characterized by somatic underdevelopment, stunting of growth, and sexual immaturity

Skeletal changes in endocrine disorders

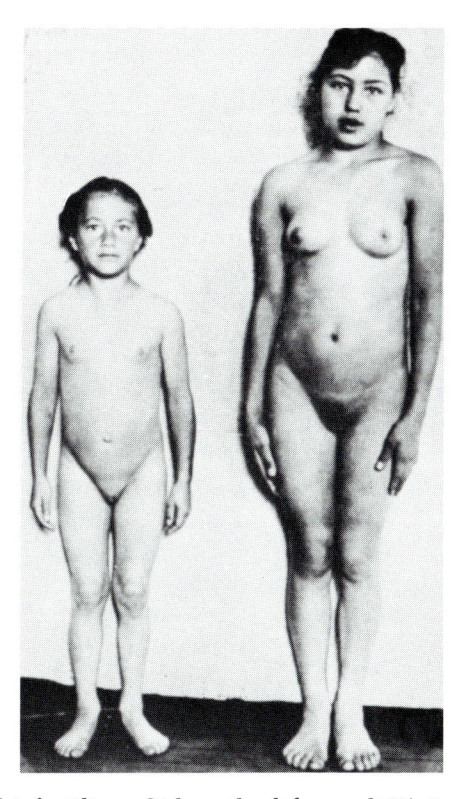

Fig. 5-3. Hypophyseal infantilism. Girl on the left, aged 15, is sexually infantile. Her normal sister on the right is 2 years younger and well matured. Patient's height was only 3 feet, 9 inches. Bone age was estimated at 10 years. This patient presents a striking example of pituitary dwarfism plus sexual infantilism. (From Lisser, H., and Escamilla, R. F.: Atlas of clinical endocrinology, ed. 2, St. Louis, 1962, The C. V. Mosby Co.)

(Fig. 5-3). The body habitus is featured by slender fragile build, thin skin, and very fine hair.

In the pituitary dwarf, normal skeletal proportions are maintained. For the first few years of life, growth proceeds at a normal rate, but then growth of all tissues lags. In the skeleton there is an arrest or retardation of ossification at the epiphyseal growth plates and in other sites as well. Ossification in the epiphyses themselves is likewise held up. Altogether, the bone age of the child lags behind the chronologic age (Fig. 5-3). However, there is no abnormality of form of the ossification centers, as there is in the epiphyseal dysgenesis of the hypothyroid dwarf.

As for the mechanism of hypopituitarism in physiologic and biochemical terms, it now appears that pituitary dwarfism is actually a heterogenous group of disorders, which may result from disturbances in any part of the hypothalamic-hypophyseal-target organ system. This unfolding complex exposition of recent developments has been summarized in an informative, brief review by Rimoin.[1]

Administration of pituitary growth hormone extracted from human glands obtained fresh at autopsy has proved to be of therapeutic value in the hands of Li and his associates[11-12] at the University of California. Hopefully, we shall before long have a potent synthetic product available for general use.

In male adolescents or preadolescents, the *Fröhlich* type of plumpness and girdlelike adiposity *(dystrophia adiposogenitalis)* is associated with somatic and skeletal underdevelopment. There is also characteristic loss of sexual libido and potency.

Complete destruction of the anterior lobe of the pituitary, whatever its cause, is incompatible with life and leads to an eventually fatal cachectic state (Simmond's disease).

ADRENAL GLANDS

With reference to skeletal changes particularly, mention should be made here of *hypercorticism* as seen in Cushing's syndrome,[13-15] which results in marked thinning of the bones, among other familiar effects. The catabolic effect on bone of excessive adrenal corticoids, whether these are produced by tumorous or hyperplastic suprarenal glands or are administered therapeutically, will be discussed in Chapter 8. It is estimated that about 40% of primary adrenocortical tumors are malignant. It is noteworthy, also, that Cushing's syndrome may develop occasionally in patients with bronchial carcinoma, ovarian tumors of various types, and thymic tumors, not necessarily manifesting adrenal metastases.

Benign or malignant cortical tumors may have other relevant effects, stemming from the fact that the adrenal cortex normally elaborates a significant quantity of androgenic hormones. In the female, these hormones generally have a masculinizing effect; in the male, exaggerated male characteristics become manifest. In the male child, sexual precocity and inordinate muscular development in these circumstances make for a little Hercules. The skeleton shows acceleration of growth at first, but the end result paradoxically is premature fusion of epiphyses and small stature. In the adolescent or adult male, a condition of virility and striking hirsutism may result.

THYROID GLAND

Hyperthyroidism (Graves' disease, Basedow's disease, exophthalmic goiter) may sometimes induce skeletal demineralization leading to clinical osteoporosis, involving the calvarium, ribs, and spine. Concomitantly, there is increased urinary excretion of calcium and phosphorus. If prolonged and untreated, the demineralization of bone can be as pronounced as that in Cushing's syndrome. The mechanism of osteoporosis in thyrotoxicosis appears to be that of excessive osteoclastic resorption, associated with the customary fibrous replacement of resorbed bone ("osteitis fibrosa"). If the onset of the condition is before the end of adolescence, there may be accelerated skeletal growth. In general, it may be said that hyperthyroidism stimulates bone growth in the young, but leads to bone wasting in the adult.

Protracted, untreated *hypothyroidism* leads to myxedema in the adult and to

Skeletal changes in endocrine disorders

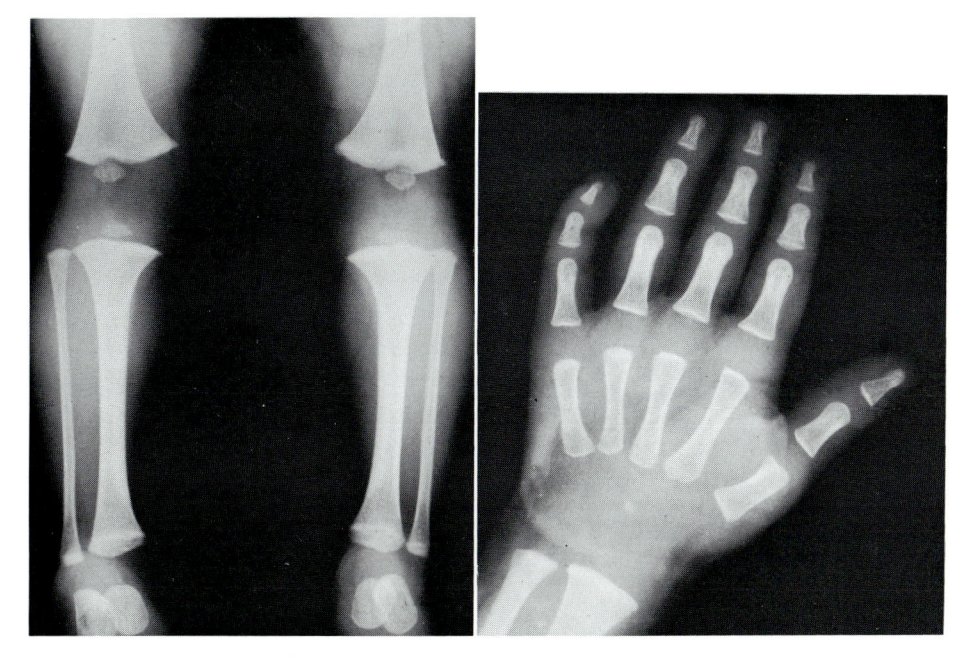

Fig. 5-4. Roentgenograms showing delayed skeletal development in a young patient with cretinism.

cretinism in young children. One of the manifestations of cretinism is dwarfism, which may result from congenital aplasia of the thyroid, from subtotal inflammatory or infectious destruction of the gland, or from endemic iodine deficiency (in mountainous regions). Occasionally it can result from one of a series of inherited enzymatic disorders of thyroid hormone synthesis. Whatever the cause, there is delayed appearance and retarded growth of centers of ossification (Fig. 5-4), retarded growth at epiphyseal cartilage plates, and persistence of growth plates and sutures beyond their usual age of disappearance and even into adult life. Eventually, deformities of the articular ends of long bones may ensue. If untreated, cretins will show a more extreme form of arrested growth than is clinically encountered in any other form of dwarfism.

Mention should also be made here of *thyrocalcitonin*, discovered by Copp in 1963. Thyrocalcitonin is a polypeptide hormone secreted presumably by interstitial or parafollicular cells of the thyroid (independently of the parathyroids), which plays a role in calcium homeostasis.[16] It has been stated that it is responsible for incorporation of calcium into bone and that it can actively lower the serum calcium and block bone resorption (essentially the reverse of the parathyroid effect on bone). The hormone has been successfully synthesized by several pharmaceutical teams, and one can therefore look forward to continued exploration of its clinical effects and therapeutic application.

In general, calcitonin provides the mechanism for fine adjustment or the precise rapid control of serum calcium levels. At this time, however, our understanding of the role of calcitonin in calcium homeostasis is still far from complete.

Diseases of bone and joints

For a detailed account of recent progress, the reader may have recourse to an informative review by Kleeman, Massry, and Coburn.[17]

GONADS

Primary hypogonadism, whether it results from castration, trauma, or infection, has no effect on the skeleton when it develops after the growth period, except insofar is it may favor osteoporosis (in women). In female children with *ovarian agenesis,* stunted growth, or *dwarfism,* which is often associated with other congenital developmental anomalies such as webbed neck or coarctation of the aorta, is found. Hypogonadism in the male child results in *eunuchism,* or eunuchoid habitus, depending on its degree. The skeleton is relatively tall, the limb bones are long and slender with thin cortices, and the epiphyseal cartilage plates persist beyond the normal age and remain active.

With reference to calcium homeostasis, estrogens and androgens produce positive calcium balance by an anticatabolic mechanism.[18]

PINEAL GLAND

Teratomas of the pineal gland and, less often, pinealomas encroaching on the third ventricle and invading the hypothalamus may be responsible in young male children for the *macrogenitosomia praecox* syndrome. As its name implies, this syndrome is featured by excessive body growth and genital development and other manifestations of precocious puberty. The skeleton shows advanced centers of ossification, so that the long bones, for example, are large and heavy in relation to the age of the subject.

PANCREAS

Hypofunction of islet tissue resulting in clinical *diabetes mellitus* may be responsible for altered skeletal development in children. Specifically, with recent onset of the disease, the centers of ossification may be advanced so that initially the body height is above average for the age of the patient. However, with a long history, the centers of ossification may eventually be retarded; the bones are then thin and narrow and even osteoporotic.

In adults, as is well known, one may see accelerated arteriosclerosis with narrowing and occlusion of peripheral arteries, as well as a tendency to gangrene and infection, particularly in the lower limbs. Also noteworthy is the yellow-brown discoloration of the bones, especially of the calvarium, to which Schmorl directed attention many years ago.

THYMUS

As Rowntree and his associates demonstrated, injection of potent thymic extract into young animals (rats) can bring about accelerated prepubertal growth and development, hastened onset of adolescence in the offspring, and increased fertility of parent animals. This is, of course, of more theoretic than practical importance.

PARATHYROID GLANDS

Parathormone, a polypeptide hormone (molecular weight about 9500) has, as its target organs, the bones, the kidney, and the gut. Accordingly, its three major actions are to mobilize calcium from the skeleton, induce phosphate diuresis, and, like vitamin D, increase absorption of calcium from the intestine. The hormone molecule is composed of an 84-amino acid chain, and the first 34-amino acid segment, synthesized by Aurbach and his associates, constitutes the biologically active portion.

The potency of the hormone produced by parathyroid adenomas, as measured by assay and by clinical observations, apparently varies within wide limits, as does its relative effect on the target organs. Thus, some adenomas may induce striking demineralization of the bones, whereas others induce relatively little skeletal resorption, or none at all that is demonstrable, and there seems to be more involved than the time factor alone. Some few parathyroid adenomas may be biologically inactive.

The mechanism of bone resorption is apparently that of dissolution of bone salt and concomitant breakdown of bone matrix. These changes can develop rapidly—susceptible animals to whom large doses of parathormone have been administered manifest osteoclasis and fibrosis (so-called osteitis fibrosa) in as short a time as 12 hours. Resorption starts mainly in spongy bone areas of the medulla, but soon extends around the haversian canals and in time leads to cancellization of the cortex. The most obvious changes are likely to be found in the cancellous bone of vertebrae, the small bones like the phalanges, the ends of long bones, and the tables of the calvarium, and on certain periosteal surfaces.

As for the kidneys, as is well known, one may observe renal stones (composed of calcium phosphate or oxalate) and nephrocalcinosis, especially in the pyramids and medulla. These are potentially dangerous sequelae of persistent hypercalcemia and, if unchecked, can lead to pyelonephritic scarring and, eventually, contracted kidneys and hypertension.

Primary hyperparathyroidism has received a tremendous amount of attention in recent years. Diagnosis of this condition is now made more often and much earlier, before irreversible renal damage from stone formation or nephrocalcinosis has developed. To make an early diagnosis, one must be alert and resourceful and have available a consistently accurate biochemical laboratory.

Clinical leads to diagnosis may be urolithiasis or nephrocalcinosis, symptoms of acute hypercalcemia (nausea, vomiting, constipation, weight loss, anorexia, abdominal pain, refractory peptic ulcer, muscular weakness, and psychosis), or evidence of skeletal resorptive changes (from knowledgeable roentgenographic examination, tracer studies of bone mineral turnover, and bone biopsy). In the presence of hypercalcemia, serum protein electrophoretic separation (showing elevation of $alpha_2$ and beta globulins) will help to rule out other conditions, such as myeloma or sarcoidosis, which may also be characterized by hypercalcemia.

It is noteworthy also that the hypercalcemia of hyperparathyroidism does not respond to large doses of cortisone, as does frequently the hypercalcemia of malignancy, hyperthyroidism, sarcoidosis, vitamin D intoxication, and Addison's disease. In addition to persistent hypercalcemia, renal phosphate leak must also be demonstrated for the correct preoperative diagnosis of hyperparathyroidism. For this, measurement of the tubular reabsorption of phosphorus (TRP) has been proved to be reliable by Gordan, Eisenberg, and their associates.[19-21]

Roentgenographic skeletal examination is also a valuable aid in diagnosis. In the large series surveyed by Steinbach,[21] some 22% of cases of subsequently proved hyperparathyroidism showed significant subperiosteal resorption of the cortex, best seen on the radial surface of the index and middle fingers. Some of these patients also showed granular mottling of bone elsewhere, notably in the calvarium; others showed localized rarefaction defects at the site of "brown tumors." Diffuse demineralization is not necessarily to be expected, although it may be a prominent feature; nor is resorption of the lamina dura of the teeth as dependable a criterion as was once thought (Figs. 5-5 to 5-8).

Bone involvement can be demonstrated in many additional patients with hyperparathyroidism by tracer studies (using nonradioactive strontium, for example) and by bone biopsy. In all these instances one may expect to find elevated serum alkaline phosphatase activity. However, there are undoubtedly cases of proved hyperparathyroidism in which biopsy (of the iliac crest) fails to show evidence of resorption. Perhaps this reflects early sophisticated clinical diagnosis and effective surgery, as contrasted with the bygone era in which the commonly observed end stage of long-standing osseous involvement was the devastating picture of "generalized osteitis fibrosa cystica," as described by von Recklinghausen in 1891.

When bone biopsy does show mild porosity and focal resorption tracts on spongy trabeculae or around enlarged vessel canals in the cortex, these are not pathognomonic, inasmuch as they may also be found in other conditions such as chronic renal insufficiency with uremia, breast cancer, and osteomalacia. All that the pathologist can and should say is that the changes observed are consistent with hyperparathyroidism, which is essentially a clinical diagnosis, at least prior to surgery.

Occasionally the pathologist has the opportunity to examine material from a *brown tumor,* surgically removed, as likely as not, because it was thought radiographically and clinically to be a giant cell tumor, an aneurysmal bone cyst, or perhaps a benign tumor of undetermined nature, before the presence of hypercalcemia was ascertained. The concept of the so-called brown tumor is also a relic of an old era in pathology—it is neither brown (but red, before fixation) nor a tumor. It represents essentially a localized area of exaggerated skeletal resorption, appearing radiographically as a circumscribed lucent defect of varying size and location (the jaw bones, calvarium, and hand bones may be affected, as well as long bones). Its distinction pathologically from giant cell tumor of bone is a subtle one at times, but it can be made with reasonable assurance by an experienced observer. Suffice it to state here that the lesion of hyperparathyroidism

Skeletal changes in endocrine disorders

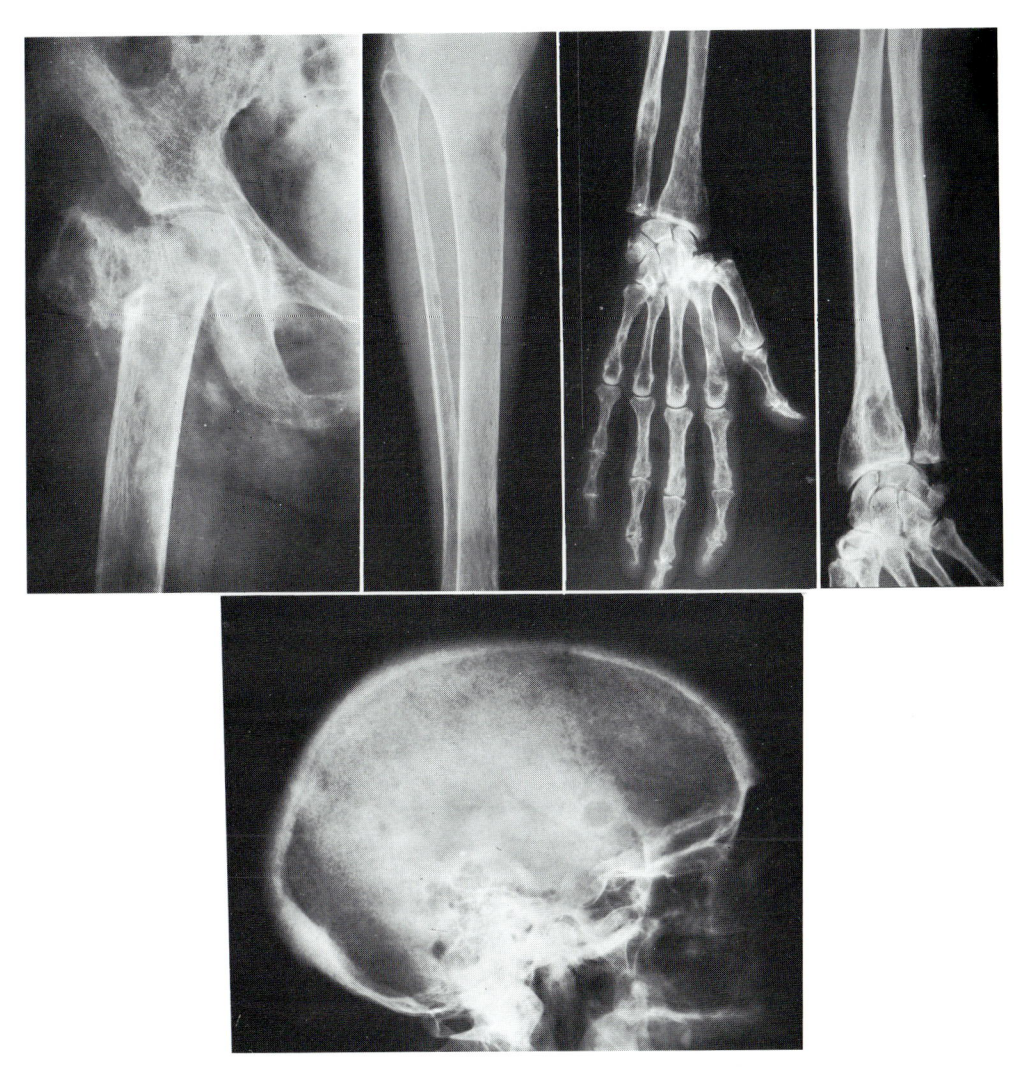

Fig. 5-5. Roentgenograms illustrating delayed recognition of hyperparathyroidism in a 60-year-old woman whose initial manifestation was fracture of the hip. Nailing of the bone did not accomplish union, and two reconstructive procedures in the course of the next 10 months were also unsuccessful. Pain in the wrist area directed attention to the presence of circumscribed lucent defects in the distal radius and other sites, and skeletal survey showed appreciable cortical thinning of the limb bones and granular porosity of the calvarium. Biopsy of the lesion in the radius pointed to hyperparathyroidism, and the serum calcium level was 16 mg. On surgical exploration (performed 15 months after fracture of the hip) a chief cell parathyroid adenoma was found, the cytology of which is illustrated in Fig. 5-10.

Diseases of bone and joints

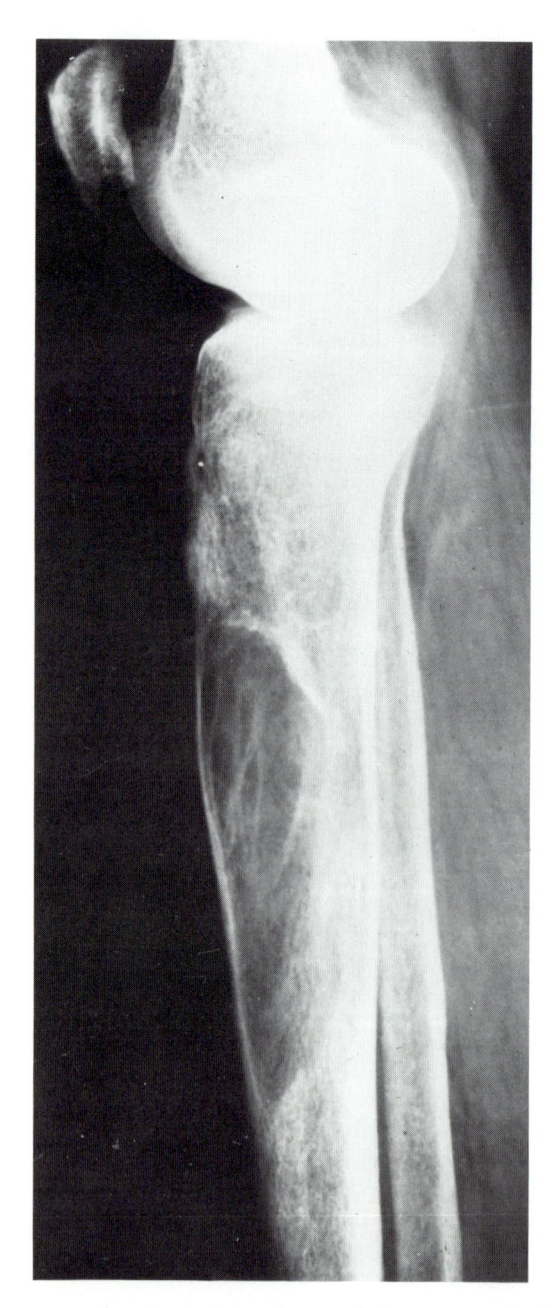

Fig. 5-6. Roentgenogram showing a large lucent defect in the shaft of a tibia, which proved to be a "brown tumor" of hyperparathyroidism. In differential diagnosis, one might also consider early resorptive Paget's disease, although the process is not extending through the cortex.

Skeletal changes in endocrine disorders

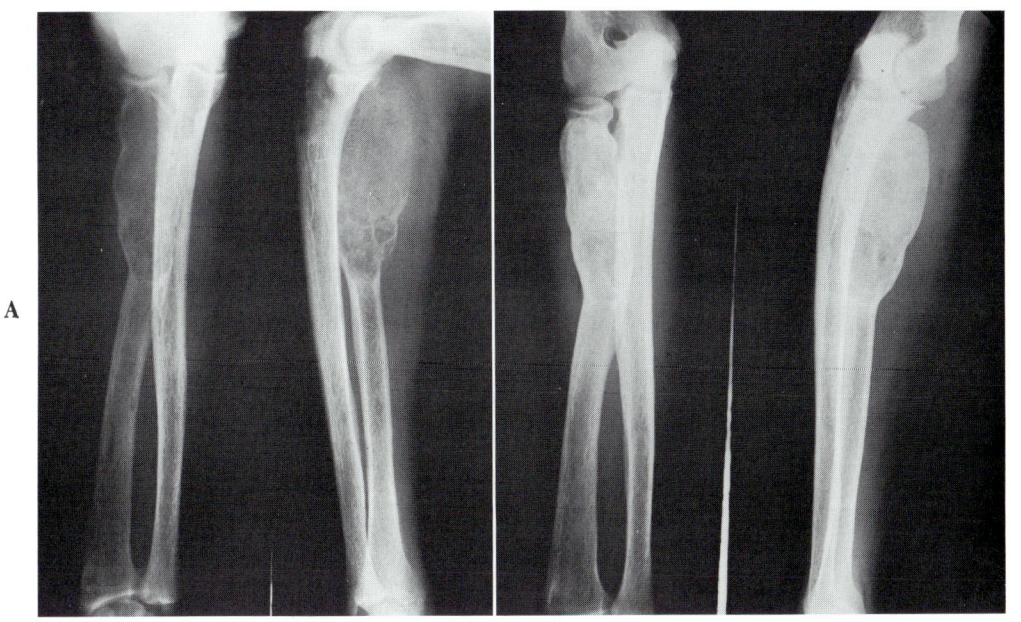

Fig. 5-7. **A,** A case of proved hyperparathyroidism in which a striking feature was the finding of a large "brown tumor" in the proximal radius. **B,** Reossification of the lesion in **A** 4 years after removal of the parathyroid tumor; the expansion and deformity of the bone persisted, however.

has a more fibrous stroma and shows some new bone formation as a rule, as an expression of attempted reconstruction. Further, its giant cells are of the nature of macrophages (rather than syncytial tumor cells), lodged for the most part within or close to vascular channels and appearing in response to blood extravasation (Figs. 5-8, *B,* and 5-9).

As for the changes in the parathyroids themselves, these have been thoroughly explored by Castleman and others on the basis of extensive material. In the great majority of instances of primary hyperparathyroidism, a single parathyroid adenoma is found (Fig. 5-10); only occasionally is more than one encountered. In a minority of cases (about 10% or less), there may be hypertrophy and hyperplasia of all four parathyroid glands, showing large water-clear cells, rather than chief cells. Only rarely is hyperparathyroidism caused by a carcinoma (although certain tumors elsewhere may cause hypercalcemia).

On the other hand, in parathyroid hyperplasia secondary to renal disease or osteomalacia, for example, all the glands are regularly enlarged. Some other less common causes of parathyroid enlargement are Paget's disease, metastatic carcinoma, myeloma, and Cushing's syndrome. The subject of secondary hyperparathyroidism, at least in relation to its most frequent causes, has been considered elsewhere (see sections on renal disease, rickets, and osteomalacia). For the sake of brevity, the observations made will not be reiterated here.

Pseudohyperparathyroidism. As is now well known, biochemical and clinical

Diseases of bone and joints

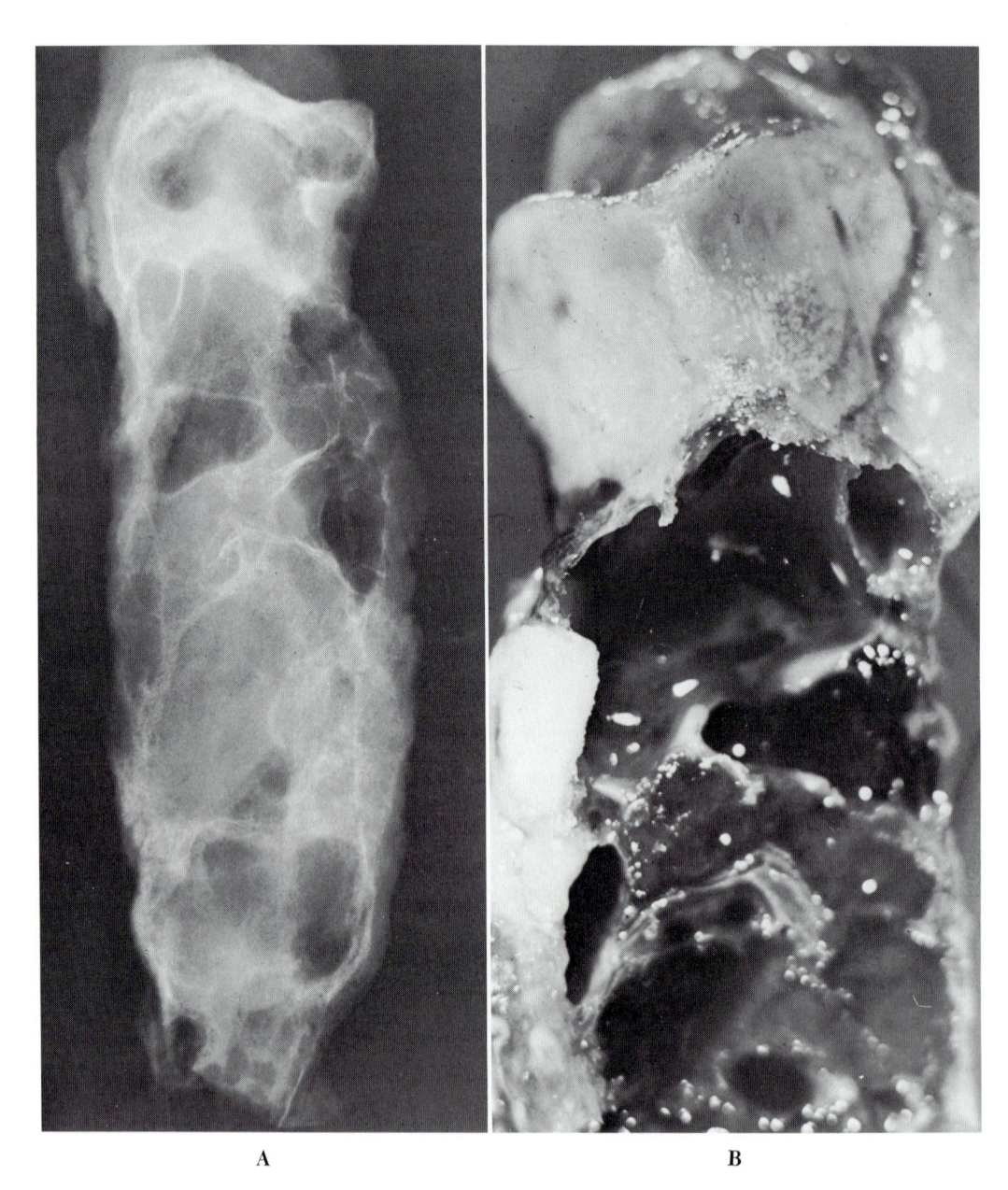

A B

Fig. 5-8. Instance of delayed recognition of hyperparathyroidism in a 57-year-old woman whose skeletal lesion in an ulna (with pain and swelling) was taken to be a giant cell tumor and resected as such. Subsequently, lucent defects were found in other bones and the serum calcium level was noted to be 14.5 mg. On exploration of the neck, a parathyroid adenoma was found. **A**, Roentgenogram of the resected portion of the ulnar bone showing expansion, marked thinning of the cortex, and cystlike rarefaction of the bone throughout. **B**, Photograph of half of the specimen, illustrating cortical thinning, reddish discoloration, and cystic transformation of its interior.

Skeletal changes in endocrine disorders

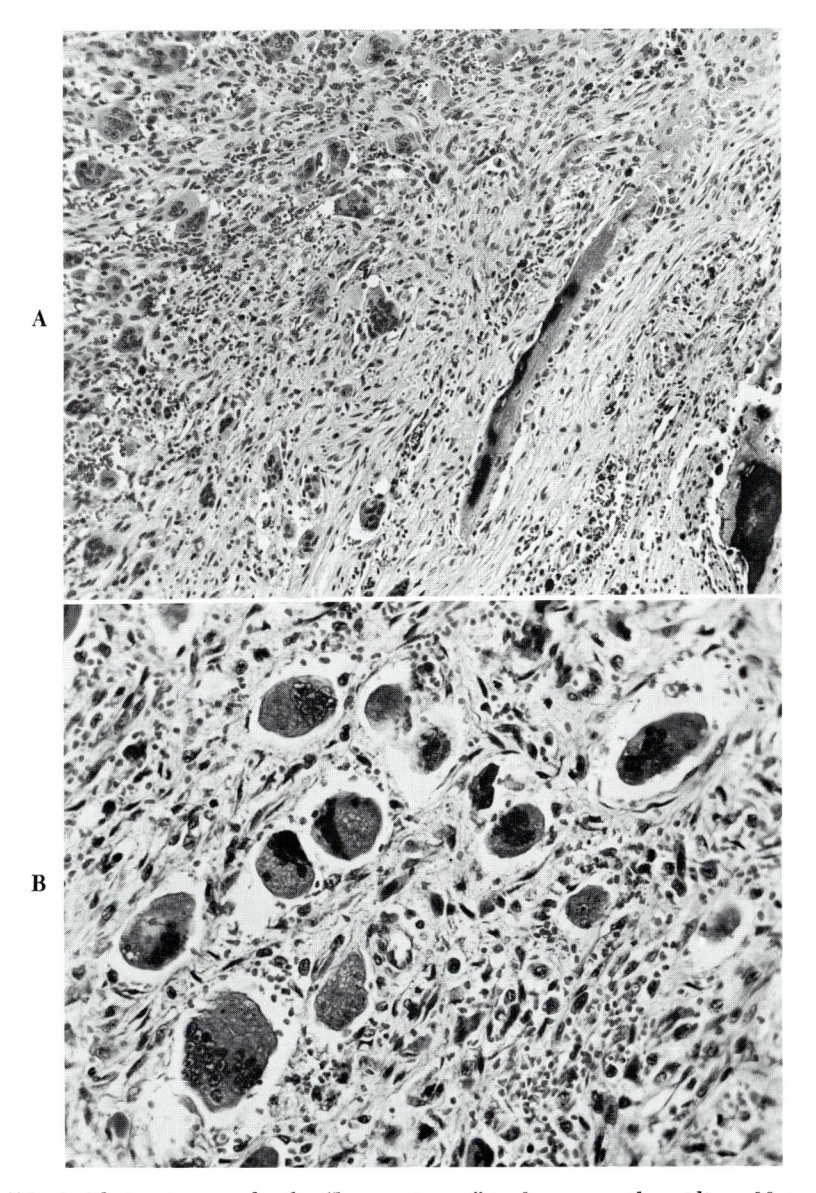

Fig. 5-9. **A,** Photomicrograph of a "brown tumor" in hyperparathyroidism. Note resorption and fibrous replacement of bone, slight new bone formation, and concentration of giant cell macrophages at a site of blood extravasation. **B,** A field from a "brown tumor" showing the osteoclastlike macrophages lodged within thin-walled vascular channels. This picture is quite different from that of neoplastic giant cell tumor of bone.

Diseases of bone and joints

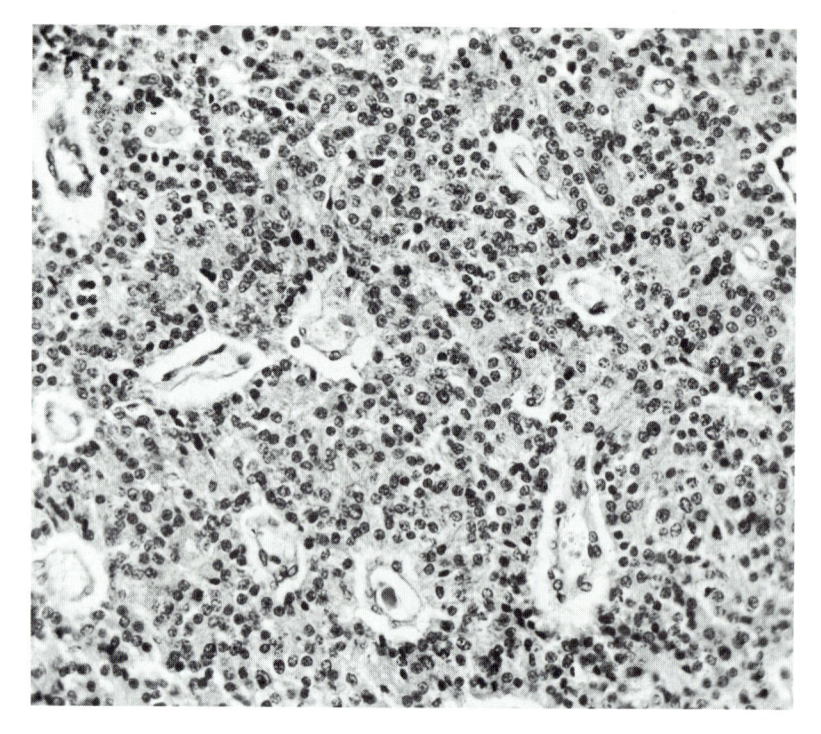

Fig. 5-10. Photomicrograph showing chief cell hyperplasia in the parathyroid adenoma removed in the case illustrated in Fig. 5-5.

manifestations of hyperparathyroidism have been observed with a wide variety of malignant tumors, including occasional carcinomas arising in the lung, kidney, pancreas, and esophagus, as well as malignant lymphoma and stromal cell sarcoma of the uterus, among other sites. The usual explanation for this simulation of hyperparathyroidism is that such tumors secrete a parathormonelike substance. The phenomenon, which can occur without bone metastases, may sometimes lead to exploration for parathyroid adenoma, if the surgeon is not wary. An occasional patient may have both cancer and a parathyroid adenoma, so good clinical judgment is required.

Also noteworthy is the observation that many patients with Zollinger-Ellison tumors (nonbeta pancreatic islet cell tumors), perhaps as many as 30% to 40%, also have hyperparathyroidism due to parathyroid adenoma, carcinoma, or hyperplasia.

As is now recognized, malignant tumors may at times be responsible for manifestations of metabolic bone disease other than hyperparathyroidism; for example, by elaboration of calcitonin; by secretion of a substance causing vitamin D–resistant rickets and osteomalacia; and, in the case of breast cancer with hypercalcemia, by elaborating osteolytic phytosterol esters.[22]

Hypoparathyroidism. Hypoparathyroidism results most often after inadvertent removal of several parathyroid glands in the course of thyroidectomy, or injury to the inferior thyroid artery with infarction of one or more parathyroids. It is less often idiopathic or spontaneous, reflecting aplasia or atrophy of the glands. It may also develop temporarily after parathyroidectomy (for adenoma), and this must be anticipated. As one might expect from the dual effect of the parathyroid hormone, the serum calcium level is low (at tetany level), while the serum phosphorus level is elevated and the tubular reabsorption of phosphorus is correspondingly high.

The major clinical manifestations relate to tetany (epilepsy or brain tumor may be simulated), cataract formation, calcification of basal ganglia, and mental deterioration (with inadequate treatment). In hypoparathyroidism of long standing, stunting of stature and a variety of other skeletal changes have been described. If the condition develops in childhood, the formation of both enamel and dentin of the teeth is impaired, and the teeth may fail to erupt or be lost prematurely.

Effective therapy is directed toward raising the blood calcium level by ingestion of calcium salts, administration of vitamin D, or both, and toward lowering the phosphate level by avoidance of phosphate-rich foods, by ingestion of aluminum hydroxide to adsorb phosphate in the gut, and by administration of vitamin D or dihydrotachysterol. The administration of parathyroid extract is not favored, since this relatively crude protein product may lead to refractoriness.

In *pseudohypoparathyroidism* (the Seabright bantam syndrome of Albright and his associates[23,24]), the manifestations of hypoparathyroidism are caused not by deficiency in the glands themselves, but by failure of the renal tubule to respond to the phosphouretic action of parathyroid hormone. The condition is a rare genetic disorder, inherited as a sex-linked recessive trait. Associated with the metabolic defect (low serum calcium and high serum phosphate unresponsive to parathormone), there are certain skeletal abnormalities, notably short stature, round face, and short metacarpal and metatarsal bones (from early epiphyseal closure). There may also be calcification in the basal ganglia and metastatic calcification in the skin. The disease may coexist with Turner's syndrome.

Some patients may have the biochemical abnormalities, but lack the skeletal manifestations. In others, the serum calcium and phosphorus levels are normal, but the skeletal alterations are present—so-called *pseudo-pseudohypoparathyroidism*.

In occasional patients with the complete syndrome of pseudohypoparathyroidism, the responsiveness of the renal end organ to parathormone is altered, but that of the bone is not, so that the usual manifestations of the disease are complicated by hyperparathyroidism developing in response to hypocalcemia. In other words, there is a dissociation of the effects of parathyroid hormone on the kidney and bone *(pseudo–hypo-hyperparathyroidism)*.[25-31]

REFERENCES

1. Rimoin, D. L.: Editorial: New knowledge about HGH, Calif. Med. 115(2): 75, 1971.
2. Asling, C. W., and Evans, H. M.: Anterior pituitary regulation of skeletal development. In Bourne, G. H., editor: The biochemistry and physiology of

bone, London, 1956, Academic Press, Inc., p. 671.
3. Atkinson, F. R. B.: Acromegaly, London, 1932, John Bale Sons & Danielsson.
4. Bailey, P.: Intracranial tumors, Springfield, Illinois, 1933, Charles C Thomas, Publisher.
5. Cushing, H.: Pituitary body and its disorders, Philadelphia, 1912, J. B. Lippincott Co.
6. Erdheim, J.: Über Wirbelsaülenveränderungen bei Akromegalie, Virch. Arch. Path. Anat. 281:197, 1931.
7. Marie, P.: Sur deux cas d'acromégalie, Rev. Méd. 6:297, 1886.
8. Marie, P., and Marinesco, G.: Sur l'anatomie pathologique de l'acromégalie, Arch. Méd. Exp. Anat. Path. 3:539, 1891.
9. Virchow, R.: Ein Fall und ein skelet von Akromegalie, Klin. Wschr. 26:81, 1889.
10. Erdheim, J.: Nanosomia pituitaria, Beitr. Path. Anat. 62:302, 1916.
11. Li, C. H., and Papkoff, H.: Preparation and properties for growth hormone from human and monkey pituitary glands, Science 124:1293, 1956.
12. Escamilla, R. F., and Forsham, P. H.: Treatment with human growth hormone (Li) for over eight years—effects of long-term therapy in a pituitary dwarf, Calif. Med. 115(6):72, 1971.
13. Knowlton, A. J.: Cushing's syndrome, Bull. N.Y. Acad. Med. 29:441, 1953.
14. Poutasse, E. F., and Higgins, C. C.: Surgery of the adrenal gland for Cushing's syndrome, J. Urol. 70:129, 1953.
15. Strickland, B.: Cushing's syndrome, Proc. R. Soc. Med. 47:341, 1954.
16. Copp, D. H.: Review: Endocrine control of calcium homeostasis, J. Endocrinol. 43:137, 1969.
17. Kleeman, C. R., Massry, S. G., and Coburn, J. W.: The clinical physiology of calcium homeostasis, parathyroid hormone, and calcitonin, Calif. Med. 114(4):19, 1971.
18. Gordan, G. S.: Recent progress in calcium metabolism, Calif. Med. 114:28, 1971.
19. Gordan, G. S.: Hyperparathyroidism, Tex. Med. 57:578, 1961.
20. Gordan, G. S., Eisenberg, E., Loken, H. F., Gardner, B., and Hayashida, T.: Clinical endocrinology of parathyroid hormone excess, Recent Prog. Horm. Res. 18:297, 1962.
21. Steinbach, H. L., Gordan, G. S., Eisenberg, E., Crane, J. T., Silverman, S., and Goldman, L.: Primary hyperparathyroidism: a correlation of roentgen, clinical and pathological features, Amer. J. Roentgen. 86:329, 1961.
22. Gordan, G. S., Lichtenstein, L., and Roof, B. S.: Metabolic bone disease associated with malignancy, Israel J. Med. Sci. 7:499, 1971.
23. Albright, F., Burnett, C. H., Smith, P. H., and Parson, W.: Pseudo-hypoparathyroidism—example of "Seabright-bantam syndrome": report of 3 cases, Endocrinology 30:922, 1942.
24. Albright, F., Smith, P. H., and Fraser, R.: A syndrome characterized by primary ovarian insufficiency and decreased stature, Am. J. Med. Sci. 204:625, 1942.
25. Editorial: Pity the twisting tongue, J.A.M.A. 205:92, 1968.
26. Costello, J. M., and Dent, C. E.: Hypo-hyperparathyroidism, Arch. Dis. Child. 38:397, 1963.
27. Watson, L.: Hypo-hyperparathyroidism, Proc. R. Soc. Med. 61:287, 1968.
28. Kolb, F. O., and Steinbach, H. L.: The syndrome of pseudo–hypo-hyperparathyroidism, First Int. Congress of Endocrinology, Copenhagen, 1960, p. 475.
29. DeMowbray, R. R., Smith, S. H. L., and Symonds, W. J. C.: Hypoparathyroidism and pseudo-hypoparathyroidism, Br. Med. J. 1:903, 1954.
30. Bronsky, D., Kushner, D. S., Dubin, A., and Suapper, I.: Idiopathic hypoparathyroidism and pseudo-hypoparathyroidism: case reports and review of the literature, Medicine, 37:317, 1958.
31. Kolb, F. O., and Steinbach, H.: Pseudo-hyperparathyroidism with secondary hyperparathyroidism and osteitis fibrosa, J. Clin. Endocrinol. Metab. 22:59, 1962.

GENERAL REFERENCES

Bortz, W., and others: Differentiation between thyroid and parathyroid causes of hypercalcemia, Ann. Intern. Med. 54:610, 1961.

Dent, C.: Some problems of hyperparathyroidism, Br. Med. J. 2:1419, 1962.

Hellstrom, J., and others: Primary hyperparathyroidism, Acta Chir. Scand. 294(Supp.): 1-113, 1962.

Hyde, R. D., Jones, R. V., McSwiney, R. B., and Prunty, F. T. G.: Investigation for hyperparathyroidism in the absence of bone disease, Lancet 1:250, 1960.

Jailer, J. W.: Virilism, Bull. N. Y. Acad. Med. 29:377, 1953.

Rasmussen, H., and Craig, L. C.: Isolation and characterization of bovine parathyroid hormone, J. Biol. Chem. **236**:759, 1961.

Rasmussen, H.: Parathyroid hormone: nature and mechanism of action, Am. J. Med. **30**: 112, 1961.

Rasmussen, H., and Reifenstein, E. C., Jr.: The parathyroid glands. In Williams, R. H., editor: Textbook of endocrinology, ed. 4, Philadelphia, 1968, W. B. Saunders Co., pp. 847-961.

Robinson, P. K., Carmichael, E. A., and Cummings, J. N.: Idiopathic hypoparathyroidism; study of 3 cases, Q. J. Med. **23**:383, 1954.

Wilkins, L.: The diagnosis and treatment of endocrine disorders in childhood and adolescence, Springfield, Illinois, 1965, Charles C Thomas, Publisher.

Wilkins, L.: Disturbances in growth, Bull. N. Y. Acad. Med. **29**:280, 1953.

Wilkins, L. and Fleischmann, W.: The diagnosis of hypothyroidism in childhood, J.A.M.A. **116**:2459, 1941.

chapter 6

Skeletal changes in metabolic disorders

This chapter will deal mainly with an assortment of conditions that have in common the fact that they result from inborn errors of metabolism. These conditions are bracketed here for convenient orientation. The main groupings, considered mainly for their skeletal effects, are: the primary disorders of lipid metabolism (especially Gaucher's disease and xanthoma tuberosum multiplex), disorders of purine metabolism (gout, in particular), abnormal amino acid metabolism (especially hereditary ochronosis, which produces significant bone and joint disease), abnormal mucopolysaccharide metabolism (gargoylism is the major condition in point), and some disorders of pigment metabolism (porphyria, mainly). Also considered briefly will be miscellaneous conditions such as amyloidosis, the effect of cachetic states on the bone marrow, and the influence of trace elements on the skeleton.

The skeletal changes in some other important metabolic disorders, most of which are not congenital, have been discussed in other chapters. For the sake of brevity, these observations will not be reiterated here. Specifically, these conditions are scurvy, rickets, and osteomalacia (discussed in Chapter 4); diabetes mellitus (Chapter 5); chronic renal insufficiency, with or without secondary hyperparathyroidism (Chapters 4, 5, and 7); aminoaciduria and other manifestations of renal tubular transport disease (Chapter 7); and sprue, steatorrhea, and pancreatic insufficiency (Chapter 4).

PRIMARY DISORDERS OF LIPID METABOLISM

After being dormant for a long time, the field of abnormal lipid metabolism has once again become the subject of active investigation. As additional observations accrue, the disorders in question become increasingly complex. Thus Niemann-Pick disease, once thought to be a lethal disease of young infants,[1] is now believed to occur in adults as well.[2-4] Collaterally, relatively new concepts of systemic infantile lipoidosis (generalized gangliosidosis[5,6]) and of mucopolysaccharidosis have developed. Gaucher's disease, once considered to be a protracted disease of adults,[7,8] is now recognized as occurring occasionally in a more acute form in infants and young children.[9,10] Amaurotic idiocy, once thought to be an entity of uniform character (Tay-Sachs disease), is now held to appear in no less than six recognized clinical types, according to Volk,[5,6] that effect older patients as well as infants. The biochemical defect is apparently a deficiency of activity of the lysosomal enzyme hexosaminidase A.[11]

As for familial hyperlipoproteinemia and the problems of fat transport by lipoproteins in general,[12] at least five different patterns of circulating lipids of varying clinical significance are now recognized, reflecting increases in the chylomicron, cholesterol, beta lipoprotein, and triglyceride fractions, respectively. While these observations are of great interest to geneticists, pediatricians, and biochemists, as well as internists concerned with the clinical management of arteriosclerosis, the brief account in this book must, of necessity, be limited to the meaningful skeletal alterations that may ensue.

Niemann-Pick disease. In Niemann-Pick disease, prominent aggregates of foam cells are found at autopsy[1] in the bone marrow, in the other reticulum-bearing organs, and in many other sites throughout the body (lungs, intestine, kidneys, and so on). These lipid-laden macrophages are stuffed with sphingomyelin and other phospholipids, and their content of cholesterol esters is also high. This abnormal shift in lipid formation is at the expense of normal body fat, which is depleted.[1] As a rule, there are no structural changes in affected bones (as there may be in Gaucher's disease), perhaps because the condition does not last long enough for them to develop. Only occasional patients survive beyond infancy or early childhood.

Niemann-Pick disease, currently classed among the sphingolipidoses, is an autosomal-recessive genetic disorder in which the hydrolytic enzyme sphingomyelinase is lacking. It has been tentatively subdivided into four groups, depending on the age of onset and its clinical manifestations; the infantile form or Crocker type A accounts for some 85% of cases. Incidentally, the cherry-red spot in the macula may be observed in a number of the lipid storage diseases and is not diagnostic of any one entity.[13]

Gaucher's disease. Gaucher's disease is another congenital, and sometimes familial, disorder of lipid metabolism. It is characterized by excessive widespread deposition of a glucocerebroside[14] long designated as kerasin,[15] notably in the spleen (which can become huge), in the liver (which may eventually undergo cirrhosis), in the bones (which undergo certain structural alterations, infarcts, and, occasionally, fractures), in the deeper lymph nodes, and, to a lesser extent, in other structures such as the skin and conjunctivae.

The condition is an autosomal-recessive genetic disorder in which there is an absence of lysosomal beta-D glucosidase, essential for the breakdown of glucocerebroside.[13]

Whatever its site of deposition, kerasin is taken up by aggregates of distinctive large, pale, foamy histiocytes with delicate fibrillar striations within their

Diseases of bone and joints

cytoplasm; these are quite different from ordinary foam cells containing cholesterol esters. In fact, their appearance is pathognomonic of Gaucher's disease. The diagnosis can be made readily by an experienced observer, whether the biopsy comes from bone, spleen, or liver tissue.

Gaucher[16] is usually credited with the first case report, under the title of "epithelioma of the spleen" (sic). Actually, our basic knowledge of the condition stems in large part from the pioneer pathologic studies of Brill, Mandelbaum, and Libman[7] and their successors[17-19] at Mount Sinai Hospital in New York. (Perhaps this explains why so many of the early case reports were of Jewish patients.)

Gaucher's disease is commonly encountered or recognized in adults and may pursue a chronic protracted course over a period of decades.[20] However, in recent years there have been a number of reports[9,10] of instances in infancy and early childhood featuring a more rapid course with cerebral involvement, so that the clinical differentiation from Niemann-Pick disease may be a problem. In this regard, the finding of Tuchman and his associates[18] that the serum acid phosphatase level is significantly elevated in Gaucher's disease may be helpful. There may be certain hematologic manifestations—specifically, hypochromic anemia, presumably from bone marrow encroachment, and leukopenia and thrombocytopenia (with a tendency to hemorrhage) from splenic involvement.

The osseous changes[8,19,21] are more relevant here. They may be demonstrable roentgenographically in many sites, but in general they are characterized by increased lucency, thinning of cortices, loss of cancellous bone markings, and sometimes expansion of the affected bone. Pathologic fracture may occasionally be observed. One of the best known changes, to which diagnostic importance is attached, is the tendency to cortical thinning and bilateral symmetrical flaring or fusiform expansion of the lower femora (Fig. 6-1, A). Comparable changes may be observed also in the distal humerus (Fig. 6-1, B). Involvement of vertebral bodies with collapse and resulting cord compression has been described, but this is unusual. Particular attention has also been directed to avascular necrosis in the femur, especially in the femoral head and neck, often followed by compression or collapse with subsequent osteoarthritic changes (Figs. 6-1, C, and 6-2, A).

There is not much that one can accomplish in the way of treatment beyond symptomatic relief, correction of anemia (if present), and appropriate orthopedic management of such complications as infarction in a femoral head or compression of one or more vertebral bodies.

Fig. 6-1. **A**, Skeletal changes in Gaucher's disease in a child. Note the cortical thinning and bilateral symmetrical flaring of the distal femur. **B**, Comparable changes in a humerus of the same patient. **C**, Another case of Gaucher's disease in a child, aged 5, with involvement of upper femora, showing collapse of one and displacement of capital femoral epiphysis.

Skeletal changes in metabolic disorders

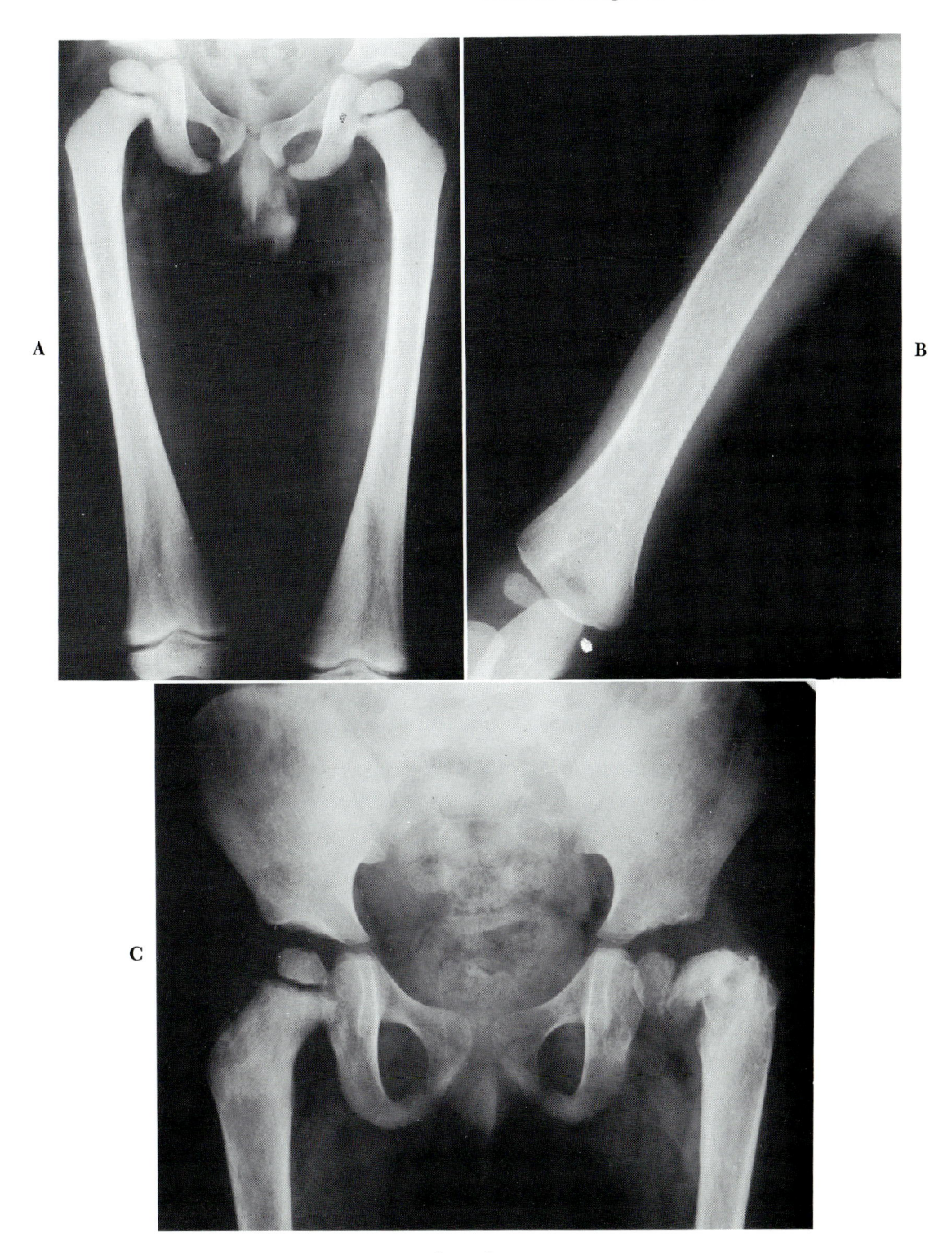

Fig. 6-1. For legend see opposite page.

Diseases of bone and joints

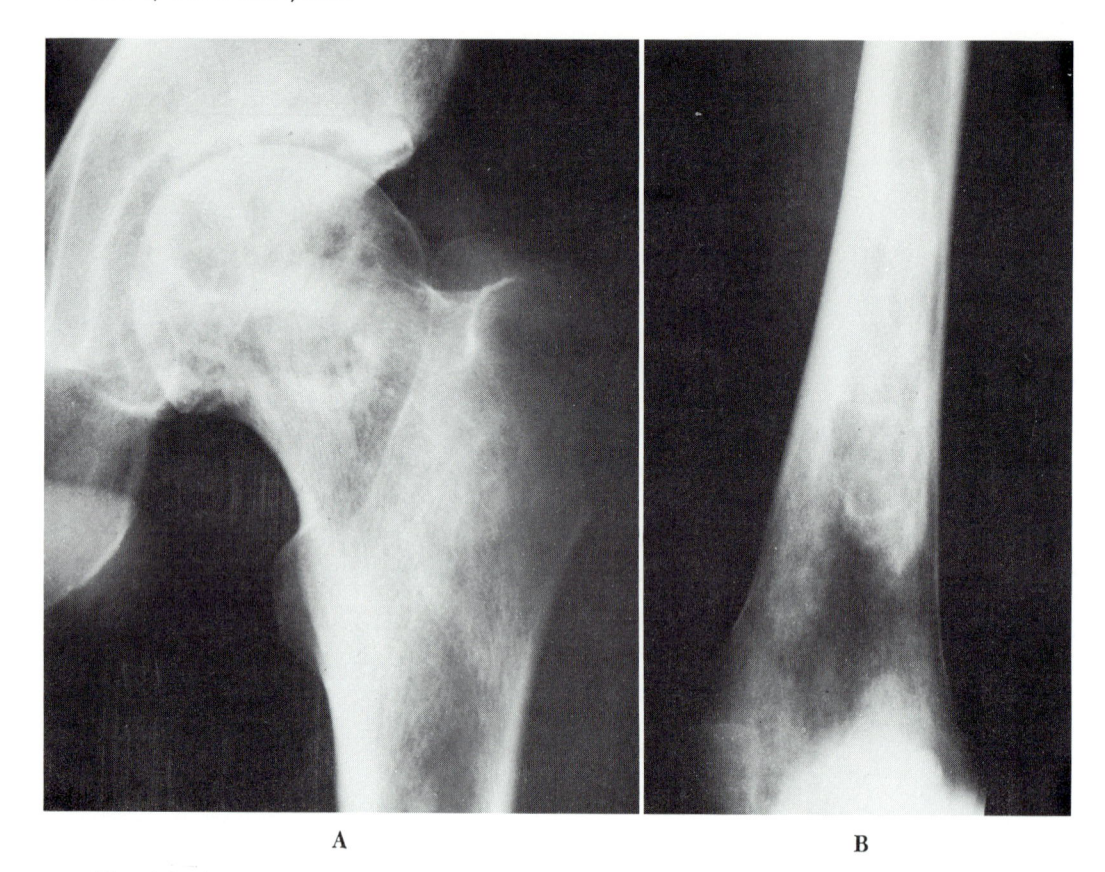

A   B

Fig. 6-2. **A**, Roentgenogram showing partial avascular necrosis (bone infarct) in the femoral head of an adult with Gaucher's disease. There were secondary osteoarthritic changes in the hip, but collapse of the head had not taken place (as it may). **B**, A bone infarct in the lower femoral shaft of the same patient. There was also a comparable old infarct in the opposite femur (not shown).

Irradiation of skeletal lesions, which enjoyed a brief vogue, is of questionable value and objectionable in principle. As for splenectomy, this should *not* be done casually, without very good indications, since removal of a major depot for lipid storage throws an added burden on the bone marrow and the liver, where the development of Gaucher's cirrhosis constitutes a serious problem.

Xanthoma tuberosum multiplex (lipid gout; essential hypercholesterolemia). Xanthoma tuberosum multiplex, a manifestation of familial hyperlipoproteinemia, is characterized by hypercholesterolemia (up to 600 mg./100 ml., or more) and multiple cholesterol deposits in the skin, subcutis, and tendons, especially of the hands and feet, where pain and tumorous swelling may be produced.[22] This latter manifestation is well known to orthopedic surgeons. In present day biochemical parlance, it is encountered mainly with type II and occasionally with type III familial hyperlipoproteinemia, in which the levels of both cholesterol and triglyceride are elevated.[23] Occasionally there may be lipid storage in bone as well.

Skeletal changes in metabolic disorders

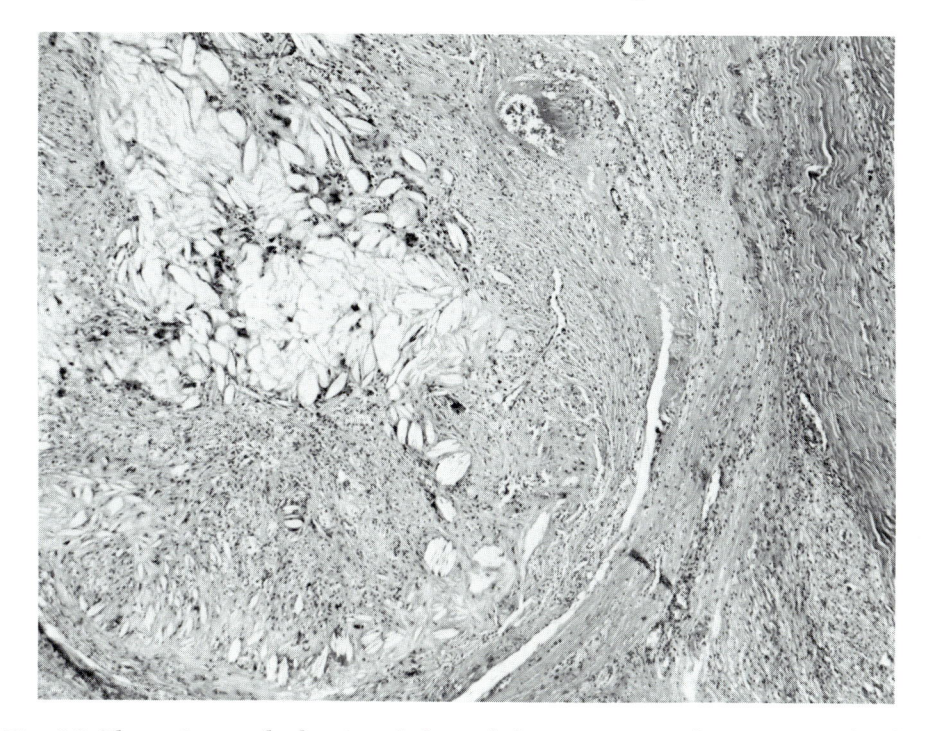

Fig. 6-3. Photomicrograph showing cholesterol deposition in tendinous tissue of a foot in xanthoma tuberosum multiplex. The pale cholesterol crystals characteristically provoke foreign-body reaction, and there is also foam cell (cholesterol ester) deposition not readily seen at this low magnification.

I have seen a case in point in which there was resulting collapse of a vertebral body.

Of greater importance is the observation that some individuals suffering from this disease may develop serious, if not fatal, coronary atherosclerosis and occlusion at a relatively early age.

Examination of a representative specimen from the skin and subcutis or from a tumorous mass in a tendon shows abundant deposition and intermingling of cholesterol as crystals and also of cholesterol esters as foam cells (Fig. 6-3). As one might expect, the cholesterol crystals provoke foreign body reaction, but otherwise there is little or no inflammatory reaction.

One occasionally sees material from painful localized lesions in bone obtained as surgical specimens, which show cholesterol crystals, foam cells, or both, within fibrous connective tissue, without any apparent basis for their deposition. As likely as not, such lesions are labeled "xanthoma" of bone for want of a more meaningful designation. I have seen a number of such puzzling instances, including several in an ulna and one in a scapula. In such cases, one should be circumspect about the possibility of familial hyperlipoproteinemia and check the serum cholesterol level, as well as the cutis and superficial tendons, for possible lipid deposition.

Diseases of bone and joints

GOUT

The term "gout" has been used loosely in the past to refer to a number of conditions, including so-called calcium gout (calcinosis), lipid gout (xanthoma tuberosum multiplex), and even oxalic gout (oxalism). The present discussion deals exclusively with classical gout, which has plagued man since antiquity. It may be defined for basic orientation as a hereditary disorder of purine metabolism characterized by hyperuricemia, irregularly recurring attacks of acute arthritic involvement, and a tendency to urate deposition, often leading to more or less severe chronic tophaceous arthritis. The biochemical basis for these manifestations of sustained hyperuricemia is apparently quite complex,[24-28] and at least five forms of gout have been postulated,[27,28] with perhaps more to come.

Many persons (the relatives of gouty patients especially) may have a latent tendency to gout, manifested only by otherwise unexplained hyperuricemia, but they may never develop clinical gout. The latter is commonly ushered in by acute gout[29] affecting not only the first metatarsophalangeal joint (podagra) but frequently other joints as well. The incidence and severity of these sporadic, excruciatingly painful attacks vary considerably from case to case, and their pathogenetic basis has long been a matter of conjecture, although it has been reported[30] that sodium urate crystals injected into the joints of volunteer gout patients caused a reaction very similar to an acute gout attack. In other words, acute gouty arthritis apparently represents microcrystalline synovitis.[27] As for the mechanism of this remarkable phenomenon, it has been shown[33] that monosodium urate crystals (among other crystalline substances, including calcium pyrophosphate) activate Hageman factor in joint fluid and produce an acute arthritis, which can be prevented by an antibody to Hageman factor. Between attacks (the so-called intercritical period), gouty patients may be ostensibly well, and many never develop significant tophaceous gout.[31] Some, however, after years of recurring episodes of acute gout, go on to develop chronic deforming changes associated with progressive urate deposition.[32] While this is ordinarily a relatively slow process, it may be remarkably accelerated at times.

It should also be noted that manifestations of gout may appear in patients with hematopoietic disorders in which the turnover of nucleic acids involved in hematopoiesis is accelerated, with excessive formation of uric acid. Whatever the reason for excessive urate formation, its accumulation is of potentially serious consequence in man (as distinct from lower mammalian species) because of enzymatic inability to convert uric acid to allantoin and because, normally, fully 80% of the glomerular urate filtrate is reabsorbed by the renal tubules. Moreover, the relatively low solubility of uric acid and its salts in tissue fluids also favors the insidious deposition of urate deposits in certain skeletal and extraskeletal sites of predilection, which will be indicated presently. It is essential to note further that in some gouty patients there is an associated tendency toward vascular disease of potentially serious import, reflected in a significantly high incidence of hypertension, severe nephrosclerosis with renal insufficiency, cardiac failure, and cerebrovascular accidents.[32]

Skeletal changes in metabolic disorders

Renewed interest has been evinced in gout in recent years, and from this clinical and biochemical research markedly improved therapeutic measures have evolved.[33] One may cite here the proved effectiveness of phenylbutazone, corticotropin, and colchicine in terminating attacks of acute gout; the use of regular colchicine prophylaxis to reduce the incidence and severity of acute episodes; the administration of new uricosuric agents (such as probenecid, sulfinpyrazone, and allopurinol [HPP]) to help prevent chronic gouty arthritis and, with long-term good clinical control, to ameliorate established deformities and disability[34]; and the use of allopurinol (an inhibitor of uric acid synthesis), especially for gouty patients with a tendency to lithiasis.

That the skeletal connective tissues, particularly the joints and periarticular structures, bear the brunt of urate deposition in tophaceous gout is common knowledge. Within an affected joint (be it a metatarsophalangeal, metacarpophalangeal, or interphalangeal joint, a knee, a hip, a shoulder, or any other), focal, chalky white or yellow, tophaceous deposits are observed on the articular surfaces. These deposits are also found in the deeper layers of the cartilage. The articular cartilage tends gradually to be destroyed and replaced by pannus (see Fig. 15-10). Eventually, in severe instances with attendant deformity and immobilization, fibrous ankylosis may ensue, as well as the usual changes of secondary osteoarthritis. Concomitantly, the synovial lining and sublining connec-

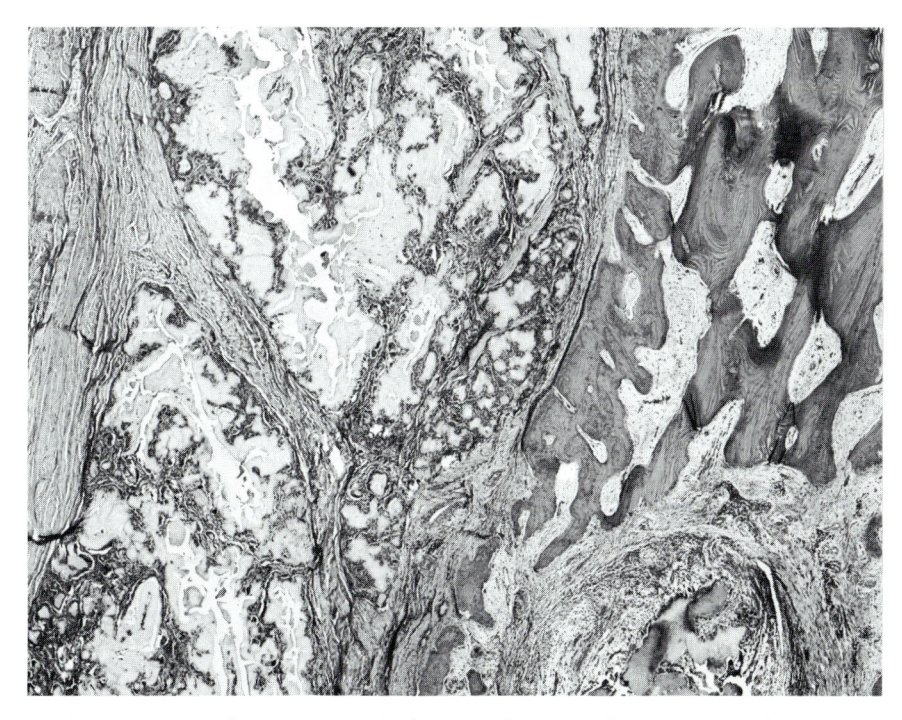

Fig. 6-4. Low-power photomicrograph showing the general appearance of urate deposits within bone. (×55.) This picture is characteristic of chronic tophaceous gout.

Diseases of bone and joints

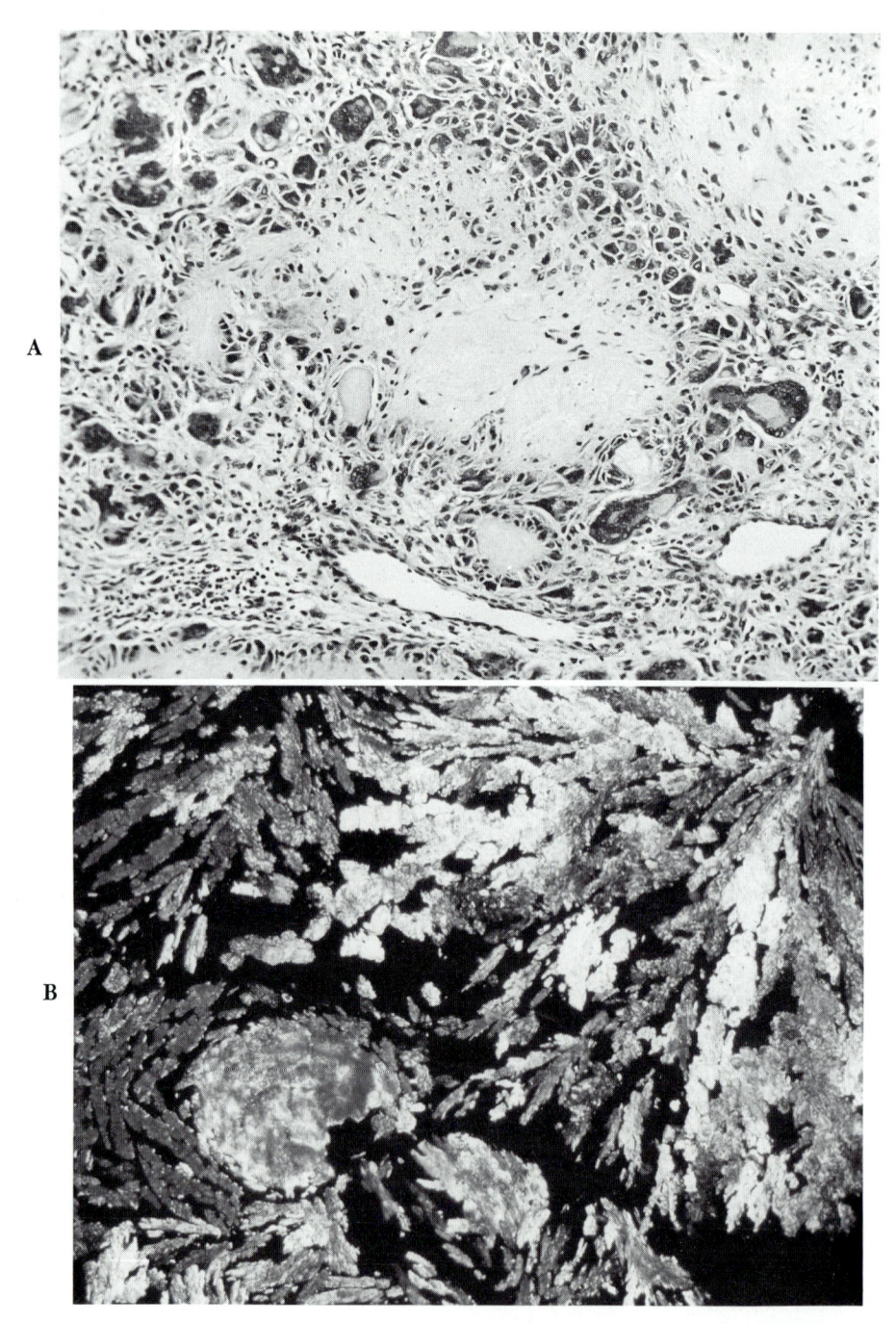

Fig. 6-5. **A**, Photomicrograph of a representative field of a gouty tophus showing urate deposits characteristically ringed by foreign body giant cells as well as smaller macrophages. This block was fixed in formalin rather than alcohol, and crystalline structure is lacking. (×250.) **B**, Photomicrograph of an autopsy specimen from a joint region of a subject with gout, fixed in absolute alcohol to preserve the crystalline structure of tophaceous deposits. Note the urate crystals, as viewed in polarized light. (×100.)

tive tissue of the affected joint capsule likewise exhibit focal impregnation by urates. Eventually, more or less extensive reactive chronic villous synovitis ensues. The articular bone ends frequently manifest urate deposits within their periosteal covering, as well as in the subchondral spongy bone (Fig. 6-4). The ligaments and tendons, too, may be more or less heavily impregnated. Similarly, certain of the periarticular bursae, especially the olecranon and prepatellar bursae, are often predilected. In the vertebral column, the intervertebral discs and the contiguous portions of the bodies may be the sites of appreciable urate deposition.[32]

As for extraskeletal urate deposits, tophaceous involvement of the skin and subcutis, especially of the hands and feet and occasionally of the ear, is commonly observed in instances of moderate severity. Urate deposits are frequently encountered at necropsy in the kidney (where they favor the development of pyelonephritis), and occasionally in the lower urinary tract as stones or gravel. Involvement of the eye, of the heart and blood vessels, of the upper and lower airways, and of many other sites has been documented,[32] although today these are unusual, if not rare.

In chronic tophaceous gout, the characteristic tissue response to urate deposits, wherever they may be encountered, is essentially that of a peculiar and distinctive foreign-body reaction (Fig. 6-5). The urate material usually appears rather amorphous in formalin-fixed specimens, and only in alcohol-fixed preparations does one regularly discern crystalline structure. On microscopic examination, one characteristically observes smaller or larger, discrete or conglomerate deposits, ringed peripherally by foreign body giant cells, mononuclear histiocytes, or both. This reaction pattern is sufficiently distinctive for reliable diagnosis, and blackening with silver is scarcely required for confirmation. The inflammatory response otherwise is usually rather inconspicuous, provided that there has not been ulceration or complicating infection (which is unusual). At times, one may see calcification of urate deposits and even conspicuous heterotopic ossification.[32]

HEREDITARY OCHRONOSIS

Since Garrod[35] introduced the concept of inborn errors of metabolism in 1923, specific gene defects producing enzymatic abnormalities have been postulated for more than a hundred syndromes, and the list will undoubtedly continue to grow. Many of these disorders result from abnormal amino acid metabolism. A substantial number may be responsible for mental retardation—phenylketonuria (PKU) is a well-known example. As with congenital disorders of skeletal development, it appears that everything that can possibly go wrong apparently does so at one time or another. The possibilities of error are so numerous that a whole cluster of diseases in point result from defects in the intermediary metabolism of phenylalanine and tyrosine alone: for example, phenylpyruvic oligophrenia, tyrosinosis, albinism, phenylketonuria, and hereditary ochronosis (alkaptonuria).

Diseases of bone and joints

The present discussion will deal briefly with only one of these disorders, hereditary ochronosis,[36] which was selected because of its striking skeletal changes. For a comprehensive account of the genetic background and detailed pathologic changes, the reader may have recourse to my paper[37] on the subject published in 1954. Alkaptonuria reflects the urinary excretion of homogentisic acid (2,5-dihydroxyphenylacetic acid) as one manifestation and usually the initial expression of hereditary ochronosis. As such, alkaptonuria is no more a disease per se than is glycosuria in relation to diabetes mellitus.

Far from being a harmless curiosity, as has often been implied, hereditary ochronosis results eventually in a more or less disabling arthritis and ankylosing spondylitis of a specific nature.[37-40] The development of calcific aortic stenosis may be another serious sequel. Still other deleterious effects of abnormal pigment deposition are severe arteriosclerosis, ochronotic nephrosis, and the formation of pigment calculi in the urinary tract.[37]

That the skeletal connective tissue structures bear the brunt of ochronotic pigment deposition is well known (Figs. 6-6 to 6-10). The bones themselves, apart from their articulations and their periosteal investment, are altered only to a limited extent. In affected synovial joints, the articular cartilage becomes hard, brittle, and pigmented and tends to break away piecemeal in the course of articular function, so that eventually the bone ends may be largely, if not entirely, denuded of cartilage (see Fig. 15-11). When the involved joint is a compara-

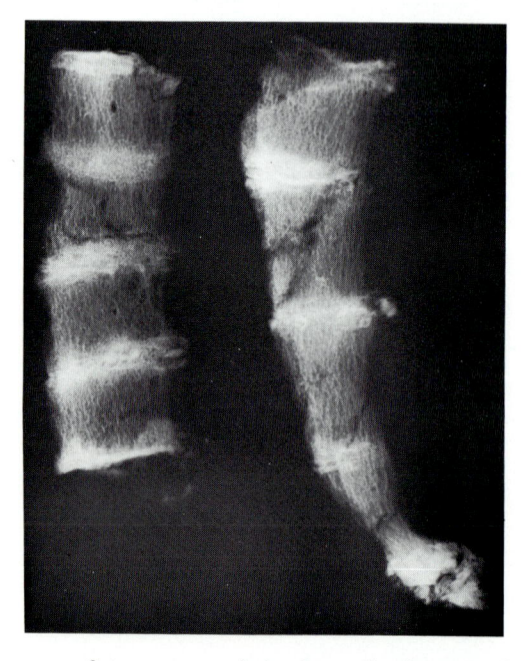

Fig. 6-6. Roentgenogram of a segment of the lower lumbar vertebral column showing conspicuous radiopacity of the intervertebral discs. Also evident are the arthritic changes in the lumbosacral joint at the distal end of the specimen.

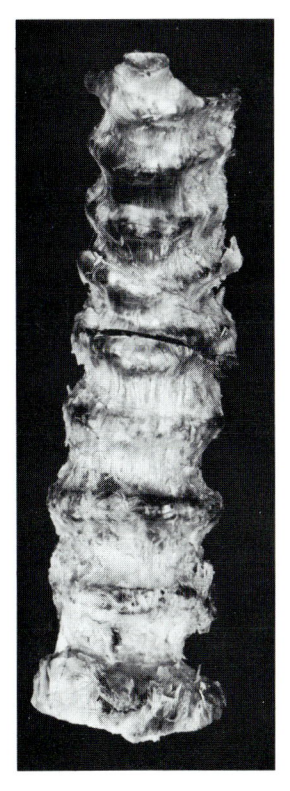

Fig. 6-7. Photograph (reduced) of a portion of the vertebral column (lower dorsal and lumbar) as viewed externally, showing blackened osteophytic rings at the levels of the intervertebral discs.

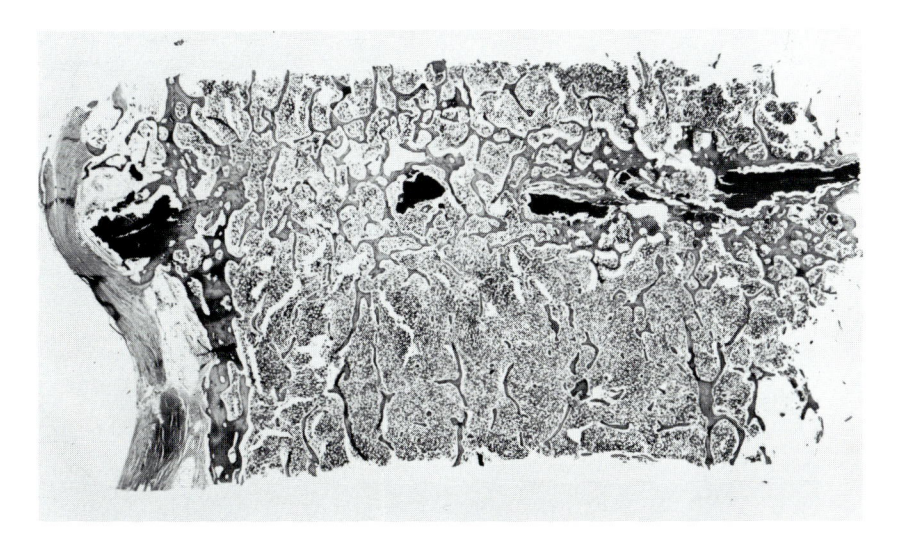

Fig. 6-8. Photomicrograph of a section of the vertebral column showing an involved intervertebral disc. Most of the impregnated disc tissue has disappeared at this level, and only discontinuous remnants of it are seen. Where the disc is defective, the contiguous vertebral bodies have fused.

129

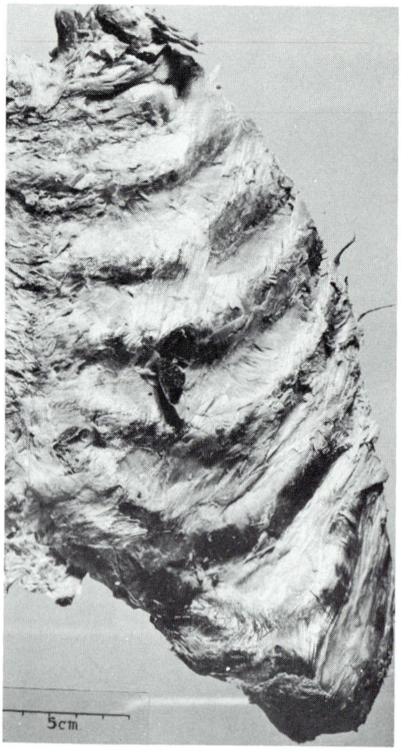

Diseases of bone and joints

Fig. 6-9. Photograph (reduced) showing conspicuous blackish discoloration of the costal cartilages and their perichondrium, as well as of the periosteum of the ribs and the intercostal ligaments.

tively large one, such as the knee, some of these pigmented cartilage fragments may constitute free joint bodies.[38] Many of them are ground into the synovium and the subsynovial connective tissue, producing the striking picture illustrated in Fig. 15-11, *B*. In these circumstances, it is not surprising that the synovium should show blackening and reactive villous synovitis or that, with continued function, marginal exostoses, conspicuous subchondral sclerosis, and other changes of secondary osteoarthritis of appreciable severity should ensue. While these changes of ochronotic arthritis develop slowly and usually become a clinical problem in middle age, pertinent cases have been recorded in which significant disability ensued long before the age of 40.

Equally important are the changes in the vertebral column; these lead eventually to a peculiar *ochronotic ankylosing spondylitis*. This has its basis in heavy impregnation of the intervertebral discs by ochronotic pigment, which is reflected roentgenographically by conspicuous radiopacity (Fig. 6-6). The pigment is deposited throughout the discs, in the anulus fibrosus, nucleus pulposus, and contiguous longitudinal ligament (where it provokes the formation of prominent, somewhat blackishly discolored, osteophytic rings; Fig. 6-7). The profoundly altered, impregnated disc tissue tends ultimately to be resorbed, and at many

Skeletal changes in metabolic disorders

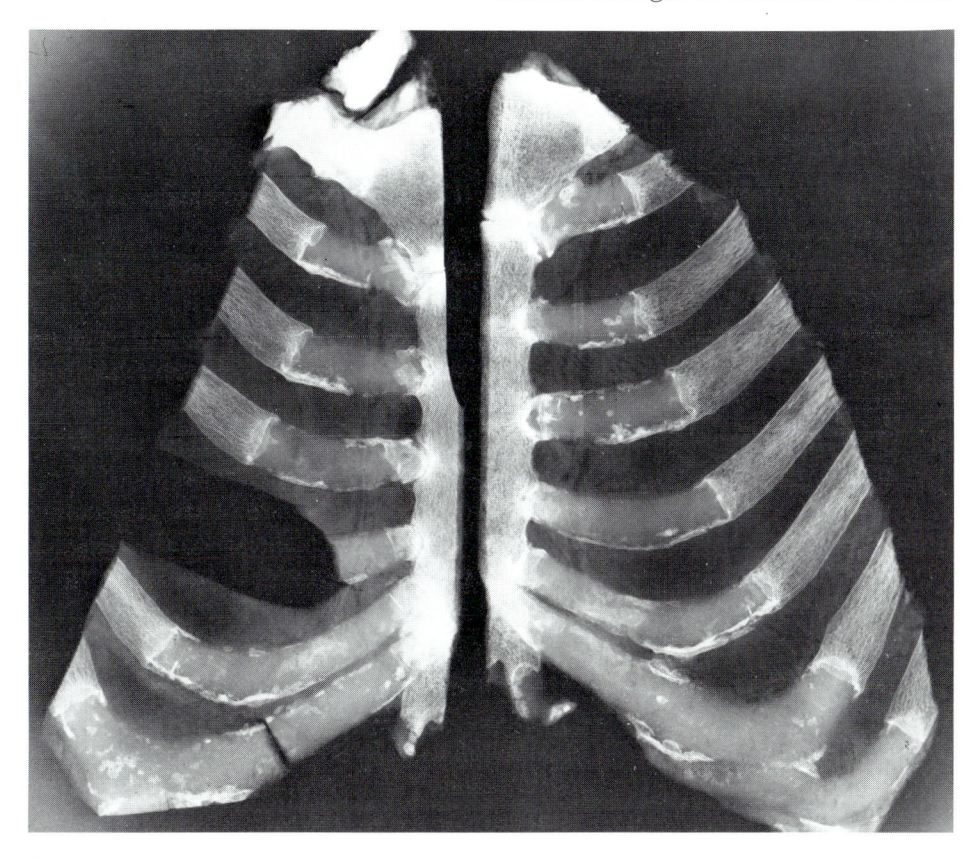

Fig. 6-10. Roentgenogram of a sternum and attached ribs (autopsy specimen) in a patient with hereditary ochronosis, emphasizing the striking radiopacity of the pigment deposits in the cartilage and at the articulations.

levels one may observe merely residual discontinuous remnants of it. The contiguous vertebral bodies manifest a tendency to fusion where the disc material is defective or absent (Fig. 6-8). The end result may be that of a substantially fused "poker" spine showing abnormal curvature. In the light of these changes, one can readily appreciate the disability commonly associated with involvement of the vertebral column in ochronosis and the singularity of gait that Osler[41] described 70 years ago.

Brief mention may be made here to two other abnormalities of amino acid metabolism in which there are incidental skeletal effects. In *cystine storage disease* (cystinosis, Lignac-Fanconi disease), which shows many of the features of renal tubular transport disease (leakage of phosphate, glucose, amino acids, and so forth), characteristic crystals are deposited in the bone marrow, cornea, and reticulum-bearing tissues.

Also, in primary hyperoxaluria (oxalosis), which is thought to reflect a defect or block in glycine metabolism, oxalate stones may form in the urinary tract and oxalate crystals may appear in the bone marrow, cartilage, kidney, heart muscle,

Diseases of bone and joints

and other sites,[42,43] where they provoke fibrous and giant cell reaction. They show up as birefringent crystals when viewed with polarized light.

PORPHYRIA

Porphyria results from an unusual inborn error of porphyrin metabolism, in which there is spontaneous excessive excretion of uroporphyrin and porphyrin precursors. The porphyrins in general are a remarkable group of pyrrole ring–containing, metalbinding, fluorescent chemical compounds found combined with protein in respiratory pigments, such as hemoglobin, cytochrome, and catalase. Another important member of the group is chlorophyll, a magnesium-porphyrin compound essential for photosynthesis in plants.

Despite the brilliant work of Hans Fischer on the chemical structure of the porphyrins over 50 years ago, we still know relatively little about their intermediary metabolism in man or about the precise nature of the enzymatic defect or aberration in human porphyria. The protean clinical manifestations of the disease, however, have been clarified, and it is now conventional[44,45] to classify cases of porphyria as falling into two types.

The first type, which constitutes a relatively small group, is *porphyria erythropoietica* (congenital), inherited as a mendelian recessive trait. It manifests itself in childhood by photosensitivity, increased hemolysis and increased erythropoiesis, red urine, reddish discoloration of teeth *(erythrodontia)*, and staining also of the bone to a red or mahogany-brown. The last apparently reflects marked increase of marrow porphyrin within the growing bones. Fluorescent microscopy of such marrow samples shows intense red fluorescence concentrated in the nuclei of normoblasts.

The second type, which accounts for most of the clinical cases, is now designated at *porphyria hepatica*. It includes as subtypes *acute intermittent porphyria* and *porphyria cutanea tarda*, as well as occasional mixed forms and latent porphyria (most often found in relatives of patients with so-called hepatic porphyria). The most common expression of the disorder, acute intermittent porphyria, usually begins in early life and is characterized by potentially serious repeated crises, often with bizarre symptoms featuring abdominal pain (simulating that of an acute surgical abdomen), varied neurologic manifestations, and psychiatric disorders. In this expression of porphyria, as in the cutanea tarda form, excessive porphyrins or their precursors are said to be concentrated in the liver rather than the bone marrow, so that there are no noteworthy skeletal changes.

SYSTEMIC DISORDERS OF MUCOPOLYSACCHARIDE METABOLISM

Mucopolysaccharides are important constituents of cartilage, subcutaneous tissue, vessel walls, and cornea, among other tissues. Chemically, they are macromolecules made up of alternating units of hexuronic (glucuronic) acid and hexosamine (glucose or galactose amine). Genetically determined disorders have

Skeletal changes in metabolic disorders

thus far been related to disturbances in the metabolism of three specific mucopolysaccharides: chrondroitin sulfate B, heparitin sulfate, and keratosulfate.

The major skeletal disease caused by a mucopolysaccharide metabolic disorder is gargoylism (Hurler's syndrome), the variants of which were discussed in Chapter 2. Morquio's disease (Morquio-Brailsford syndrome), once thought to be a separate anomaly of skeletal development, is now classed[46,47] as a varient of gargoylism (MPS IV).

Another unusual storage disease that has some resemblance to gargoylism and that perhaps belongs here also has been described in several infants at autopsy by Farber, Cohen, and Uzman[48] under the title of "Lipogranulomatosis: a new lipo-glyco-protein 'storage' disease." In this condition, as in gargoylism, the excessive abnormal storage material was found on chemical analysis to have a large polysaccharide residue (forming a complex with a polypeptide). Its anatomic distribution, however, apart from comparable central nervous system neuron involvement, was different. Specifically, in the cases cited there were widespread storage deposits within macrophages, predilecting the joints, the subcutaneous and periarticular tissues (featuring goutlike nodules, especially on the hands), the juxtaarticular bone, the larynx (hoarseness), the lymph nodes, and eventually the viscera, particularly the central nervous system and the lungs. Some ten cases of this peculiar inbred disorder of metabolism have now been reported.[49]

It seems likely that this category is still far from being completely delineated[50] and that, in time, still other comparable disorders may be recognized by astute observers. For detailed consideration of this as yet poorly defined group of inherited disorders, cited under many obscure eponyms, the reader may have recourse to the valuable review of the genetic mucopolysaccharidoses by McKusick and his associates[51] and to McKusick's subsequent astute discussion of the nosology of the mucopolysaccharidoses.[46] The latter article is part of a symposium on mucopolysaccharidoses,[47] and is recommended for general orientation in this burgeoning field of investigation.

SOME MISCELLANEOUS CONSIDERATIONS

In long-standing, terminal cachectic states, one may commonly observe gelatinous atrophy of the fat cells in the bone marrow. For example, it is often possible to suspect that a patient died of carcinomatosis from examination of a section of the bone even before one learns of the clinical history.

In some long-standing infections, especially chronic osteomyelitis and tuberculosis, *amyloid* may be deposited in the parenchymatous organs, particularly the liver, spleen, adrenal glands, and kidneys. In contrast to this conventional pattern of distribution, one may occasionally find amyloid deposited in large quantities in bones, muscles, joint capsules, and skeletal connective tissues generally, as well as in the skin and subcutis, buccal and mucous membranes, tongue, heart, lungs, intestines, genitourinary tract, and other tissues. The basis for this atypical amyloidosis may be unsuspected multiple myeloma, but sometimes there is no apparent predisposing cause (idiopathic).

Diseases of bone and joints

Influence of trace elements on the skeleton. As Asling and Hurley[52] have emphasized in their comprehensive survey of the various elements found in trace amounts in animal tissues, four elements—manganese, zinc, copper, and iodine—are clearly required for normal skeletal growth and development. A fifth, molybdenum, produces skeletal abnormalities when it is present in the diet in excess. Serious consequences to the epiphyseal cartilage plate may result from both manganese and zinc deficiencies, while copper deficiency appears to cause a defect in osseous replacement of cartilage. Moreover, in animals at least, manganese and zinc are required for normal elongation of the bones. As Asling points out further, in all of these deficiencies gross malformations of bone shape (especially in weight-bearing bones), of epiphyseal structure, or of joint relationships are reported frequently. The abnormalities may be recognized at several sites or may be more localized; this apparently varies with different species.[52-54]

The primary role of iodine is influencing activity of the thyroid gland, although it is also necessary for normal skeletal development.

Whether the abnormalities resulting from manganese, zinc, and copper deficiencies have their counterpart in humans, especially in young children, is a matter of conjecture. It is conceivable that they might in certain areas with mineral-deficient soils or under conditions of severe deprivation. However there are few, if any, relevant observations on which to base a judgment.

REFERENCES

1. Sobotka, H., Epstein, E. Z., and Lichtenstein, L.: The distribution of lipoid in a case of Niemann-Pick's disease associated with amaurotic family idiocy, Arch. Path. **10**:677, 1930.
2. Crocker, A. C., and Farber, S.: Niemann-Pick disease, Medicine **37**:1, 1958; ibid., Am. J. Clin. Nutr. **9**:63, 1961.
3. Lynn, R., and Terry, R. D.: Lipoid histochemistry and electron microscopy in adult Niemann-Pick disease, Am. J. Med. **37**:987, 1964.
4. Terry, R. D., Sperry, W. M., and Brodoff, B.: Adult lipoidosis resembling Niemann-Pick's disease, Am. J. Pathol. **30**:263, 1954.
5. Volk, B. W.: Tay-Sachs disease, New York, 1964, Grune and Stratton, Inc., pp. 36-67.
6. Volk, B. W., Adachi, M., Schneck, L., Saifer, A., and Kleinberg, W.: G_5—ganglioside variant of systemic late infantile lipoidosis, Arch. Pathol. **87**:393, 1969. (For recent literature.)
7. Brill, N. E., Mandelbaum, F. S., and Libman, E.: Primary splenomegaly, Gaucher type, Am. J. Med. Sci. **129**:491, 1905.
8. Pick, L.: Die skelettform des Morbus Gaucher, Jena, 1927, Gustav Fisher Verlag.
9. Stein, M., and Gardner, L. I.: Acute infantile Gaucher's disease, Pediatrics **27**:491, 1961.
10. Harrison, W. E., Jr., and Louis, H. J.: Osseous Gaucher's disease in early childhood, J.A.M.A. **187**:997, 1964.
11. Okada, S., and O'Brien, J. S.: Tay-Sachs disease; generalized absence of a beta-D-N-acetylhexosaminidase component, Science **165**:698, 1969.
12. Frederickson, D. S., Levy, R. I., and Lees, R. S.: Fat transport in lipoproteins—an integrated approach to mechanisms and disorders, New Eng. J. Med. **276**:34, 1967.
13. Yatsu, F. M.: Sphingolipidoses, Calif. Med. **114-4**:1, 1971.
14. Frederickson, D. S.: Cerebroside lipoidosis: Gaucher's disease. In Stanbury, J. B., Wynngarden, J. B., and Frederickson, D. S., editors: The metabolic basis of inherited disease, ed. 2, New York, 1966, McGraw-Hill Book Co., pp. 565-580.
15. Rosenberg, A., and Chargoff, E.: Reinvestigation of cerebroside deposited in Gaucher's disease, J. Biol. Chem. **233**:1323, 1958.

16. Gaucher, P. C. E.: De l'epithéliome primitif de la rate, Thèse de Paris, 1882.
17. Arkin, A. M., and Schein, A. J.: Aseptic necrosis in Gaucher's disease, J. Bone Joint Surg. **30-A**:631, 1948.
18. Tuchman, L. R., Suna, H., and Carr, J. J.: Elevation of serum acid phosphatase in Gaucher's disease, J. Mount Sinai Hosp. N. Y. **23**:227, 1956.
19. Welt, S., Rosenthal, N., and Oppenheimer, B. S.: Gaucher's splenomegaly with special reference to skeletal changes, J.A.M.A. **92**:637, 1929.
20. Knox, J. H., Wahl, H. R., and Schmeisser, H. C.: Gaucher's disease, Bull. Johns Hopkins Hosp. **27**:1, 1916.
21. Milch, H., and Pomeranz, M.: Bone changes in Gaucher's splenomegaly, Ann. Surg. **89**:552, 1929.
22. Glueck, C. J., Levy, R. I., and Frederickson, D. S.: Acute tendinitis and arthritis: a presenting symptom of familial type II hyperlipoproteinemia, J.A.M.A. **206**:2895, 1968.
23. Wessler, S., and Avioli, L. A.: Classification and management of familial hyperlipoproteinemia, J.A.M.A. **207**:929, 1969.
24. Editorial: Hyperuricemia and gout, Bull. Rheum. Dis. **18**:465, 1967.
25. Emerson, B. T.: An enzyme defect in metabolic gout, Ann. Intern. Med. **68**:707, 1968.
26. Gutman, A. B.: Some recent advances in the study of uric acid metabolism and gout: the musculoskeletal system: a symposium, presented at New York Academy of Medicine, October, 1950, New York, 1952, The Macmillan Co.
27. Editorial: Gout and hyperuricemia, Calif. Med. **110**:258, 1969.
28. Klinenberg, J. R.: Current concepts of hyperuricemia and gout, Calif. Med. **110**:231, 1969.
29. Sydenham, T.: A treatise on the gout (Tractatus de podagra et hydrope), London, 1683.
30. Medical news: Gout—no longer among the rheumatic aristocracy, J.A.M.A. **186**:40, 1963.
31. Talbott, J. H.: Gout and gouty arthritis, New York, 1953, Grune and Stratton, Inc.
32. Lichtenstein, L., Scott, H. W., and Levin, M. H.: Pathologic changes in gout: survey of eleven necropsied cases, Am. J. Path. **32**:871, 1956.
33. Medical Staff Conference, University of California, San Francisco: Hyperuricemia—pathogenesis and treatment, Calif. Med. **111**:38, 1972.
34. Thompson, G. B., Duff, I. F., Robinson, W. L., Mikkelsen, W. M., and Galindez, H.: Long term uricosuric therapy in gout, Arthritis Rheum. **5**:384, 1962.
35. Garrod, A. E.: Inborn errors of metabolism, ed. 2, London, 1923, Hodder and Stoughton Ltd., pp. 43-64.
36. Virchow, R.: Ein fall von allgemeiner Ochronose der Knorpel und Knorpelähnlichen Teile, Virch. Arch. Path. Anat. **37**:212, 1866.
37. Lichtenstein, L., and Kaplan, L.: Hereditary ochronosis: pathologic changes observed in two necropsied cases, Am. J. Pathol. **30**:99, 1954.
38. Sutro, C. J., and Anderson, M. E.: Alkaptonuric arthritis: cause for free intra-articular bodies, Surgery **22**:120, 1947.
39. La Du, B. N., Seegmiller, J. E., Laster, L., and Zannoni, V.: Alcaptonuria and ochronotic arthritis, Bull. Rheum. Dis. **8**:163, 1958.
40. O'Brien, W. M., Banfield, W. G., and Sokoloff, L.: Studies on the pathogenesis of ochronotic arthropathy, Arthritis Rheum. **4**:137, 1961.
41. Osler, W.: Ochronosis: the pigmentation of cartilages, sclerotics and skin in alkaptonuria, Lancet **1**:10, 1904.
42. Dunn, H. G.: Oxalosis: report of a case with review of the literature, Am. J. Dis. Child. **90**:58, 1955.
43. Edwards, D. L.: Idiopathic familial oxalosis, Arch. Pathol. **64**:546, 1957.
44. Schwartz, S.: Clinical aspects of porphyrin metabolism, Vet. Admin. Tech. Bull. TB10-94, December 1, 1953.
45. Seide, M. J.: Porphyria: report of nine cases diagnosed in the greater Hartford area, including a family with three affected, N. Engl. J. Med. **258**:630, 1958.
46. McKusick, V. A.: The nosology of the mucopolysaccharidoses, Am. J. Med. **47**:730, 1969. (Extensive bibliography.)
47. Symposium on mucopolysaccharidoses, Am. J. Med. **47**:661, 1969.
48. Farber, S., Cohen, J., and Uzman, L. L.: Lipogranulomatosis: a new lipo-glycoprotein "storage" disease, J. Mount Sinai Hosp., N. Y. **24**:816, 1957.
49. Moser, H. W., Prensky, A. L., Wolfe, H. J., and Rosman, N. P.: Farber's lipogranulomatosis: report of a case and demonstration of an excess of ceramide

and ganglioside, Am. J. Med. **47**:869, 1969.
50. Klenk, E.: The pathological chemistry of the developing brain. In Waelsch, H., editor: Biochemistry of the developing nervous system, New York, 1955, Academic Press, Inc., pp. 397-410.
51. McKusick, V. A., and others: The genetic mucopolysaccharidoses, Medicine **44**:445, 1965.
52. Asling, C. W., and Hurley, L. S.: The influence of trace elements on the skeleton, Clin. Orthop. **27**:213-264, 1963. (Extensive bibliography.)
53. Comar, C. L., and Bronner, F., editors: Mineral metabolism—an advanced treatise, vol. 2B, New York, 1962, Academic Press, Inc.
54. Underwood, E. J.: Trace elements in human and animal nutrition, New York, 1956, Academic Press, Inc.

chapter 7

Skeletal changes in renal disease

We are concerned here with bone disease that may follow in the wake of primary disorders of glomerular or tubular renal function, or both. This is an important field in which active investigation still continues, with a shift in emphasis to the changes following prolonged hemodialysis and also following successful renal transplants.

For convenient orientation, these skeletal changes may be logically grouped as falling into one of two major categories, as Collins[1] emphasized: those resulting from chronic renal insufficiency of long standing, and those associated with failure of tubular reabsortion (phosphaturia, renal tubular acidosis, Fanconi's syndrome). It is true that not all patients with azotemic renal failure will in time manifest discernible skeletal changes, but a significant percentage do, and estimates[2] range from 55% to 80%. In children with tubular reabsorption defects, on the other hand, the skeletal deformities may be the most obvious clinical abnormality, overshadowing the underlying renal disease itself.[3-5]

The skeletal manifestations are of widely varying nature, depending on the age of the patient and the type of renal disease that is present, as will be indicated presently. Notwithstanding, it has been customary to bracket them collectively under the heading of "renal osteodystrophy."* In azotemic renal failure (but not in renal tubular disease), the changes in bone are mediated in part by parathyroid gland hyperplasia (secondary hyperparathyroidism). In patients with renal disease in general, there also appears to be a relative deficiency of vitamin D function, reflected in reduced calcium absorption from the gut, although the role of vitamin D in precise physiologic terms has not yet been clearly elucidated. This metabolic disturbance may afford an explanation, or

---

*This designation is calculated to raise the hackles of a perceptive pathologist, but since some convenient broad term of reference is evidently needed, it will have to do until a better one meets with general acceptance. It seems to me that "renal osteopathy" might be somewhat less objectionable.

a partial explanation at least, for the fact that dwarfism and rickets develop so often in growing children with renal disease, as does osteomalacia occasionally in older patients. These generalizations are not intended to imply that the sequence of events is simple and straightforward. On the contrary, the interplay of the factors involved is complex, and there are still unanswered questions relating to the action of vitamin D, and calcium homeostasis particularly, that perplex the physiologists and endocrinologists.[2] However, after 40 years or more of investigation, the broad outlines of what may and does happen pathologically seem clear enough.

BONE DISEASE ASSOCIATED WITH CHRONIC RENAL INSUFFICIENCY *(failure of renal excretion, uremic or azotemic osteodystrophy)*

A major manifestation of chronic renal insufficiency is the resorptive changes in bone attributable to secondary hyperparathyroidism and possibly chronic acidosis.

Some 30 years ago, Rutishauser and his associates,[6] Ginzler and Jaffe,[7] and other investigators showed that in cases of protracted renal insufficiency in adults (resulting from chronic glomerulonephritis, pyelonephritis, hydronephrosis, or pyonephrosis), one can consistently find *resorptive skeletal changes.* Such patients clinically manifest azotemia, phosphate retention, depressed serum calcium level, and lowered carbon dioxide–combining power, reflecting acidosis. Although the bones may appear normal grossly at the time of autopsy, the spongy trabeculae, especially of vertebral bodies, are likely to show at least occasional resorption lacunae on their surfaces. These lacunae are usually filled with connective tissue and possibly a few osteoclasts (Fig. 7-1).

When the changes are more advanced, these resorption tracts are more prominent (Fig. 7-1, *B*), and may also involve the cortical bone around the haversian canals. At the same time, reparative new bone apposition may be evident; this is usually slight, but occasionally it may overshadow the resorptive changes so that the end result can be a closely compacted spongiosa, or "renal osteosclerosis."[7] As Collins[1] has indicated, this osteosclerosis may have a patchy distribution and affect only a few or several bones.[8] In vertebral bodies particularly, there is a tendency for the zones adjacent to the intervertebral discs to become abnormally dense, giving them a banded appearance radiographically.

In such cases, the parathyroid glands usually show slight to moderate enlargement with chief cell hyperplasia, or only microscopic hyperplasia without obvious enlargement of the glands. Ginzler and Jaffe felt, as had Rutishauser, that there was no compelling reason to invoke a factor of functional secondary hyperparathyroidism. They believed rather that the osseous changes noted could be plausibly explained on the basis of *chronic acidosis* induced by the renal insufficiency. This seems to be a moot point. As many investigators have pointed out,[9-14] there are other instances of chronic renal insufficiency in which the parathyroid glands are distinctly enlarged and in which there is convincing

Skeletal changes in renal disease

clinical, biochemical, and roentgenographic evidence of *secondary hyperparathyroidism*. In such instances, sections of the bones show extensive resorption, fibrous replacement, and conspicuous osteoclastic activity, that is, the fullblown picture of so-called osteitis fibrosa (Fig. 7-1, *B*). In fact, it should be emphasized that chronic renal insufficiency is by far the most common cause of secondary hyperparathyroidism. The latter, in turn, may cause renal damage from nephrocalcinosis (Fig. 7-1, *C*), so a good history of primary renal disease is necessary to unravel the complex picture that may eventually ensue.

In children with chronic renal failure, the underlying kidney disease may be chronic nephritis or pyelonephritis, but is more likely to be a congenital obstructive defect, polycystic kidneys, or renal hypoplasia. In addition to the manifestations of azotemia and secondary hyperparathyroidism, there may be

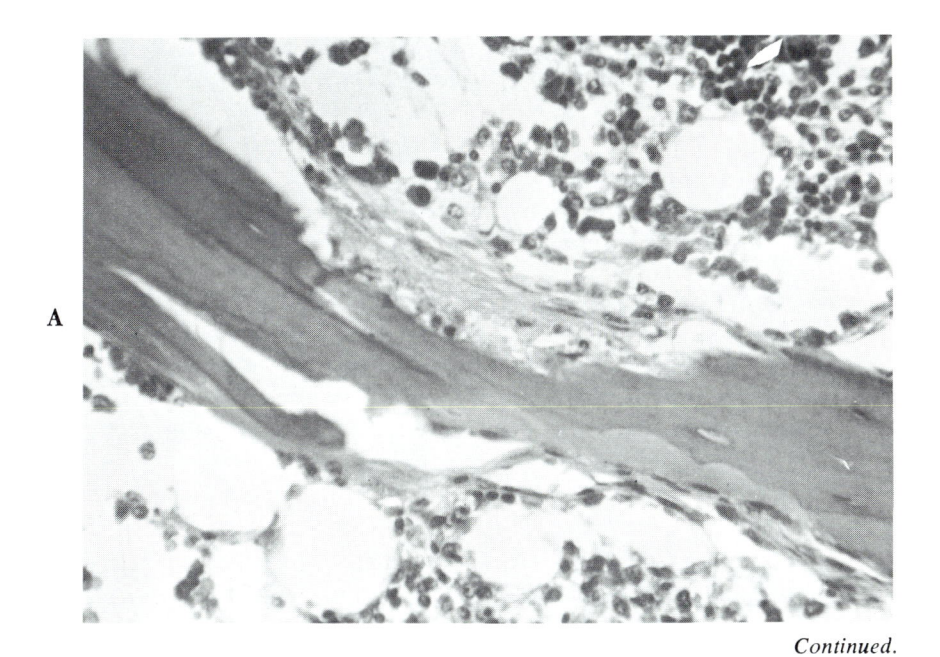

Continued.

Fig. 7-1. **A**, Photomicrograph showing skeletal resorptive changes associated with long-standing, chronic renal insufficiency. The spongy trabeculae (vertebral body) are undergoing resorption and fibrous replacement. **B**, Photomicrograph showing the changes of so-called osteitis fibrosa in an adult with secondary hyperparathyroidism, complicating long-standing renal insufficiency due to chronic pyelonephritis. In this instance, resorption of the spongy trabeculae and of associated fibrosis is much more extensive than that illustrated in **A**. The osteoclasts in proximity to trabeculae undergoing resorption are present in moderate number, but they are relatively small and inconspicuous. (×75.) **C**, Photomicrograph of a section of a kidney from the case illustrated in **B**, showing pyelonephritic scarring and (to the left) conspicuous calcium deposits from secondary hyperparathyroidism. The parathyroid glands showed chief cell hyperplasia (not illustrated). (×50.)

Diseases of bone and joints

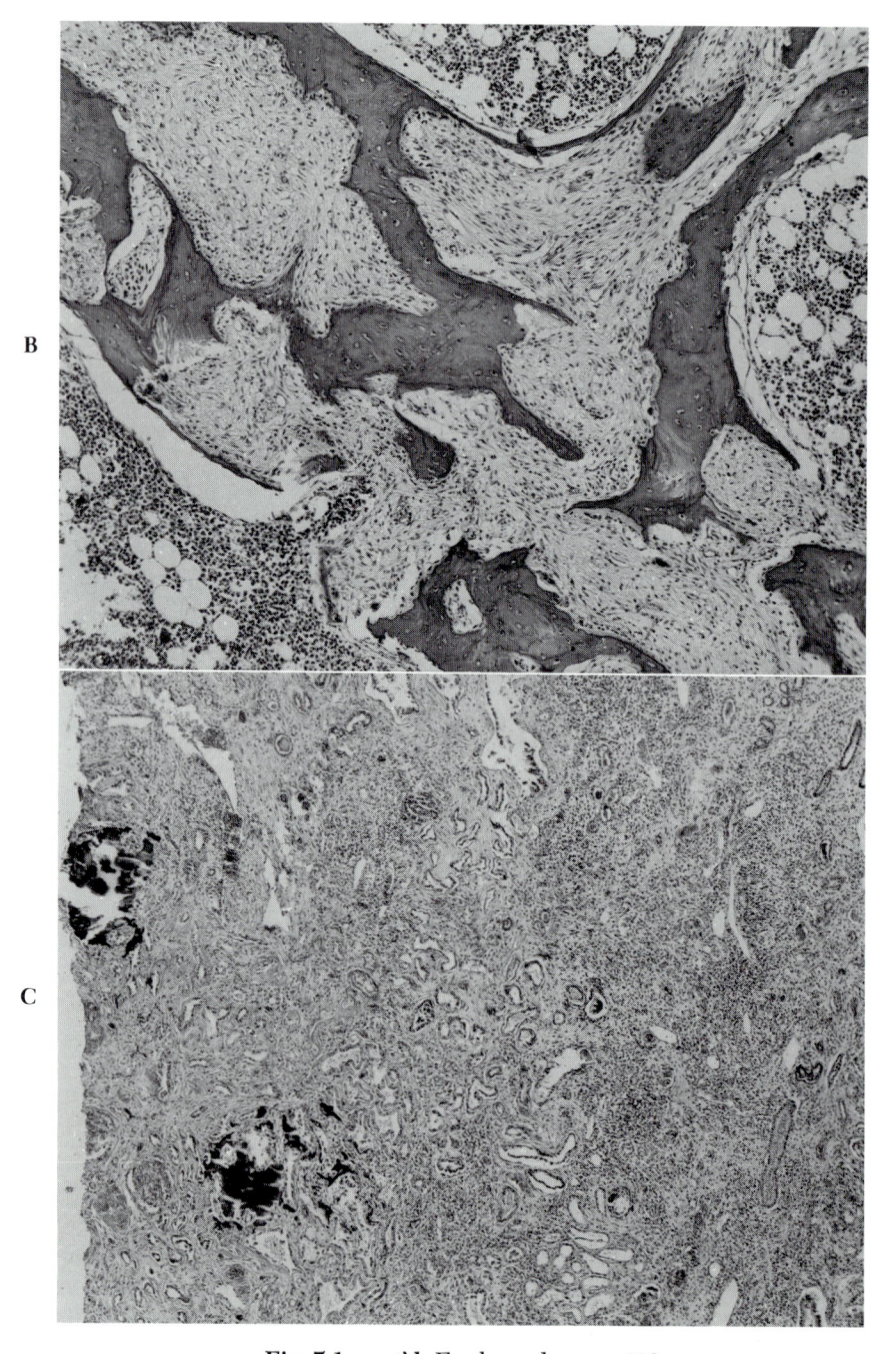

Fig. 7-1, cont'd. For legend see p. 139.

Skeletal changes in renal disease

stunted growth from arrest of endochondral ossification (renal dwarfism). Also, osseous changes clinically and pathologically resembling those of infantile vitamin D deficiency rickets may develop[15] (Fig. 7-2). In the older literature, such cases were called "renal rickets."[16] As a rule, the condition manifests itself in older children (7 to 12 years of age is the usual range). Later in the course of the disease or terminally, one may sometimes see calcific deposits in the arteries, in the soft tissues near the joints, and in the skin and subcutaneous tissue.

In comparable circumstances in older patients, one may see manifestations of osteomalacia, rather than rickets. Follis and Jackson,[17] in a study of vertebral bodies of some 39 adult subjects dying of chronic renal failure, found osteoid seams indicative of osteomalacia in more than half the cases examined.

Following prolonged hemodialysis for chronic renal failure, a striking increase in skeletal complications has been noted, despite control of the uremia. Florid renal osteodystrophy and soft tissue calcification have become important life-threatening complications of therapy by mechanical means. Acute (aseptic) periarthritic inflammation associated with soft tissue calcification has been noted during treatment with maintenance hemodialysis.[18] Mild to severe calcification is also found in the lungs, heart, stomach, and kidneys of such subjects at autopsy.[19] Pathologic fractures may be a feature in some instances. It is noteworthy that the manifestations of secondary hyperparathyroidism do not appear to be reversed by maintenance hemodialysis.

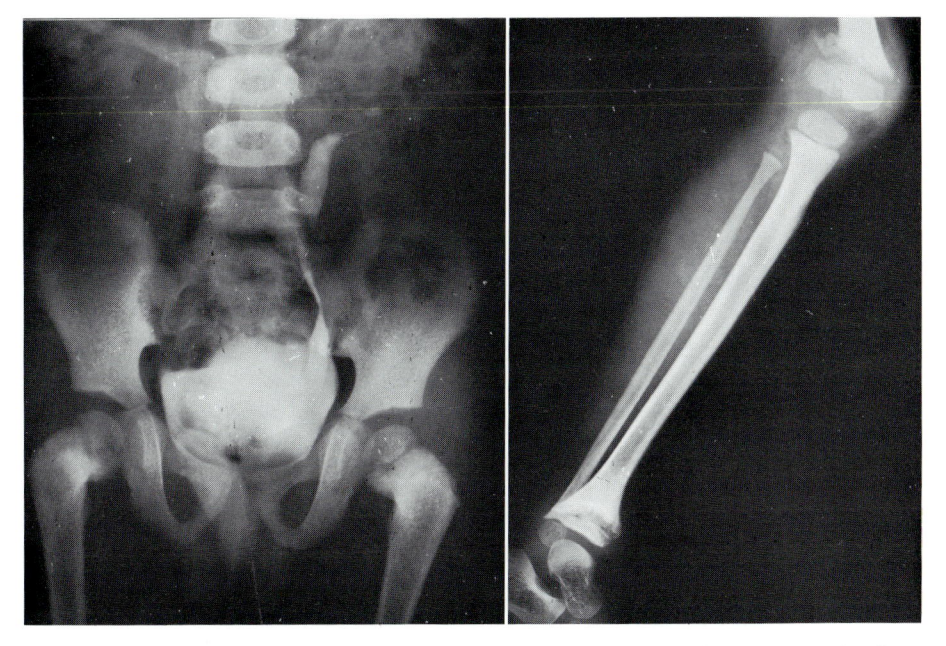

Fig. 7-2. Roentgenogram showing the changes of so-called renal rickets in the femur and lower tibia. (See also Fig. 4-6.) This child had long-standing renal insufficiency with secondary hyperparathyroidism.

Diseases of bone and joints

Successful renal homotransplantation, on the other hand, preferably from a living related donor, is usually followed by resolution of bone disease and the disappearance of metastatic calcification.[20] Hypercalcemia may persist, however, and autonomous function of chronically stimulated parathyroid glands has been suggested (tertiary or autonomous hyperparathyroidism), but this appears to be an unusual event.[20]

BONE DISEASE ASSOCIATED WITH RENAL TUBULAR REABSORPTION DEFECTS

As previously indicated (Chapter 4), when osteomalacia or late rickets develop from a renal disorder (see Fig. 4-7, C), the latter is much more likely to be in the nature of a defect of tubular reabsorption in which the kidneys leak excessive amounts of phosphate, glucose, serum protein, certain amino acids, or possibly other metabolites *(de Toni-Debré-Fanconi syndrome)*.[21] This inability of the proximal convoluted tubules to reabsorb essential components of the glomerular filtrate may result from a number of noxious chemical agents—such as copper (as in Wilson's disease) and lead—or from such conditions as myeloma and sarcoidosis. However, it more often reflects a congenital, sometimes familial, enzymatic defect. The significant persistent loss of phosphate in an affected child leads to rachitic changes requiring very large, if not massive, doses of vitamin D for effective control (so-called metabolic rickets or hypophosphatemic vitamin D–resistant rickets). In these circumstances, stunting of stature, reflecting short lower limb bones, and bowing deformities often requiring surgical correction are commonly observed.[22] The bone lesions may heal with appropriate therapy, but the serum phosphorus remains low, and relapses occur if treatment is stopped. However, one must guard against the hazard of hypervitaminosis D, manifested by hypercalcemia and nephrocalcinosis.

In some cases in point, there is *glycosuria* as well (so-called renal diabetes), but this can be readily overcome. More serious manifestations may result from concomitant *aminoaciduria,* notably cirrhosis of the liver with hepatic insufficiency, the pathogenesis of which is not clear. Certain amino acids have been implicated, particularly cystine and glycine. Specifically, it appears that in cystine storage disease,[23] tubular reabsorption may be impaired and that there may eventually be failure of renal excretory function. The cases in which cystinosis is combined with other features of aminoaciduria have been designated as showing the *Lignac-Fanconi syndrome*.[24,25] Glycine leakage in the urine has also been described[26] as an unusual cause of muscle weakness associated with osteomalacic skeletal changes (in somewhat older children or young adults). Mental retardation and glaucoma are still other unusual complications of tubule reabsorption disease that have been noted.[27]

Renal tubular acidosis, first described by Albright and his associates,[28] is another, comparatively rare expression of intrinsic tubular disease.[29] The condition is characterized by osteomalacia (histologically), nephrocalcinosis (from calciuria), potassium depletion, and the presence of acidosis.

TABLE 1. Bone changes in renal disease *(renal osteodystrophy)*

	In children	In adults
Bone disease associated with chronic renal insufficiency	Resorptive changes of secondary hyperparathyroidism (osteitis fibrosa) Stunted growth (renal dwarfism) Rickets (renal rickets) Metastatic calcification in the kidneys and arteries	Resorptive changes of secondary hyperparathyroidism (osteitis fibrosa) Osteomalacia Osteosclerosis (occasional) Metastatic calcification in the kidneys and arteries
Bone disease associated with failure of renal tubular reabsorption (renal leaks)	Persistent phosphaturia (sex-linked dominant trait) Rickets, with severe deformities (requiring very large doses of vitamin D) Renal tubular acidosis (rare) Fanconi syndrome (genetic defect in proximal convoluted tubule) Dwarfism Rickets (late) or Aminoaciduria Glycosuria Proteinuria Cystine storage in tissues (Lignac-Fanconi syndrome)	Osteomalacia Osteomalacia, with calciuria, nephrocalcinosis, potassium depletion, and acidosis Osteomalacia (requiring large doses of vitamin D)

Apparently there can be many possible factors in varying combination in this disorder, and any attempt at this time to classify them beyond a very provisional working hypothesis seems premature. Inasmuch as available clinical material for further investigation is limited, it may be quite a while before the entire picture is fully elucidated.

By way of summary, the osseous manifestations in renal disease may be tabulated as above, using the outline devised by Collins,[1] with slight modification.

REFERENCES

1. Collins, D. H.: Pathology of bone, London, 1966, Butterworth & Co. (Publishers) Ltd.
2. Rasmussen, H., The parathyroids. In Williams, R. H., editor: Textbook of endocrinology, Philadelphia, 1968, W. B. Saunders Co., pp. 949-956.
3. Dent, C. E., and Harris, H.: Hereditary forms of rickets and osteomalacia, J. Bone Joint Surg. **38-B**:204, 1956.
4. Hange, B. N.: Vitamin D resistant osteomalacia, Acta Med. Scand. **153**:271, 1956.
5. Pedersen, H. E., and McCarroll, H. R.: Vitamin-resistant rickets, J. Bone Joint Surg. **33-A**:203, 1951.
6. Rutishauser, E.: Ostéodystrophie nephrogène, Ann. Anat. Pathol. **13**:999, 1936.
7. Ginzler, A. M., and Jaffe, H. L.: Osseous findings in chronic renal insufficiency in adults, Am. J. Pathol. **17**:293, 1941.

8. Crawford, T., Dent, C. E., Lucas, P., Martin, N. H., and Nassun, J. R.: Osteosclerosis associated with chronic renal failure, Lancet **2**:981, 1954.
9. Stanbury, S. W., and Lumb, G. A.: Parathyroid function in chronic renal failure, Q. J. Med. **35**:1, 1966.
10. Albright, F., Drake,, T. G., and Sulkowitch, H. W.: Renal osteitis fibrosa cystica: review of a case with discussion of metabolic aspects, Bull. Johns Hopkins Hosp. **60**:377, 1937.
11. Carnot, P., and Lafitte, A.: Chronic nephritis, hyperparathyroidism and skeletal changes, J.A.M.A. **110**:1683, 1938.
12. Castleman, B., and Mallory, T. B.: Parathyroid hyperplasia in chronic renal insufficiency, Am. J. Pathol. **13**:553, 1937.
13. Highman, W. J. Jr., and Hamilton, B.: Hyperparathyroidism in kidney disease, J. Clin. Invest. **16**:103, 1937.
14. Pappenheimer, A. M., and Wilens, S. L.: Enlargement of the parathyroid glands in renal disease, Am. J. Pathol. **11**:73, 1935.
15. Follis, R. H.: Renal rickets and osteitis fibrosa in children and adolescents, Bull. Johns Hopkins Hosp. **87**:593, 1950.
16. Shelling, D. H., and Remsen, D.: Renal rickets: report of a case showing four enlarged parathyroids and evidence of parathyroid hypersecretion, Bull. Johns Hopkins Hosp. **57**:158, 1935.
17. Follis, R. H., and Jackson, D.: Renal osteomalacia and osteitis fibrosa in adults, Bull. Johns Hopkins Hosp. **72**:232, 1943.
18. Mirahmadi, K. S., Coburn, J. W., and Bluestone, R.: Calcific periarthritis and hemodialysis, J.A.M.A. **223**:548, 1973.
19. Hammond, W. S., Alfrey, A. C., and Huffer, W. E.: Metastatic calcification and bone disease in chronic dialysis patients: abstract, meeting of American Association of Pathologists and Bacteriologists, March 12, 1972.
20. Johnson, J. W., and others: Secondary hyperparathyroidism in chronic renal failure: effects of renal homotransplantation, J.A.M.A. **215**:478, 1971.
21. De Toni, G.: Renal rickets with phosphoglucoamino renal diabetes (de Toni-Debré-Fanconi syndrome), Ann. Pediatr. **16**:479, 1933; ibid. **187**:42, 1956.
22. Tapia, J., Stearns, G., and Ponseti, I. V.: Vitamin D resistant rickets: a long-term clinical study of 11 patients, J. Bone Joint Surg. **46-A**:935, 1964.
23. Worthin, H., and Good, R.: J. Dis. Child. **95**:653, 1958.
24. Bickel, H., and Harris, H.: The genetics of Lignac-Fanconi disease, Acta Paediatr. **42**(Suppl. 90):22, 1952.
25. Bickel, H., and Smellie, J. M.: Cystine storage disease with amino-aciduria, Lancet **1**:1093, 1952.
26. Dent, C. E., and Harris, H.: Hereditary forms of rickets and osteomalacia, J. Bone Joint Surg. **38**:204, 1956.
27. Lowe, C. U., Terry, M., and MacLachlan, E. A.: Organic-aciduria, decreased renal ammonia production, hydrophthalmas, and mental retardation; clinical entity, Am. J. Dis. Child. **83**:164, 1952.
28. Albright, R., Burnett, C. H., Parson, W., Reifenstein, E. C., and Roos, A.: Osteomalacia and late rickets, Medicine **25**:399, 1946.
29. Foss, G. L., Perry, C. B., and Wood, F. J. Y.: Renal tubular acidosis, Q. J. Med. **25**:185, 1956.

chapter 8

Osteoporosis

Osteoporosis is probably the most common of all metabolic bone disorders, as Urist[1] has emphasized, and it is discussed here in a separate chapter because of its frequency and clinical importance.

It has been traditional for pathologists[2-4] to classify osteoporosis as being of two distinct types—the primary involutional atrophy of aging individuals, and secondary osteoporosis, in which some other disorder, commonly an endocrine disturbance, plays a significant role—and, accordingly, to interpret cases in point as falling into one category or the other. It seems to me that this separation is arbitrary and that there is often too much overlapping for the distinction to be useful or valid in formulating a comprehensive concept of pathogenesis. In this discussion osteoporosis will be considered as a single disorder (or end result), often complex in its causation, concerning which there is still some uncertainty and speculation, as will be indicated presently.

In the great majority of instances, the condition develops in individuals who are over 60 years of age, although it may be observed occasionally in younger adults with special problems and rarely in children. I have seen generalized osteoporosis in a girl of 12 who did not have osteogenesis imperfecta. Incidentally, these remarkable instances of so-called juvenile osteoporosis in the 10- to 15-year age group may be distinct from the more common disorder seen in the elderly,[5] and Dent and Friedman[6] have described marked improvement in the bones by combined vitamin D and sex hormone therapy. Women 10 years or more past menopause are especially vulnerable, comprising more than 60% of all cases. An estimated 20% of men over 65 years of age also suffer from osteoporosis.[7] These estimates may actually be low, for, as Collins[2] has emphasized, vertebral osteoporosis exists undetected in many elderly individuals of both sexes who do not present themselves for clinical diagnosis.

The bones first involved are those of the axial skeleton and more particularly those of the weight-bearing vertebral column, especially the cancellous areas of the lower thoracic and lumbar vertebrae, so that pain in the lumbar spine is a common complaint. It is only when the condition is far advanced or severe,

Diseases of bone and joints

as in Cushing's syndrome, that one sees comparable changes in the long bones, pelvis, ribs, and occasionally the skull. In such severely affected patients, osteoporosis may be a significant contributing cause of the hip fractures (transcervical and intertrochanteric femoral fractures) that hospitalize so many older people for long periods and bring about their physical decline. Thus, it is one of the major causes of physical disability in old age, especially in women.[7]

In the milder grades of osteoporosis, it is essential to establish that the apparent loss of bone observed radiographically is genuine and not the reflection of various technical factors. This is easier said than done, however, and radiologists have long experienced difficulty in establishing reliable criteria for the determination of early or relatively mild osteopenia (up to 30% of bone loss). Some success in coping with this problem indirectly has been achieved recently by in vivo measurement of bone mass, through the estimation of the photon energy absorbed by bone from a monochromatic gamma ray source. The distal radius is the site selected for examination by this device, which is now commercially available (General Electric Co.), and the findings are said to reflect the loss of bone mass from the vertebral column.[8]

The pathogenesis of osteoporosis has been the subject of discussion and investigation for a long time. As MacCallum[3] stated 50 years ago in his remarkable textbook of pathology, "The processes of building up and breaking down of bone go on constantly through life, and it is apparently the result of a disproportion between these, that the constructive processes are in old age overshadowed by the otherwise normal destructive processes. The result is the senile osteoporosis which attenuates the bony structures until the bone becomes very much rarefied and easily broken." Rasmussen[5] has aptly expressed the same concept in modern parlance by defining osteoporosis as primarily a disorder of skeletal homeostasis. Incidentally, MacCallum was aware, as was Erdheim, the great Viennese pathologist, of the role that certain endocrine glands play in the regulation of bone formation and resorption, but the information available to him was still vague and indefinable in any precise physiologic and biochemical terms.

The premise generally accepted at present is that osteopenia in most instances results basically from decreased bone formation, associated with diminution in the production of anabolic sex hormones, especially estrogen. The imbalance, or bone deficit, may be achieved more dramatically by excessive bone resorption resulting from hyperfunction of the catabolic thyroid and adrenal hormones or from the therapeutic administration of a whole range of adrenal corticoids, for whatever reason.[9-11] It is noteworthy that osteoporosis has also been noted in young diabetic patients with hypoinsulinism, as well as in rats with alloxan-induced diabetes.[12,13] Osteoporosis is known to occur in some patients with primary hyperparathyroidism.[5] It is noteworthy also that an appreciable number of individuals maintained on heparin anticoagulation therapy, and given daily doses exceeding 20,000 units, develop osteoporosis. The mechanism here appears to be one of increased lysis of collagen in the ground substance of involved

Osteoporosis

bones.[5] Another factor that has been invoked in some instances is that of a long-term deficit in dietary calcium, which may be aggravated by hypercalciuria or by malabsorption of calcium and vitamin D from the gut. According to Rasmussen,[5] osteoporosis, with or without associated osteomalacia, is a common accompaniment of malabsorption syndromes. Finally, and this is a well-known clinical observation, a certain amount of physical activity is essential for normal osteoblastic function and calcium balance; immobilization of a part, or of the entire body, may lead rather quickly to thinning of the bones (disuse atrophy) Fig. 8-1. Interestingly, this was a problem in relatively inactive, weightless astronauts, as Berry has shown, so that on later flights a special program of exercises for them was devised. We are not concerned here with the (osteoporotic) atrophy of bone that is associated with severe arterial insufficiency or occlusive vascular disease, notably in the lower extremity.

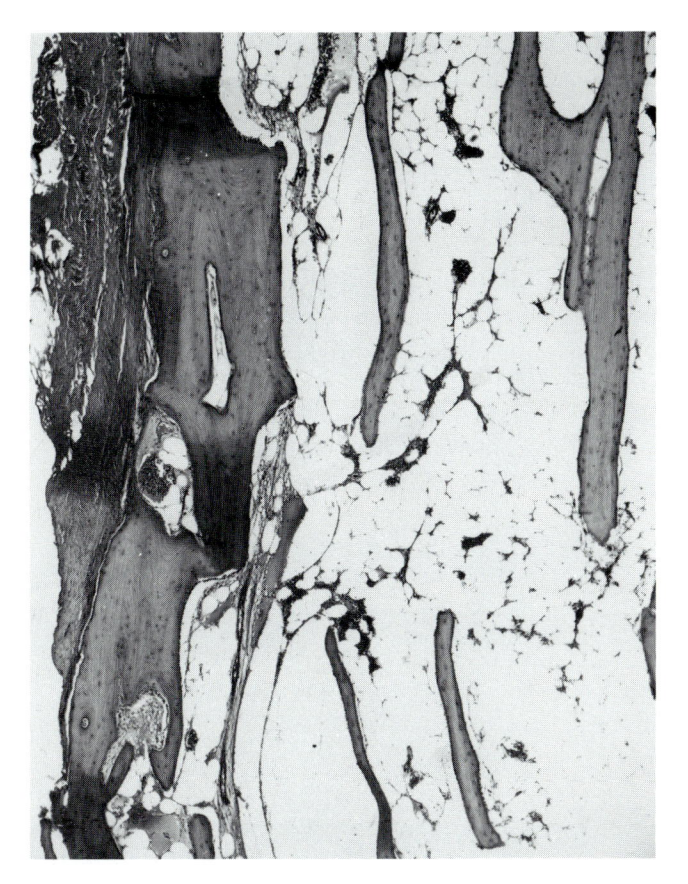

Fig. 8-1. Photomicrograph of a section through a femoral stump showing extreme osteoporosis. The attenuated cortical bone (on the left) is undergoing vascular resorption and cancellization. The longitudinal spongy trabeculae are thin and sparse. The transverse trabeculae appear to have dropped out. (×30.)

Diseases of bone and joints

Substantive proof and further insight into the rather complex mechanism of osteoporosis has been gained through the use of (strontium) tracer techniques.[10,14] It has been demonstrated that there are two basic mechanisms in osteoporosis. One is associated with decreased bone formation, as seen in postmenopausal women, in whom the mineral pool is small, as is the turnover of bone-seeking mineral. The other, associated with Cushing's disease as a prime example, shows the same phenomenon more intensively, together with increased urinary excretion of bone-seeking mineral not compensated for over a period of time.

In keeping with these physiologic and pathologic observations, it may be stated by way of summary that the most common causes of osteoporosis clinically fall into three major categories: disuse atrophy from immobilization; diminution or loss of anabolic (or anticatabolic) sex hormones, especially in women 10 years or more past spontaneous menopause, but also in eunuchoid states, senility, and gonadal dysgenesis (Turner's syndrome); and excess of catabolic hormones, specifically in thyrotoxicosis[15] or in Cushing's syndrome,[16] occurring either spontaneously (unusual) or after the therapeutic administration of large doses of cortisone or other corticoids. As Gordan[9] has emphasized, all

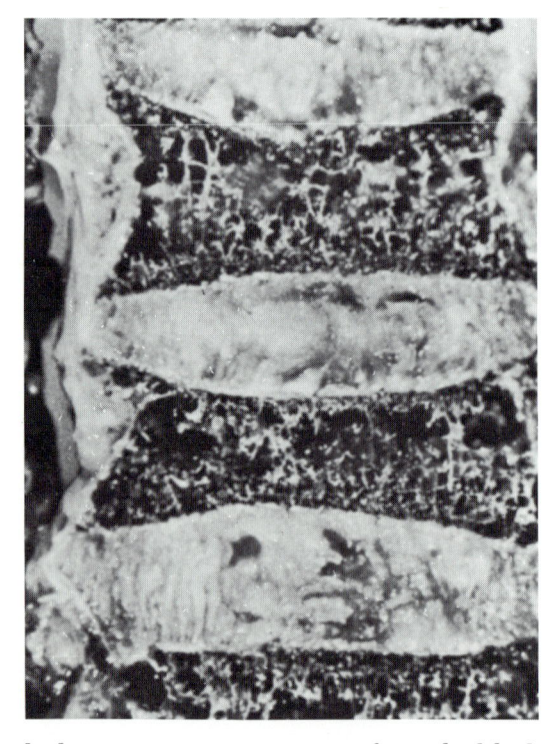

Fig. 8-2. Photograph showing severe osteoporosis of vertebral bodies developing after the therapeutic administration of large doses of steroids. Note open-meshed, porous spongy bone, compression of vertebral bodies, and corresponding expansion of the intervertebral discs.

Osteoporosis

the available corticoids rapidly produce calcium wasting and can cause clinical osteoporosis (Fig. 8-2). At autopsy, in subjects who had spontaneous Cushing's disease the bones generally have become so soft and thin that one is able to cut them with a knife, without any decalcification.

Apart from these three major categories there are a number of other relatively infrequent or unusual causes of osteoporosis that warrant brief consideration for the sake of completeness. Osteoporosis may be associated with malnutrition of long standing, perhaps because of insufficiency or abnormality of protein bone matrix, although hunger osteopathy usually takes the form of osteomalacia (p. 95). Osteoporosis has been observed after *gastrectomy*, presumably as a special malabsorption problem, and I have seen the osteoporotic bone sections (Fig. 8-3) of a young man in his thirties in whom the only ostensible cause was a gastrectomy several years previous. It occasionally is a

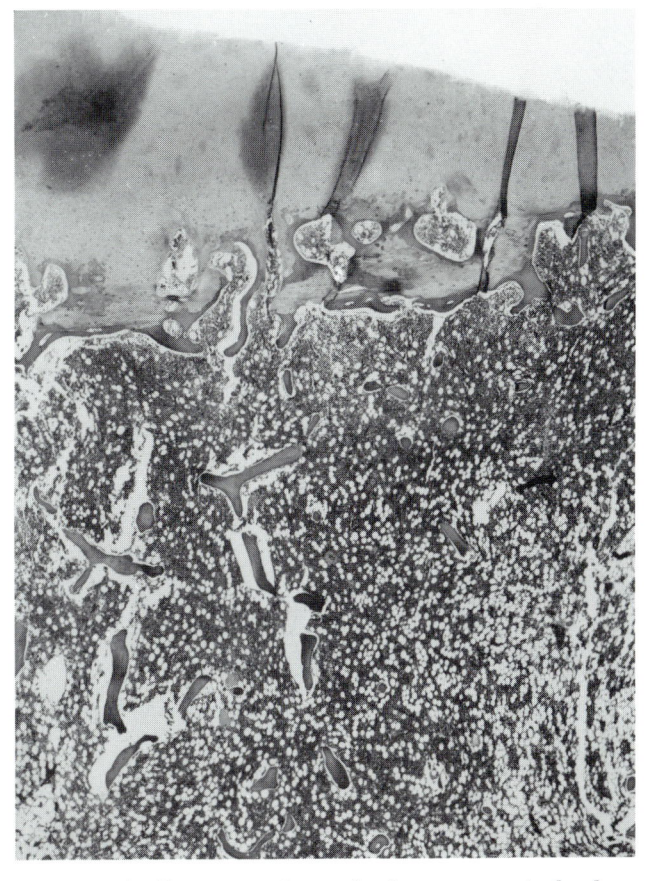

Fig. 8-3. Photomicrograph (low magnification) of an osteoarticular bone end showing advanced osteoporosis. Note the sparse, small, thin trabeculae of spongy bone in an area where the bone structure is normally sturdy. The patient was a young adult in his thirties who had had a gastrectomy some years previously. At autopsy, no other possible cause of osteoporosis was found. (×20.)

Diseases of bone and joints

manifestation of *acromegaly*, perhaps as a calcium-wasting side effect of persistently high levels of growth hormone.[9] The precise cause of osteoporosis in *biliary cirrhosis*[17] is still a subject of speculation, but again this may be a malabsorption problem. When it occurs in *scurvy*, it could conceivably be a sequel of immobilization resulting from weakness and painful hemorrhages in bones and joints, although lack of adequate collagen bone matrix has also been inculpated. The development of osteoporosis in the third trimester of pregnancy[18] could conceivably result from increased production of corticoids at that time.

Whatever the complexities of pathogenesis may be in any given instance, the pathologic alterations appear to be much the same in all of them, varying only in the severity and extent of involvement, the stage of evolution, and the presence (or absence) of such complications as fractures.[19] In the vertebral

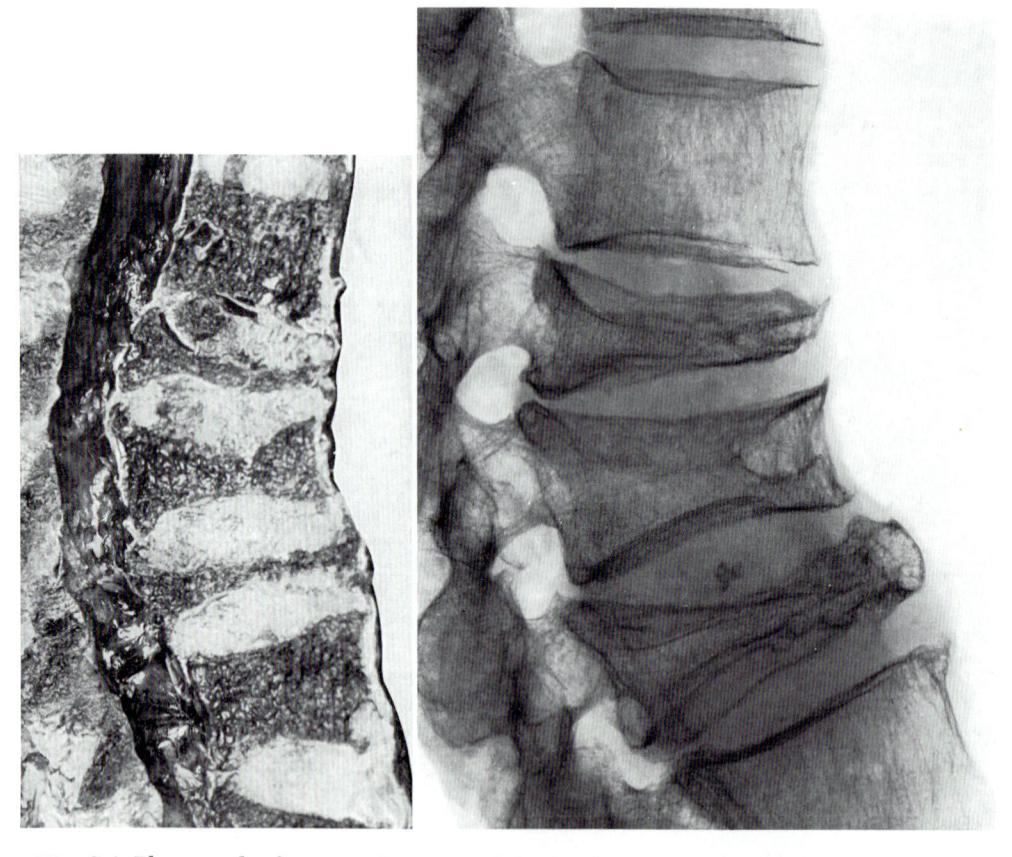

Fig. 8-4. Photograph of a sagittal section of the lumbar vertebral column of a 77-year-old woman showing the changes of marked osteoporosis. Note compression of three contiguous vertebral bodies, expansion and degeneration of their intervertebral discs, and mild kyphosis. *Right*, Roentgenogram of the specimen on the left. There is a small focus of calcification in one of the IV discs. (From Schmorl, G., and Junghanns, H.: Die Gesunde und die Kranke Wirbelsäule in Rontgenbild und Klinik, ed. 4, Stuttgart, 1972, Georg Thieme Verlag.)

Osteoporosis

column particularly, kyphotic deformity, shortening of stature, and so forth, are sequelae of thinned and weakened bone structure (Figs. 8-4 and 8-5). One seldom has the opportunity, at least in American hospital practice, to examine the entire skeleton of osteoporotic patients, as was once done in the old German institutes of pathology. However, for convenient orientation, the reader may have recourse to the excellent photographs of the gross anatomic changes in the spine (the major site of involvement) and corresponding roentgenograms of these specimens, contained in the monograph by Schmorl and Junghanns[20] on disorders of the vertebral column. Also, a detailed, well-illustrated account of the gross and microscopic pathologic alterations in these and other ostoporotic bones, including the tubular bones, may be found in the presentation of Jaffe,[4] who had access to the valuable pathologic collection of Erdheim.

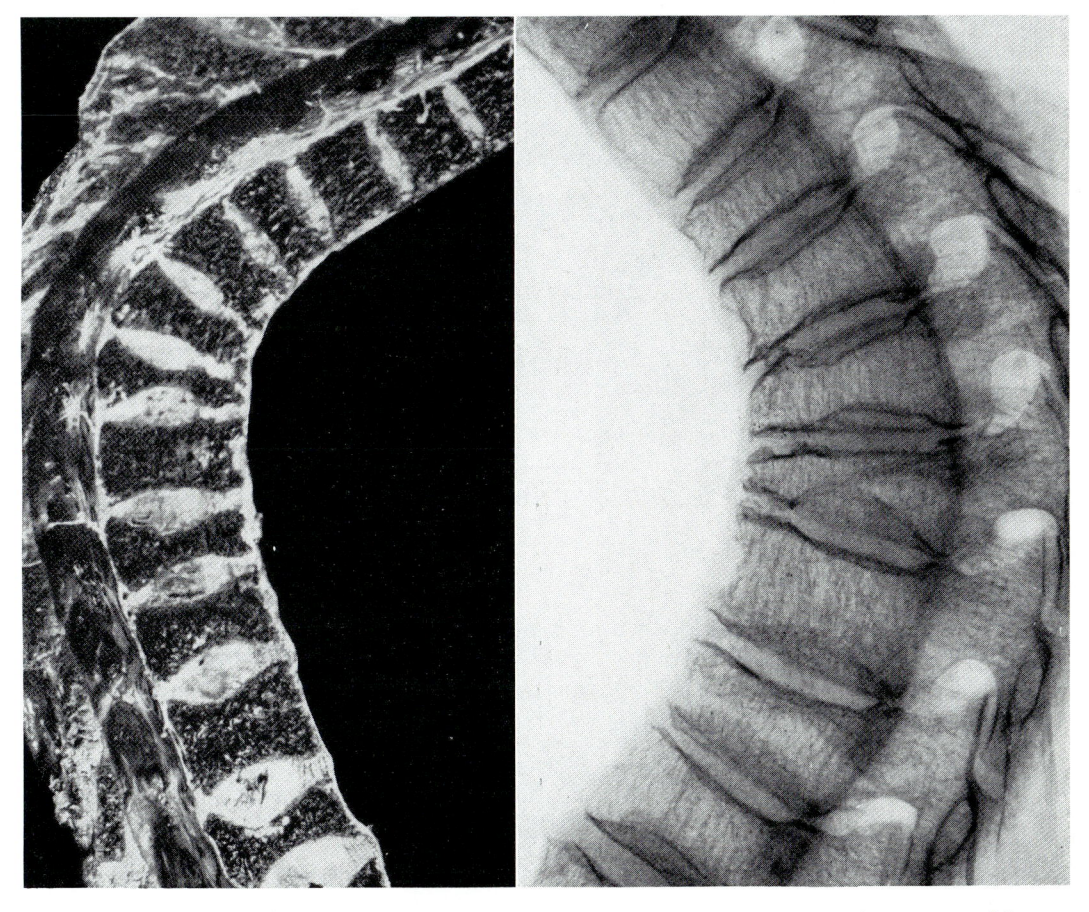

Fig. 8-5. Sagittal section of the osteoporotic thoracic vertebral column of a 63-year-old woman showing kyphosis associated with compression of the bodies of D-6 and D-7. Note also the biconcave expansion of the lower thoracic and upper lumbar discs. *Right*, Roentgenogram of the midportion of the specimen illustrated on the left. (From Schmorl, G., and Junghanns, H.: Die Gesunde und die Kranke Wirbelsäule in Rontgenbild und Klinik, ed. 4, Stuttgart, 1972, Georg Thieme Verlag.)

Diseases of bone and joints

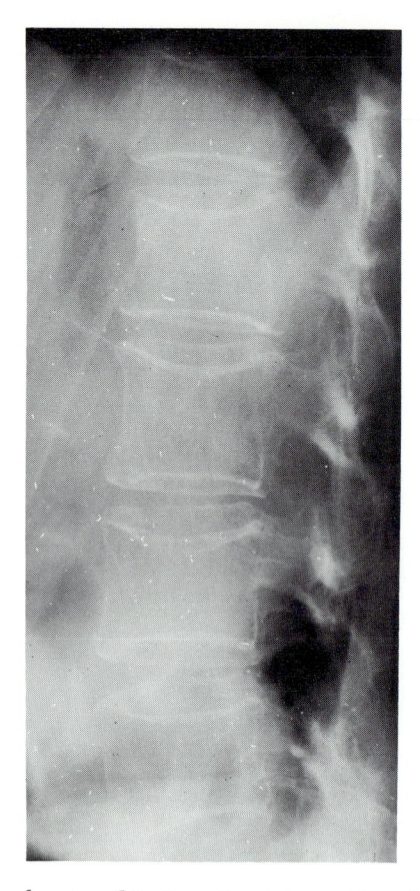

Fig. 8-6. Roentgenogram showing thinning of vertebrae (dorsal and lumbar) and expansion of intervertebral discs. Osteoporosis developed spontaneously for no apparent cause. The washed-out appearance of the spine reflects significant loss of spongy bone substance.

In vertebral bodies, in keeping with their more or less washed-out roentgenographic appearance (Fig. 8-6), one finds that the spongy trabeculae have become thinner and sparser and that many of the transverse trabeculae, especially, have disappeared. The resulting abnormally open texture of the cancellous bone can be brought out, par excellence, in macerated preparations (Fig. 8-7). Some of the bodies may be narrowed in their longitudinal direction or wedged from old or recent compression fractures, especially in the thoracic region. Concomitantly, there is biconcave expansion of the intervertebral discs, producing a picture reminiscent of fish vertebrae (Fig. 8-8). Also, as noted, the narrowing of thoracic vertebrae accentuates the normal curvature of the spine at this level and may produce more or less pronounced kyphotic deformity (Fig. 8-5).

In other bones, such as the ribs and tubular bones, one may likewise observe loss of spongy trabeculae, at least in more severe instances. Thinning of cortical bone is seen as a relatively late alteration in such cases, starting on

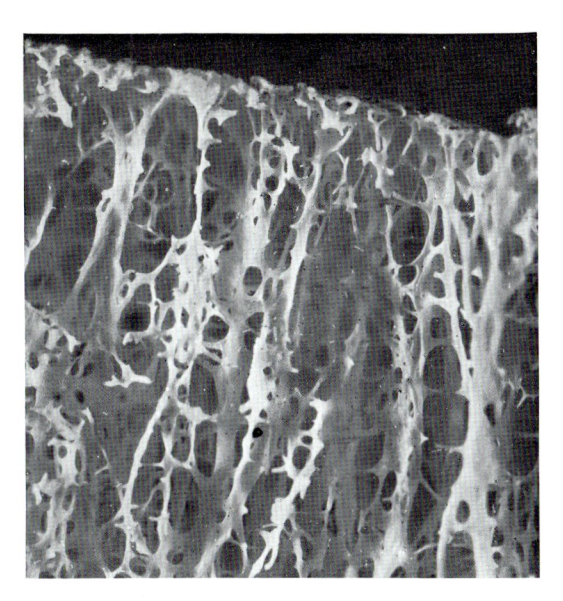

Fig. 8-7. Macerated preparation (somewhat enlarged) of a portion of a vertebral body of an elderly woman with osteoporosis. The cancellous bone plates are reduced in number and thickness, and the spaces between them are correspondingly enlarged. (From Schmorl, G., and Junghanns, H.: Die Gesunde und die Kranke Wirbelsäule in Rontgenbild und Klinik, ed. 4, Stuttgart, 1972, Georg Thieme Verlag.)

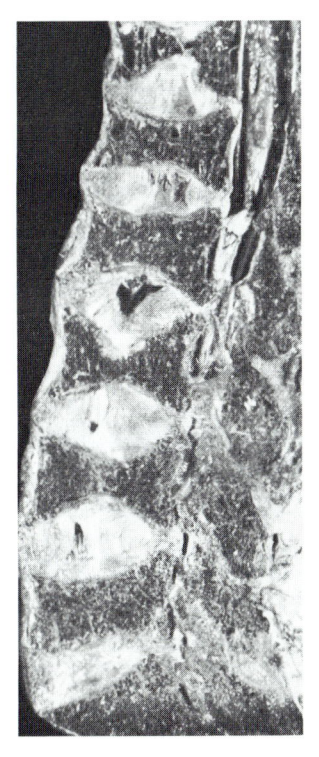

Fig. 8-8. Photograph of sagittal section of lower dorsal and lumbar vertebral column of a woman past 70 showing the changes of advanced osteoporosis. Compression of vertebral bodies and biconcave expansion of the intervertebral discs are conspicuous features.

the medullary face and proceeding outward. Here, the haversian canals enlarge as the cortex becomes porotic and perceptibly thinned and, as Collins[2] expressed it, the compact cortical bone undergoes cancellous transformation.

Much information of value in differential diagnosis can be elicited from needle-core bone biopsy specimens taken from the iliac crest[21] or a lumbar vertebral body of a patient thought to have osteoporosis. One finds, as previously noted, that the cortex is relatively thin (as compared with that of normal controls) and that the spongy bone trabeculae are relatively thin and sparse (Fig. 8-1). The osteoblasts on their surface are quiescent and inconspicuous. This loss of bone substance is not the result of vascular or osteoclastic resorption, such as one finds in hyperparathyroidism or Paget's disease, nor is there any fibrosis of the marrow. Also, there are no osteoid borders or seams on the surface of the spongy trabeculae, as one sees in osteomalacia. Bone biopsy also helps to rule out the presence of (osteolytic) malignant tumors, especially myeloma and metastatic carcinoma. Apart from their quantitative diminution, the spongy trabeculae do not appear abnormal in any way, at least as viewed by light microscopy. If there is any significant alteration in the collagen or mucopolysaccharide components of the ground substance or matrix, as has been suggested,[22] this is not evident in sections stained with hematoxylin and eosin, nor is it demonstrable by the special stains currently employed.

Reflecting these findings, the serum calcium and phosphorus levels are ordinarly within the normal range, and since there is no appreciable stimulus to new bone formation, serum alkaline phosphatase activity is likewise unaltered unless there has been a recent fracture.

In the matter of clinical management, one must stress the necessity for reliable diagnosis by exclusion of other causes of rarefying bone disease, especially in the vertebral column, as well as recognition of the specific causes of osteoporosis in any given patient and its correction whenever possible. Thus, adrenal cortical tumors can be removed, and thyrotoxicosis, immobilization, or malnutrition can be corrected. As Gordan and his associates[9,10] have emphasized, the most important single cause that can be treated effectively is hormonal deficiency in the postmenopausal or hypogonadal patient. For this they have used cyclically administered estrogens for their anabolic (or anticatabolic) effect, without inducing carcinoma in a single instance. Estrogen therapy provides positive calcium balance and halts further bone resorption, so that the tendency to fractures and loss of height is brought under control. It has its limitations, however, and does not induce restoration of bone that has already been lost.

Some have advocated supplemental calcium and vitamin D, in addition to sex hormone therapy; but if this is done, the amounts administered must be carefully controlled to avoid hypercalcemia, hypercalciuria, and nephrolithiasis. Phosphate supplements and the adjunct use of sodium fluoride have also been tried, but experience with them is still too limited to advocate their general use. As Rasmussen[5] has suggested, another therapeutic possibility is the long-term use of thyrocalcitonin, but it is not yet generally available for clinical investigation.

REFERENCES

1. Urist, M.: Observations bearing on the problem of osteoporosis. In Rodahl, K., Nicholson, J., and Brown, M. Jr., editors: Bone as a tissue, New York, 1960, McGraw-Hill Book Co., p. 18.
2. Collins, D. H.: Pathology of bone, London, 1966, Butterworth & Co. (Publishers) Ltd.
3. MacCallum, W. G.: A textbook of pathology, ed. 3, Philadelphia, 1924, W. B. Saunders Co.
4. Jaffe, H. L.: Metabolic, degenerative and inflammatory diseases of bones and joints, Philadelphia, 1972, Lea & Febiger, Chapter 14.
5. Rasmussen, H., The parathyroids. In Williams, R. H., editor: Textbook of endocrinology, ed. 4, Philadelphia, 1968, W. B. Saunders Co., p. 957.
6. Dent, C. E., and Friedman, M.: Idiopathic juvenile osteoporosis, Q. J. Med. 34:177, 1965.
7. Facts about osteoporosis, Bethesda, Md., 1970, National Institute of Arthritis and Metabolic Diseases.
8. Smith, D. M., Johnston, C., Jr., and Yu, P-L.: In vivo measurement of bone mass: its use in demineralized states such as osteoporosis, J.A.M.A. 219:325, 1972.
9. Gordan, G. S.: Osteoporosis: diagnosis and treatment, Tex. Med. 57:740, 1961.
10. Gordan, G. S., and Eisenberg, E.: The effects of estrogens, androgens and corticoids on skeletal kinetics in man, Proc. R. Soc. Med. 56:1027, 1963.
11. Soloman, G. F., Dickerson, W. J., and Eisenberg, E.: Psychologic and osteometabolic responses to sex hormones in elderly osteoporotic women, Geriatrics 15:46, 1960.
12. Hernberg, C. A.: Skelettveränderungen bei Diabetes mellitus der Erwachsenen Acta. Med. Scand. 143:1, 1952. The bone structure in alloxan-induced diabetes mellitus in rats, ibid. 142:274, 1952.
13. Boulet, P., and Mirouze, J.: Les ostéoses diabetiques (osteoporose et hyperostose), Ann. Med. 55:674, 1954.
14. Eisenberg, E., and Gordan, G. S.: Skeletal dynamics in man measured by nonradioactive strontium, J. Clin. Invest. 40:1809, 1961.
15. Williams, R. H., and Morgan, H. J.: Thyrotoxic osteoporosis, Int. Clin. 2:48, 1940.
16. Howland, W. J., Pugh, D. G., Jr., and Sprague, R. G.: Roentgenologic changes of the skeletal system in Cushing's syndrome, Radiology 71:69, 1958.
17. Atkinson, M., Nordin, B. E. C., and Sherlock, S.: Malabsorption and bone disease in prolonged obstructive jaundice, Q. J. Med. 25:299, 1956.
18. Nordin, B. E. C., and Roper, A.: Postpregnancy osteoporosis: a syndrome? Lancet 1:431, 1955.
19. Gershon-Cohen, J., Bechtman, A. M., Schraer, H., and Blumberg, N.: Asymptomatic fractures in osteoporotic spines of the aged, J.A.M.A. 153:625, 1953.
20. Schmorl, G., and Junghanns, H.: Die Gesunde u die kranke Wirbelsäule in Roentgenbild und Klinik, ed. 4, Stuttgart, 1957, Georg Thieme Verlag, p. 71.
21. Beck, J. W., and Nordin, B. E. C.: Histological assessment of osteoporosis by iliac crest biopsy, J. Pathol. 80:391, 1960.
22. Kelley, M., Little, K., and Courts, A.: Bone matrix and osteoporosis, Lancet 1:1125, 1959.

GENERAL REFERENCES

Casuccio, C.: An introduction to the study of osteoporosis: biochemical and biophysical research in bone aging, Proc. R. Soc. Med. 55:663, 1962.

Sissons, H. A.: The structural pathology of osteoporosis, Proc. R. Soc. Med. 48:566, 1955.

chapter 9

Skeletal changes in neurotrophic disorders

The major neurotrophic disorders associated with spinal cord disease are Charcot neuroarthropathy from tabes dorsalis, which mainly affects the joints of the lower extremity and the spine, and comparable changes in the upper extremity from syringomyelia. The concept of joint destruction as a neurotrophic manifestation dates back fully a century to the observations of the brilliant French neurologist, Charcot.[1]

There are many other conditions, however, that should be cited here. On occasion, destructive neurotrophic changes in the foot may be observed in neglected or poorly controlled diabetes mellitus of long standing (Fig. 9-1). Comparable involvement of other joint regions has been described, but it is distinctly unusual.[2] This subject has received considerable attention in recent years, and an awareness of it is important because the process can often be halted or even substantially improved by adequate diabetic treatment and corrective orthopedic measures.[3-5] Also noteworthy is the observation that spinal cord damage associated with spina bifida or severe multiple sclerosis, or resulting from cord injury with irreparable paraplegia,[6] may predispose to parosteal ossification, particularly in the vicinity of the hip and knee joints (Fig. 9-2).

Neuroarthropathy has also been said to be a sequel of injury to peripheral nerves (from trauma or tumor compression); for example, neuroarthropathy of an ankle joint may result from severance of the sciatic nerve,[7] although this is distinctly unusual. The classical example of extensive neurotrophic changes resulting from peripheral nerve disease is the neural form of leprosy in which there may be loss of digits and other mutilating deformities of the hands or feet, especially in patients whose disease is not controlled by sulfone therapy (Fig. 9-3). For a comprehensive list of still other unusual or rare causes of neuropathies of bones and joints (and the responsible disease foci may be in the brain, spinal cord, or peripheral nerves), the reader may have recourse to the old article of Shands,[8] which is still useful for orientation (Fig. 9-4).

By far the most common cause of neuroarthropathy is *tabes dorsalis*[9] (old-

Skeletal changes in neurotrophic disorders

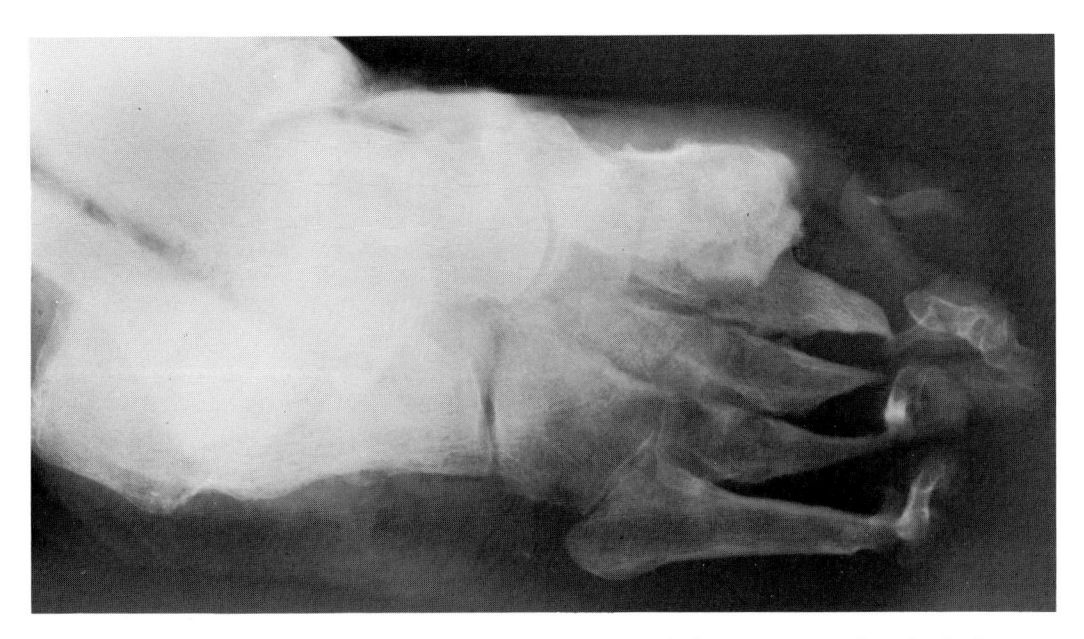

Fig. 9-1. Roentgenogram of a neurotrophic foot in a diabetic patient who also had a long-standing refractory trophic ulcer (not evident in this picture). Note the atrophy and partial disappearance of the phalanges and metatarsal bones.

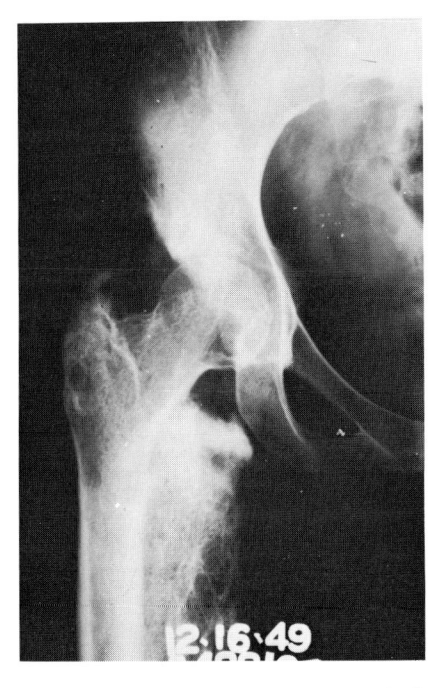

Fig. 9-2. Metaplastic ossification contiguous to the upper shaft of a femur in a patient with multiple sclerosis with extensive severe spinal cord damage. (Comparable lesions are observed more often in paraplegic patients.)

Diseases of bone and joints

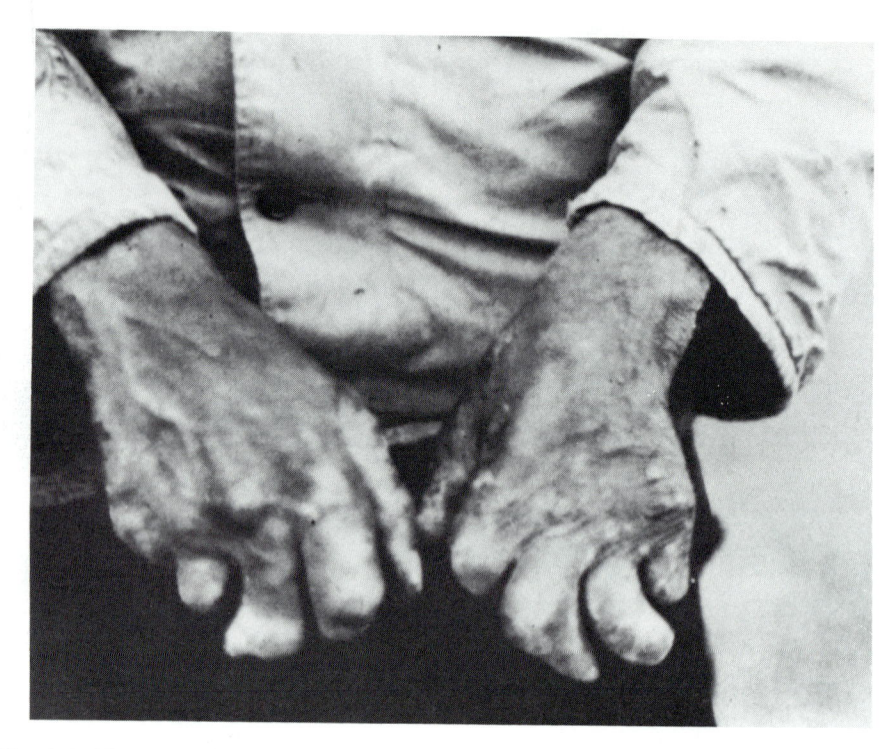

Fig. 9-3. Photograph showing mutilating changes in the hands in the neural form of leprosy (see also p. 67).

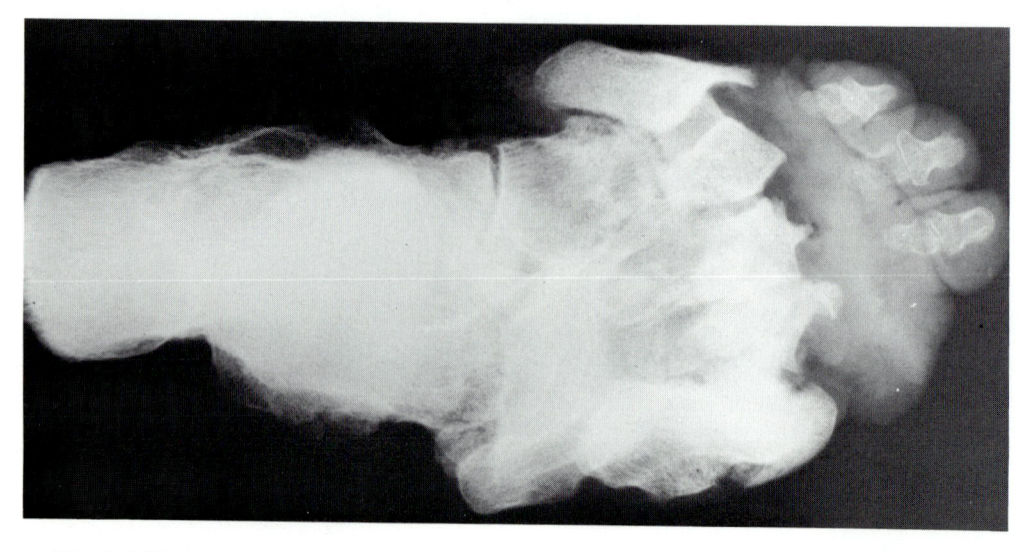

Fig. 9-4. Roentgenogram of an amputated foot showing advanced neurotrophic changes caused by a spinal cord defect (possibly congenital, although not spina bifida). The metatarsal bones have disappeared, and there is atrophy of the remaining phalanges.

Skeletal changes in neurotrophic disorders

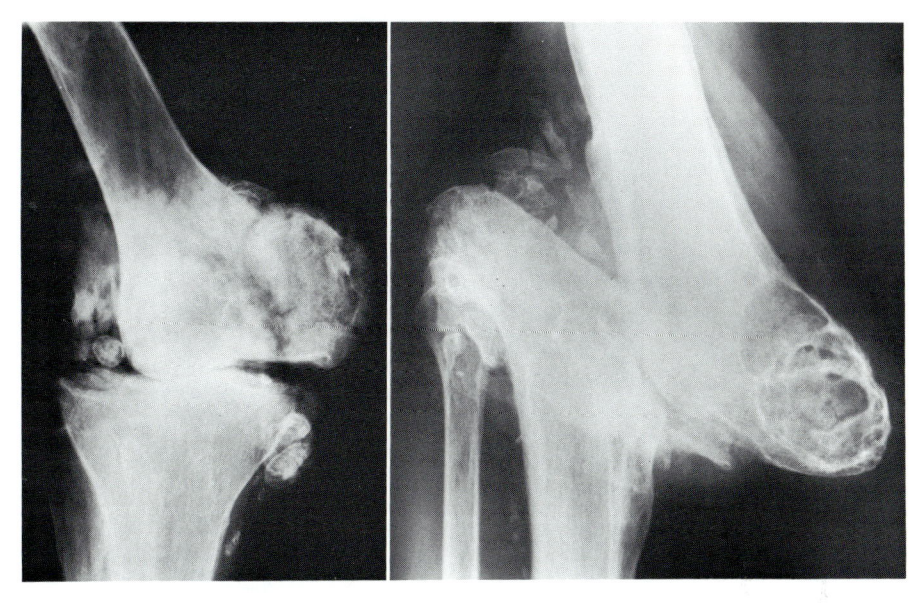

Fig. 9-5. Roentgenograms showing two Charcot knee joints in an advanced stage. In both instances, there was an old history of untreated syphilis.

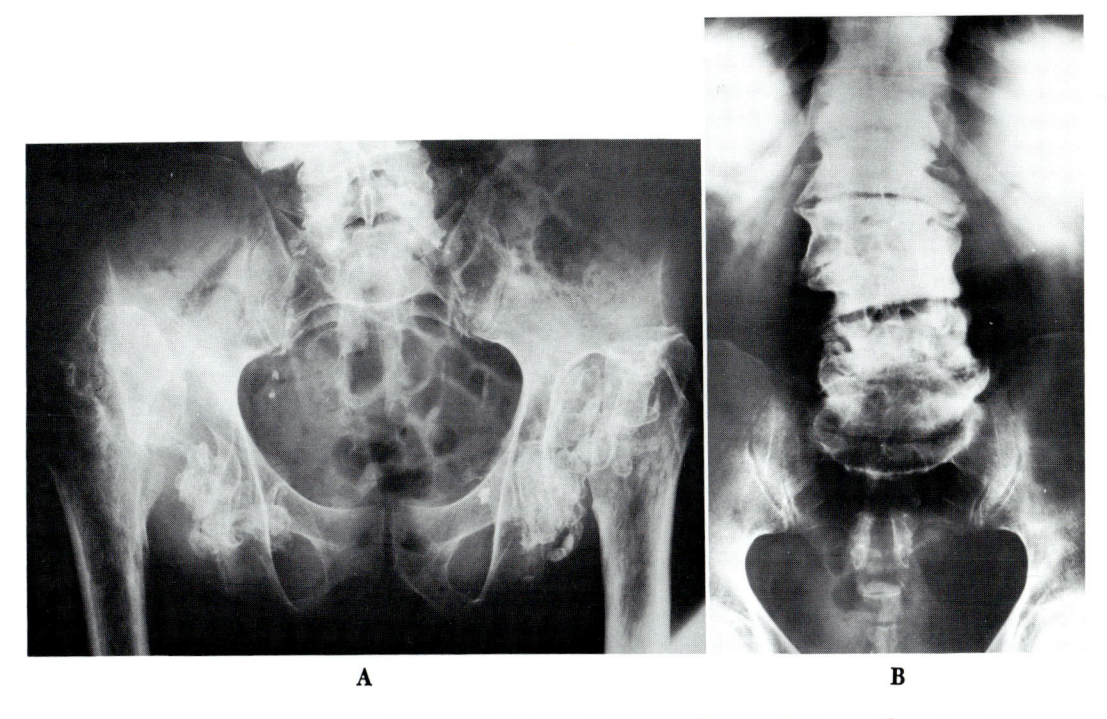

A B

Fig. 9-6. Roentgenograms showing, **A,** bilateral Charcot hips and also a Charcot spine (lumbar), and **B,** another Charcot spine.

Diseases of bone and joints

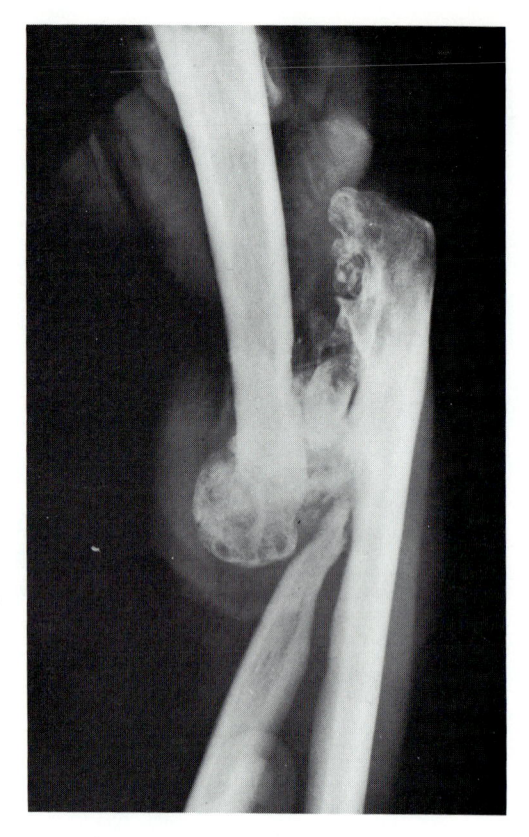

Fig. 9-7. Roentgenogram of an unusual Charcot elbow joint in a man of 58 with tabes dorsalis. At autopsy, evidence of cardiovascular syphilis was also found.

fashioned locomotor ataxia), an expression of untreated or inadequately treated syphilis that has resulted in sclerosis of the posterior or dorsal columns of the spinal cord. The knee joint is commonly involved in this condition (Fig. 9-5), although the hip joints and the vertebral column may also be affected (Fig. 9-6). Only occasionally does one observe comparable involvement of a joint in the upper extremity, such as an elbow (Fig. 9-7). While Charcot joints are usually painless, there are enough exceptions to this rule so that the diagnosis cannot be dismissed because of the presence of pain.

Painless, spontaneous fractures through the shafts of bones, rather than their articular ends, have also been described and designated as "neuropathic," but we are not particularly concerned with them here.

There has been much speculation in the past about the pathogenesis of the striking destructive changes in a Charcot joint. In my opinion, what apparently happens is that, with loss of proprioceptive muscle sense resulting from dorsal column disease, there is malalignment of the bone ends of the affected joint in the course of articular function. The repeated trauma, in time, results in multiple osteoarticular fractures with breaking off of numerous fragments, some of

Skeletal changes in neurotrophic disorders

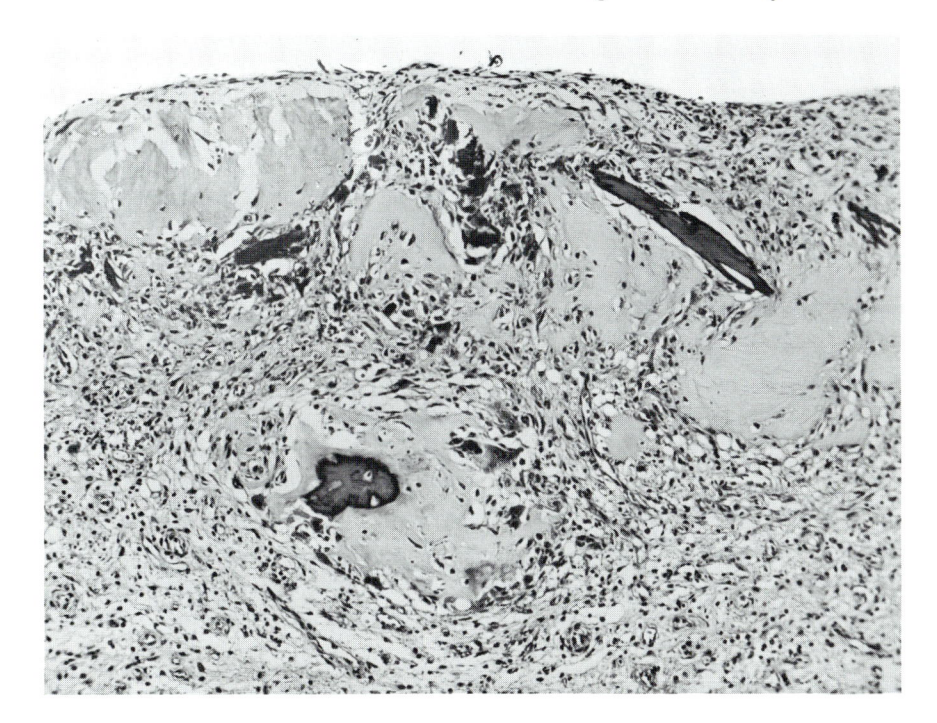

Fig. 9-8. Photomicrograph (at low magnification) showing the characteristic changes in the synovial lining of a Charcot knee. Note the numerous fragments of articular cartilage and bone detritus ground into the membrane, which is thickened and chronically inflamed. Only in a neuropathic joint does one observe so much cartilage and bone debris in the synovial membrane.[10] From a picture such as this, one would have good reason to suspect that the patient had tabes.

Fig. 9-9. A, Roentgenogram showing neuroarthropathy of a shoulder joint in a patient with syringomyelia. **B,** Neuroarthropathy at the wrist of another patient with syringomyelia.

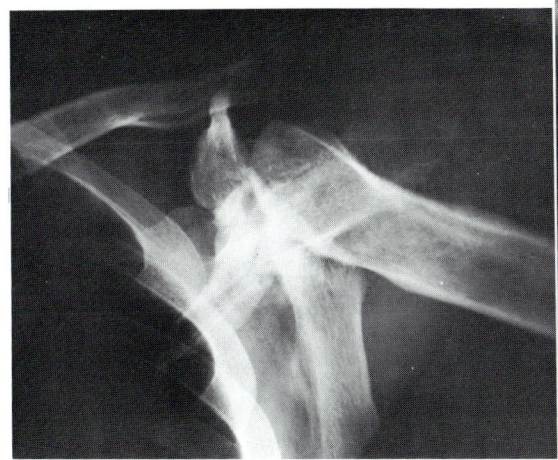

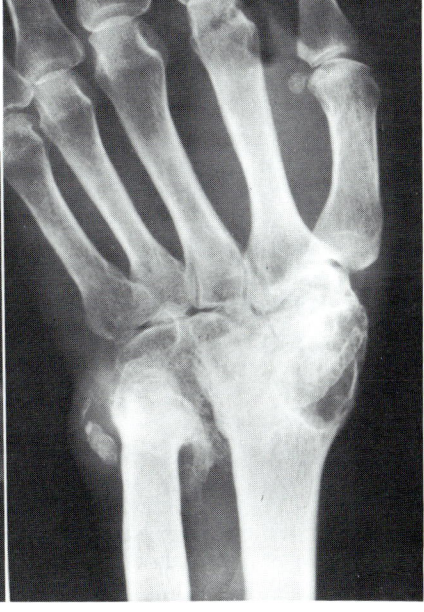

Diseases of bone and joints

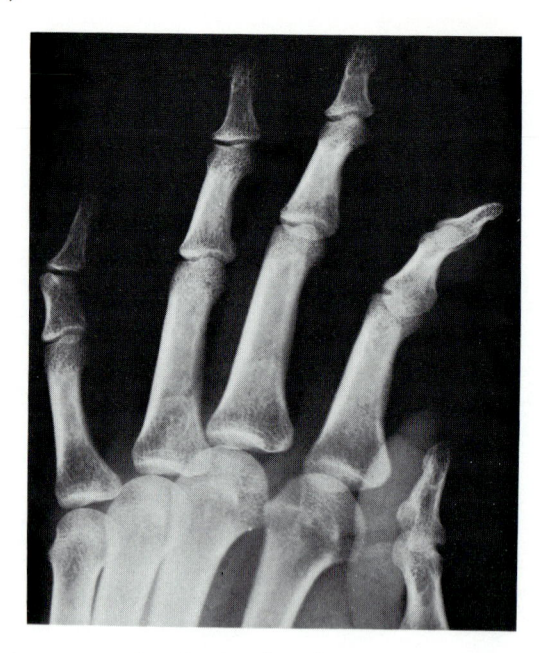

Fig. 9-10. Roentgenogram showing trophic changes in the hand in syringomyelia.

which float as joint bodies, while others are ground into the joint capsule (Fig. 9-8). Each of the osseous fragments embedded within or deep to the synovium acts as a nidus around which new bone may be formed. As a result, the synovium becomes thickened and chronically inflamed, while the joint capsule as a whole tends to become distended, boggy, and fluid-filled. Eventually, marked destruction, deformity, and luxation of the articular bone ends ensues (Figs. 9-5 to 9-7). In the process of traumatic damage to articular cartilage, extensive changes of secondary osteoarthritis inevitably develop. This, of course, is a prominent feature of the fully developed lesion. When the arthropathy is well advanced, the ligaments as well as the joint capsule are quite loose, and this undoubtedly contributes to the deformity and malfunction. Occasionally, secondary infection may be a complicating factor.

Another important though far less frequent cause of neuroarthropathy, especially in the upper extremity, is *syringomyelia* (syrinx of the spinal cord at the cervical level). This too is an old observation,[11] dating back about 80 years. It is estimated[12] that in some 25% of cases of syringomyelia, changes comparable to those described may develop in the shoulder, elbow, or wrist joints (Fig. 9-9). On occasion there may be trophic changes in the hand as well (Fig. 9-10).

REFERENCES

1. Charcot, J. M.: Sur quelques arthropathies qui paraissent d'ependre d'une lésion du cerveau ou de la moelle épinière, Arch. Physiol. Norm. Path. 1:161, 1868.
2. Feldman, M. J., Becker, K. L., Reefe, W. E., and Longo, A.: Multiple neuropathic joints including the wrist, in a patient with diabetes mellitus, J.A.M.A. 209:1690, 1969.
3. Bailey, C. C., and Root, H. F.: Neuro-

pathic foot lesions in diabetes mellitus, N. Engl. J. Med. **236**:397, 1947.
4. Martin, M. M.: Charcot joints in diabetes mellitus, Proc. R. Soc. Med. **45**:503, 1952.
5. Degenhardt, D. P., and Goodwin, M. A.: Neuropathic joints in diabetics, J. Bone Joint Surg. **42-B**:769, 1960.
6. Liberson, M.: Soft tissue calcifications in cord lesions, J.A.M.A. **152**:1010, 1953.
7. Kerwein, G., and Lyons, W. F.: Neuroarthropathy of the ankle joint from complete severence of the sciatic nerve, Ann. Surg. **115**:267, 1942.
8. Shands, A. R.: Neuropathies of the bones and joints, Arch. Surg. **20**:614, 1930.
9. Steindler, A., Williams, L. A., and Puig, J.: Tabetic arthropathies, Urol. Cut. Rev. **46**:633, 1942.
10. Horwitz, T.: Bone and cartilage debris in the synovial membrane: its significance in the early diagnosis of neuro-arthropathy, J. Bone Joint Surg. **30-A**:1579, 1948.
11. Schlesinger, H.: Die Syringomyelie, Vienna, 1895, Verlag Franz Deuticke.
12. Luck, J. V.: Bone and joint diseases, Springfield, Illinois, 1950, Charles C Thomas, Publisher, p. 255.

chapter 10

Skeletal changes in certain blood diseases

This section will deal primarily with a number of blood disorders in which the skeletal alterations are noteworthy or important. These disorders are, specifically, hemophilia (and other coagulation deficiency diseases producing comparable effects) and the chronic hemolytic anemias, particularly sickle cell anemia, thalassemia major, and spherocytic anemia. For a comprehensive discussion of these conditions and an appreciation of this rapidly developing frontier in molecular biology and genetics, the reader may have recourse to the last edition of the encyclopedic monograph of Wintrobe.[1] For more detailed consideration of the roentgenographic changes that may be observed, the text of Caffey[2] is valuable for orientation.

To avoid repetition, only brief mention is made here of myelosclerosis, mastocytosis, multiple myeloma, and the skeletal manifestations of malignant lymphoma, since these conditions have been discussed in my book, *Bone Tumors*.[3]

HEMOPHILIA

Hemophilia has been known since ancient times as a congenital disease of bleeders. In modern genetic parlance, it results from the hereditary trasmission of a sexlinked recessive mendelian trait to affected males. The frequency of hemophilic male births has been estimated[4] to be about one in 10,000, so the condition is by no means rare.

Hematologic research has shown that there are several types of hemophilia. In classic type A, blood-clotting factor VIII (platelet cofactor [AHF]) is either not present in adequate concentration or is inhibited. There are all grades of clinical severity, depending on the blood level of factor VIII. In hemophilia B, or Christmas disease, there is a deficiency of factor IX (plasma thromboplastin component [PTC]). Other conditions resembling hemophilia and presenting essentially the same clinical manifestations result from deficiency of still other

Skeletal changes in certain blood diseases

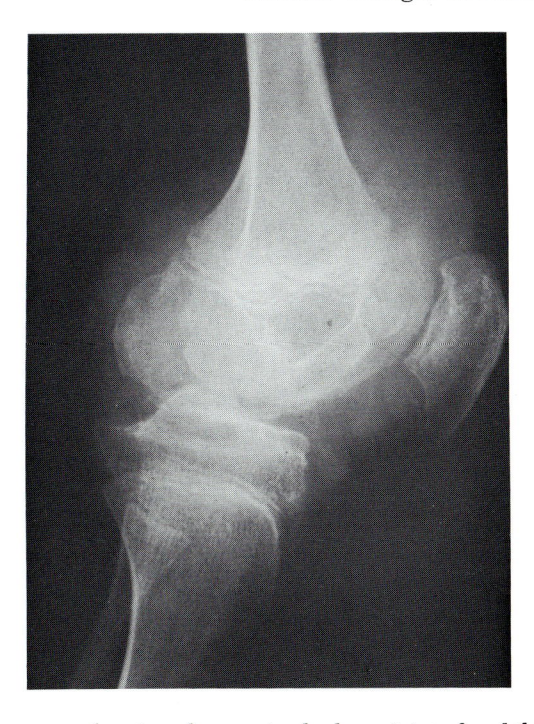

Fig. 10-1. Roentgenogram showing changes in the knee joint of a child with hemophilia—specifically, thickening of the joint capsule, narrowing of the joint space (reflecting erosion of articular cartilage), irregularity of the articular bone ends (presumably from secondary osteoarthritis), and the presence of lucent defects within the epiphyseal bone (suggesting intramedullary hemorrhage).

components involved in blood clotting (plasma thromboplastin antecedent [PTA], factor XII, and so on) or from the action of certain anticoagulants.[1,5]

However one pinpoints the coagulation deficiency in any given instance (and this is still an active area of investigation[6]), the tendency to prolonged and excessive bleeding usually appears in early childhood and may lead to repeated episodes of hemorrhage into skin and mucous membranes, muscles, eyes, various internal sites, bones, and joints. More than half of all hemophiliacs bleed into their joints.[7] The knee is most often involved (Fig. 10-1), although the hip, ankle, elbow, and other joints may be affected.[8] Rapidly developing hemarthrosis in hemophilia is likely to be painful and disabling, presumably from increased intraarticular pressure and distension of the joint capsule. Initially, the blood is resorbed, but repeated (untreated) episodes over a period of years can lead to irreparable joint damage.[9]

In small joints, substantial osteoarticular destruction may result. In a large joint like the knee (Fig. 10-1), more or less pronounced capsular swelling ensues from villous hypertrophy and fibrous thickening. Eventually the synovial lining becomes a deep forestlike web or tangled mat of brownishly discolored villi. Its gross appearance may resemble that seen in diffuse pigmented villo-

Diseases of bone and joints

nodular synovitis, although (histiocytic) nodules are lacking. In time, the articular cartilage may be overgrown and eroded; then the changes of secondary osteoarthritis come into play. In a late stage, muscle atrophy, contracture, fibrous ankylosis, and permanent deformity may be sequelae of chronic, long-standing hemarthrosis.

The potential long-term seriousness of these manifestations underscores the importance of prevention. For control of bleeding, the prompt administration of factor VIII in sufficient amount to achieve a hemostatic level (a concentration of 25% or more of estimated normal) is indicated.[1] Type-specific whole blood or plasma may be used, but fresh frozen plasma is preferable, and high-potency antihemophilic factor (AHF) concentrate is now also available.[10] Under

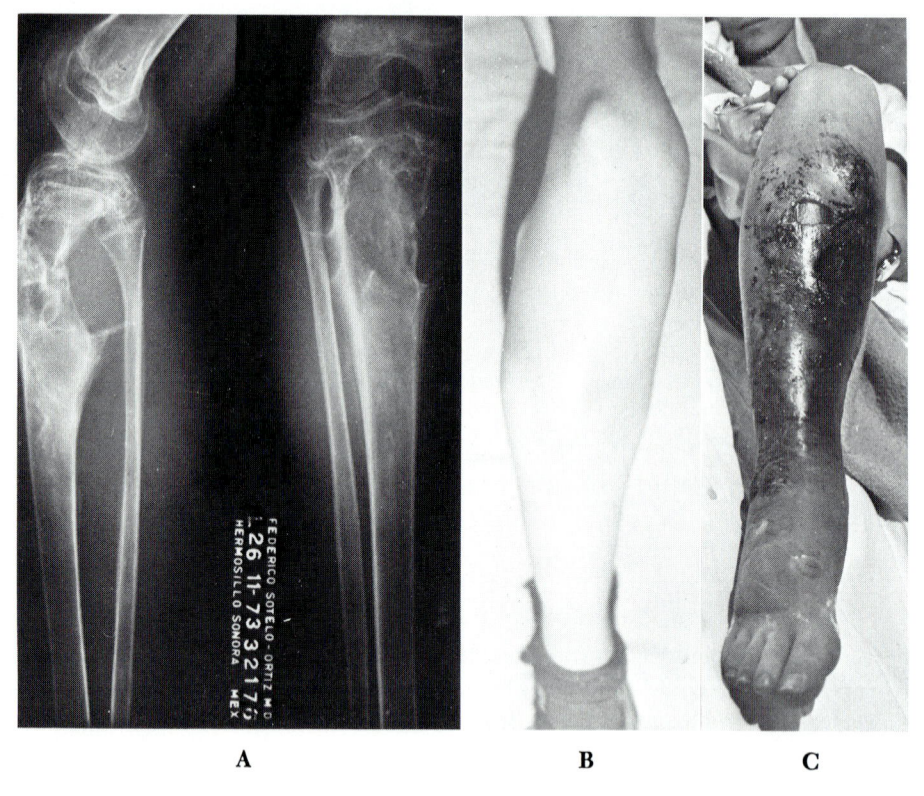

Fig. 10-2. A, Roentgenograms (lateral and anteroposterior views) of a large pseudotumor in the upper tibia of a boy of 16 with hemophilia. There is also rarefaction in the distal femoral epiphysis, indicating intramedullary hemorrhage there as well. One year previously, he had struck the upper part of the leg; a small swelling (hematoma) developed, which continued to enlarge until it attained the size illustrated in B. Concentration of factor VIII in the blood was estimated at only 10%. Some three weeks elapsed before antihemophilic factor (VIII) could be obtained and administered; by this time, the swollen leg had become black and dry gangrene had set in, C, with loss of arterial circulation in the foot. Above-knee amputation was done under cover of factor VIII, with uneventful recovery. (Courtesy Dr. F. Sotelo-Ortiz, Hermosillo, Mexico.)

this protective cover repeated aspiration of blood from a joint and even surgery can be performed safely,[11,12] as required.

At times, hemorrhage in bone or its periosteum, apart from joint involvement, may also have serious consequences for hemophiliacs if it is not controlled or well managed, although this is encountered less often. It is usually the shaft of a large limb bone, notably the femur or the tibia, that is the site of massive hemorrhage, but other bones may also be affected. Frequently there is a large hematoma in muscle as well. Extensive hemorrhage within or beneath the periosteum is followed by organization and periosteal new bone formation, much as it is in scurvy. It appears from published reports[8] that in old neglected cases there may also be more or less extensive ragged or moth-eaten erosion of the bone cortex. In such circumstances there is a great hazard of pathologic fracture. Radiographically discernible, intramedullary hemorrhage may likewise be a prominent feature. Altogether, it is not surprising that such patients are sometimes operated on for suspected malignant tumor (the diagnosis is later changed to "pseudotumor") (Fig. 10-2). In the old days, without adequate preparation or treatment, not a few succumbed to fatal hemorrhage or infection.

CHRONIC HEMOLYTIC ANEMIAS

In the chronic hemolytic anemias, as Caffey[2] has emphasized, the skeletal changes, in children at least, may be pathognomonic and often are among the most characteristic features. As indicated, the major conditions in point are sickle cell anemia, thalassemia, and spherocytic anemia. All of them are transmitted as mendelian traits and appear in a major, clinically significant form when homozygous. In each of them, the defect or abnormality in the red blood cells responsible for increased hemolysis, anemia, and sometimes icterus is specific and unique, as will be indicated presently. In general, however, this may be said with a view to understanding better the bone changes in all of them. In response to increased destruction of erythrocytes, the bone marrow becomes markedly hyperplastic. Within expansile, young growing bones, the marrow overgrowth causes widening of their medullary cavities and pressure atrophy of cortical and spongy bone, reflected radiographically in certain distinctive patterns. To be sure, the relative incidence, extent, and distribution of these skeletal alterations are variable.

Sickle cell anemia. In sickle cell disease (sicklemia), the red blood cells tend to assume a sickle (or oat) shape when oxygen pressure is reduced. The disease is caused by a dominant allele that occurs in variable frequencies, as high as 28% in different African Negro races[4] and about 8% in American Negroes. Sicklemia, or sickle cell trait, may produce few, if any, clinical manifestations. However, a small percentage of individuals with this disease (about one in forty) develops potentially serious, hemolytic, sickle cell anemia.[13] In the black population of the United States, this comes to as many as 50,000 who may suffer from the disease in a homozygous state. The condition may therefore be considered one of the more common long-term illnesses of black children, having significant economic as well as medical implications.[14] With a view to public education, investigation of the effective treatment of crises, and possible genetic counselling, a variety of rapid, low-cost screening tests for the diagnosis of sickle cell anemia have been devised.

In this connection it is important to be aware also of the interaction of the sickle hemoglobin gene with those of other red cell abnormalities, particularly hemoglobin C trait and β-thalassemia. The combined incidence of sickling disorders due to hemoglobin S-C disease and hemoglobin S–β-thalassemia is probably greater than that of hemoglobin SS disease.[15]

It was in connection with sickle cell anemia that the search for abnormal hemoglobins was started by Pauling[13] and his associates some 20 years ago. This is still an active field of investigation. More than eighty abnormal hemoglobins have now been identified,[1] with more undoubtedly to be discovered. Apparently, every alteration in the polypeptide chain structure gives rise to another addition to the wide range of abnormal hemoglobins.

Sickle cell anemia is characterized clinically by symptoms of anemia, arthritic manifestations (aching in the joints or elsewhere in the extremities, often ascribed to "rheumatism"), chronic leg ulcers (common in adolescents and adults, especially over the malleoli), and acute attacks of pain (abdominal cramps). As previously noted, bone infarcts may develop, especially in the capital femoral epiphysis (often with residual joint damage), the hand and foot bones, and even vertebral bodies (leading to compression). Curiously enough, osteomyelitis due to *Salmonella* appears to be a special hazard (Fig. 10-3, *A*).

In response to the hemolytic anemia, the bone marrow undergoes compensatory hyperplasia. As many as 50% to 70% of the nucleated cells may be nucleated red cells. On the whole, however, as contrasted with thalassemia, marrow hyperplasia is less pronounced, bone changes are less constant, symptoms often appear at a later age, and even severely affected patients survive longer.

When osseous changes occur in childhood (and they are often absent), one may observe involvement of metacarpals and proximal phalanges (so-called sickle cell dactylitis) or of the corresponding foot bones. If the long limb bones are affected, these may show cortical thinning and widening (Fig. 10-3, *B*). Sometimes the only demonstrable alterations may be in the skull bones, especially the parietal and frontal bones; on occasion, the nasal, facial, and jaw bones may also be involved. The essential changes in the calvarium are thickening from widening of the diploë, as well as the formation of spicules of new bone, oriented perpendicularly to the inner table. Bone deformities such as kyphosis, scoliosis, saber shins, and oxycephaly are also observed at times, though not as often as in thalassemia. In adults, one may find evidence of previous bone infarcts, hemorrhage and fibrosis of the marrow, patchy osteosclerosis, and endosteal bone apposition, so that the cortices of large limb bones may actually be thickened.

Skeletal changes in certain blood diseases

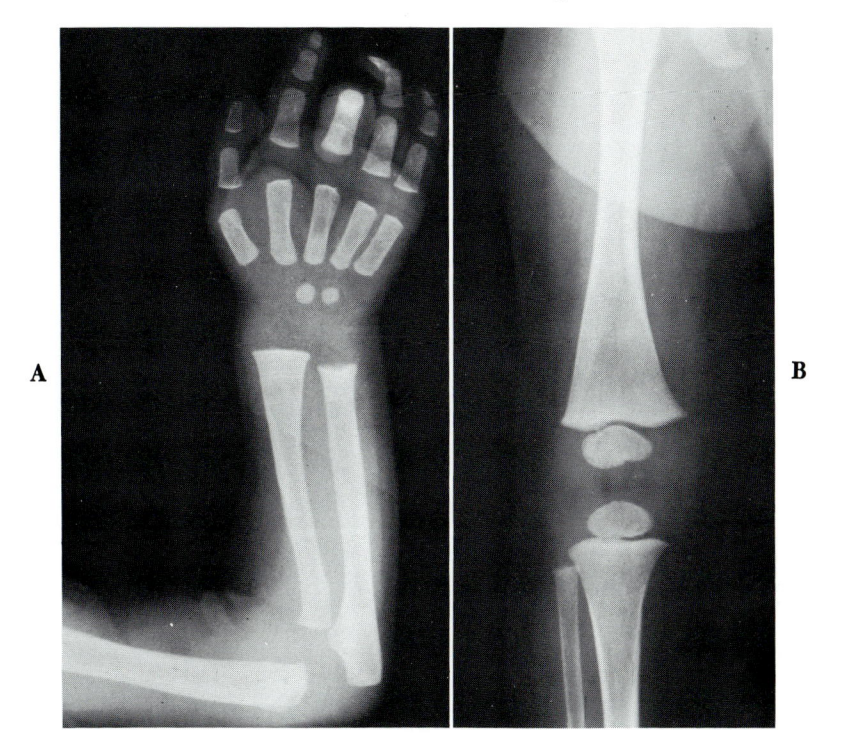

Fig. 10-3. **A**, Roentgenogram of a child with sickle cell anemia showing widening of the bones, especially of the metacarpals and proximal phalanges, and thinning of their cortices. The loss of the middle and distal phalanges of the third finger was a sequel of *Salmonella* osteomyelitis. **B**, Same case illustrated in **A**, showing cortical thinning and flaring (from marrow hyperplasia) in the distal metaphysis of the femur.

Thalassemia. Thalassemia major (from the Greek word *thalassa*, meaning sea), also designated in the older literature as Cooley's erythroblastic anemia and Mediterranean anemia, is caused by a specific, recessive allele that occurs in low frequency in various Mediterranean groups (it appears to be absent in central and northern European populations). Accordingly, the condition is largely confined either to people living on the Mediterranean shores, mainly Greeks, Italians, Syrians, and Armenians, or to their descendants, wherever they may be. In these groups, the frequency of carriers of the thalassemia trait has been estimated[4] at about one in twenty-five persons.

Like sickle cell anemia, thalassemia represents a molecular disease of abnormal hemoglobin. Recent hematologic research[16] has indicated that there are several genetic subtypes of thalassemia, featuring the presence of significantly increased amounts in erythrocytes of fetal hemoglobin, hemoglobin A_2, or both.

The clinical (homozygous) disease state (thalassemia major) may be manifested as early as the first year of life, is usually progressive in the growing child, and in severe cases may terminate life before adolescence. It is characterized by persistent anemia (responding temporarily to transfusions), icterus

Diseases of bone and joints

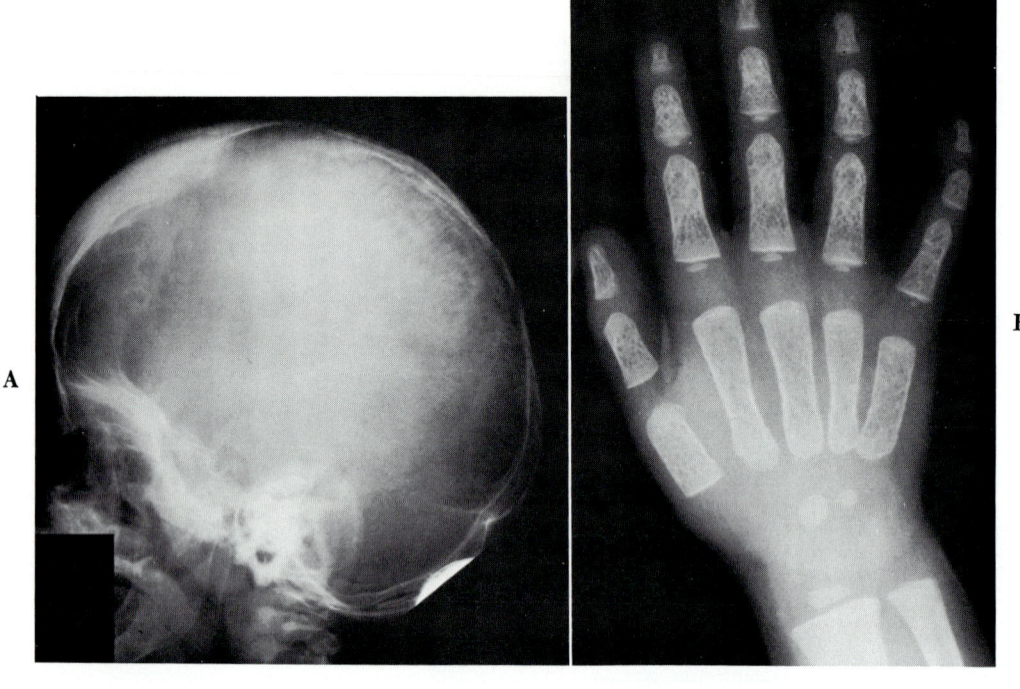

Fig. 10-4. **A,** Roentgenogram of the skull of a child with thalassemia major (Cooley's anemia) showing pronounced thickening of the anterior portion of the calvarium and, in the parietal area particularly, striae of new bone oriented perpendicularly to the outer table. **B,** The hand bones of the same patient, illustrating uniform cortical thinning of the metacarpals and phalanges and peculiar alteration of their spongy bone architecture. The metacarpal bones in particular have a rectangular contour in their projection (see also Fig. 10-5, *B*).

(reflecting elevated serum bilirubin from increased destruction of erythrocytes), elevated serum iron, hepatosplenomegaly, and certain bone changes (whose roentgenographic appearance is of diagnostic value). The bone marrow is hyperplastic and contains many immature forms, including numerous normoblasts and megaloblasts. It also contains hemosiderin-laden macrophages and foam cells as a sequel of erythrocytic destruction.

The striking skeletal changes in the skull, long bones, hand bones, vertebral column, and other sites have already been mentioned. Some of the more distinctive alterations are illustrated in Figs. 10-4 and 10-5 and are highlighted in the accompanying legends. It should be noted also that associated skeletal developmental anomalies are not infrequent and that premature fusion of epiphyses may be a feature of the disorder.[17]

Spherocytic anemia. Spherocytic anemia, also designated hereditary spherocytosis, familial hemolytic anemia, and chronic hemolytic jaundice, is characterized by spherocytosis; increased fragility of the red cells to hemolytic agents, especially to hypotonic salt solution; moderate hemolytic anemia; icterus (slight

Skeletal changes in certain blood diseases

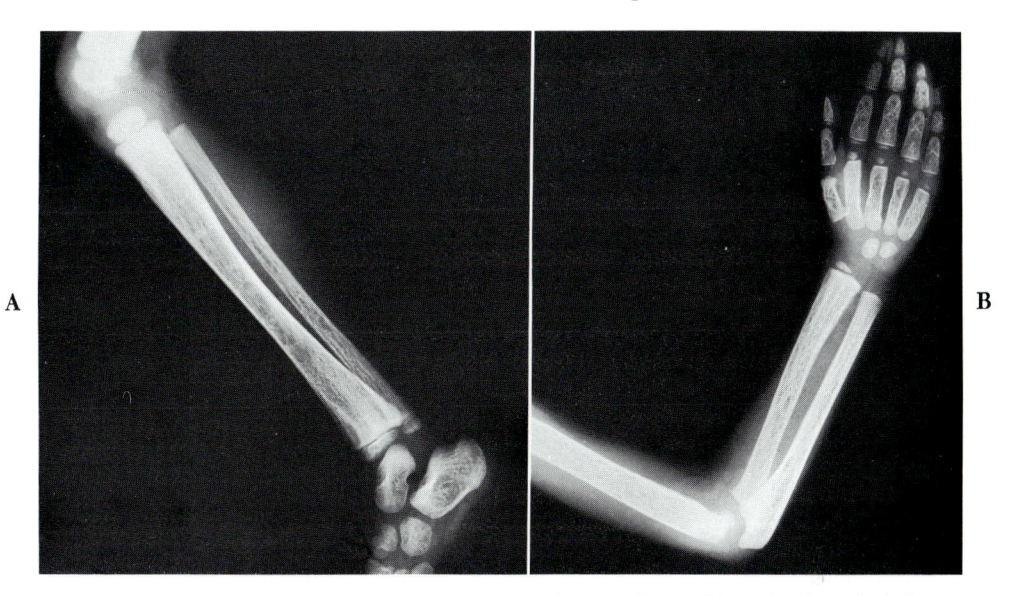

Fig. 10-5. **A**, Roentgenograms of the lower limb bones of a child with clinical thalassemia. Also evident here are thinning of the cortices of the tibia and fibula, some distension or flaring of the metaphyseal portions of the tibia, and distinct alteration of architecture of the cancellous bone. The changes are present in all the bones, but are more pronounced in the long limb bones and in the metatarsals (not shown). **B**, The upper limb bones in the case illustrated in **A**. The changes already cited are again evident in all the bones, but are particularly striking in the metacarpals and phalanges.

to moderate, except after hemolytic crises); and splenomegaly, often quite marked.

As its various names indicate, the disorder is chronic, congenital, and often familial. There are records of many families in which jaundice has existed through several generations. While the condition is transmitted through male and female descendants alike, not all of the children in a family are affected. Although the disease has been known clinically for a long time, the precise nature of the erythrocytic defect or abnormality in biochemical terms has not yet been elucidated. The jaundice may be noted shortly after birth or at any time during childhood, but it may be so slight as to escape recognition until adult life. Many affected persons live to an advanced age.

In keeping with the relative mildness of the disorder, as compared with the other chronic hemolytic anemias, skeletal changes of the nature previously described (Figs. 10-3 to 10-5) are absent or equivocal in most cases, although some instances have been recorded in which alterations in the skull and limb bones were as pronounced and extensive as in thalassemia. Also noteworthy are certain developmental anomalies that occur often enough to suggest that they are not fortuitous, but rather result from the gene defect. Oxycephaly (tower skull, turmschädel) in particular has often been noted, as have abnormalities in the eyes, the root of the nose, the palate, the teeth, and the fingers.

REFERENCES

1. Wintrobe, M. M.: Clinical hematology, ed. 6, Philadelphia, 1967, Lea & Febiger.
2. Caffey, J.: Pediatric x-ray diagnosis, ed. 5, Chicago, 1967, Year Book Medical Publishers.
3. Lichtenstein, L.: Bone tumors, ed. 4, St. Louis, 1972, The C. V. Mosby Co.
4. Stern, C.: Principles of human genetics, San Francisco, 1949, W. H. Freeman & Co.
5. Brinkhous, K. M., editor: Hemophilia and other hemorrhagic states, Chapel Hill, 1959, University of North Carolina Press.
6. Seegers, W. H.: Blood coagulation in hemophilia B, Bull. Pathol., October 1968, p. 199.
7. Thomas, H. B.: Some orthopaedic findings in 98 cases of hemophilia, J. Bone Joint Surg. 18:140, 1936.
8. Ghormley, R. K., and Clegg, R. S.: Bone and joint changes in hemophilia with report of cases of so-called hemophilic pseudotumor, J. Bone Joint Surg. 30-A: 589, 1948.
9. Freund, E.: Die Gelenkerkrankung der Bluter, Virch. Arch. Path. Anat. 256:158, 1925.
10. Brinkhous, K. M., Shanbrom, E., Roberts, H. R., Webster, W. P., Fekete, L., and Wagner, R. H.: A new high-potency glycine-precipitated antihemophilic factor (AHF) concentrate, J.A.M.A. 205:615, 1968.
11. Schaaf, W. J.: Early aspiration of joint in Christmas disease, J.A.M.A. 175:509, 1961.
12. George, J. N., and Breckenridge, R. T.: The use of factor VIII and factor IX concentrates during surgery, J.A.M.A. 214:1673, 1970.
13. Pauling, L., Itano, H. A., Singer, S. J., and Wells, T. C.: Sickle cell anemia, a molecular disease, Science 110:543, 1949.
14. Editorial: Sickle cell anemia, J.A.M.A. 214:749, 1970.
15. Kellon, D. B., and Bentler, E.: Editorial: Physician attitudes about sickle cell disease and sickle cell trait, J.A.M.A. 22:71, 1974.
16. Gabuzda, T. G., Nathan, D. G., and Gardner, F. H.: Thalassemia trait: genetic combinations of increased fetal and A_2 hemoglobins, N. Engl. J. Med. 270: 1212, 1964.
17. Currarino, G., and Erlandson, M. E.: Premature fusion of epiphyses in Cooley's anemia, Radiology 83:656, 1964.

GENERAL REFERENCE

Moseley, J. E.: Bone changes in hematologic disorders (roentgen aspects), New York, 1968, Grune and Stratton, Inc.

chapter 11

Paget's disease of bone
(osteitis deformans)

PAGET'S DISEASE OF BONE

Paget's disease is a not uncommon condition that has tantalizingly eluded full clarification, although we have learned a great deal about its manifestations over the years. We know from physiologic investigation that active lesions of Paget's disease show significant hypervascularity and, collaterally, from radioisotope tracer studies (^{45}Ca), that they manifest greatly accelerated metabolic turnover. This may have its reflection clinically in wide pulse pressure and peripheral signs of high cardiac output.[1] We know, on the other hand, from the valuable investigation of Schmorl,[2] that subclinical lesions of limited extent, involving particularly portions of the sacrum, lumbar vertebrae, or both, actually outnumber those in the pelvis, skull, long limb bones, and other sites producing symptoms. (The incidence of Paget lesions, including the silent ones in the vertebral column, was over 3% in a sizable series of subjects past 40 years of age, whose skeletons were thoroughly examined at autopsy.)

We have learned to recognize most lesions of Paget's disease roentgenographically, although some of the early lesions and those in unusual locations may present a problem at times (Figs. 11-1 and 11-2). We are well aware that sarcoma may develop in established clinical lesions of Paget's disease, with significant though not alarming frequency,[3] and that, curiously enough, benign giant cell tumors may make their appearance, especially in the calvarium and facial bones.[4,5]

We know that, pathologically, the initial expression of the disorder is a localized area of resorption (whether it be in the calvarium, tibia, humerus, or some other bone). This initial phase of resorption is followed by repeated alternating cycles of bone formation and renewed resorption over a period of several or many years, leading eventually to readily recognizable gross alterations of architecture and, microscopically, to a unique complex structural pattern of bone designated "mosaic" by Schmorl[2] (see Fig. 11-9, C). However, when it comes

Diseases of bone and joints

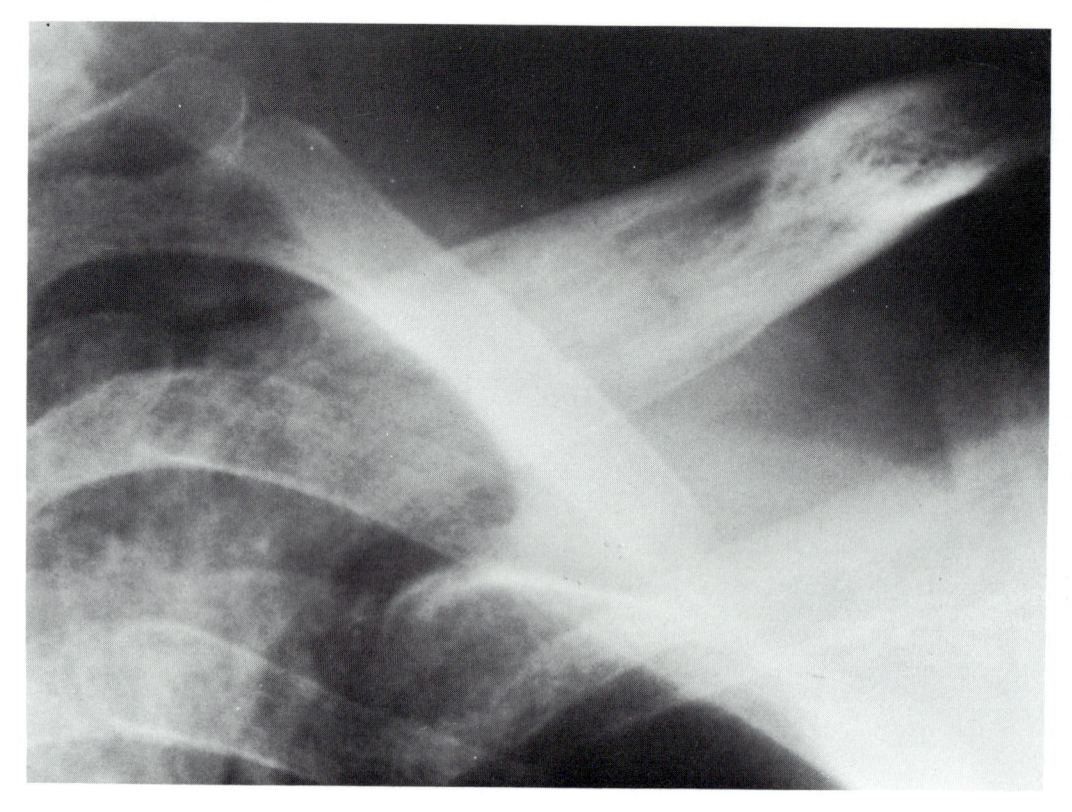

Fig. 11-1. **A,** Roentgenogram showing an expanded lesion of Paget's disease in the sternal end of a clavicle. Note the widening of the bone and early transformation of its architecture. **B,** Roentgenogram showing changes in Paget's disease in a metacarpal bone, another unusual site. Note the expansion of the bone and the presence of lucent areas within it. Coarse trabecular alteration is not yet discernible.

to the basic question of what initiates or is responsible for this sequence of changes, we actually know little more than did Sir James Paget[6] in 1877 when he described a group of advanced cases in point as "osteitis deformans," and we have not advanced beyond the stage of speculation[7] (Fig. 11-3).

Clinical considerations. Paget's disease is observed mainly in middle-aged or older patients, although occasional instances may be encountered in individuals below the age of 40.[4,8] I have seen a remarkable set of roentgenograms showing well-developed, unmistakable changes of Paget's disease in the long limb bones of both upper and lower extremities, pelvis, and lumbar spine of a young man, aged 18, who had complained of bone pain for some 3 years previously (Fig. 11-4). It may be noted, on the other hand, that most cases of so-called juvenile Paget's disease in the older literature apparently represent instances of fibrous dysplasia. Familial incidence has been observed but is exceptional.[9]

The only laboratory aid to diagnosis is estimation of serum alkaline phosphatase activity, which is consistently elevated in Paget's disease, even when it

Paget's disease of bone (osteitis deformans)

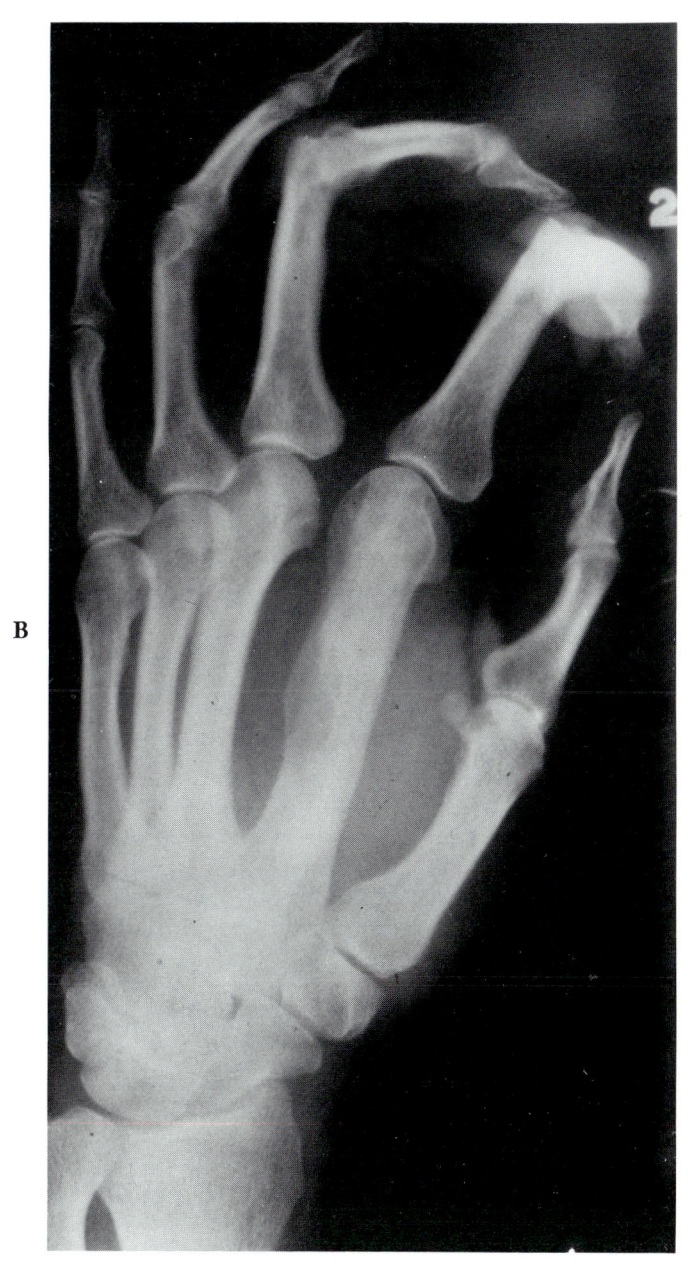

Fig. 11-1, cont'd. For legend see opposite page.

Diseases of bone and joints

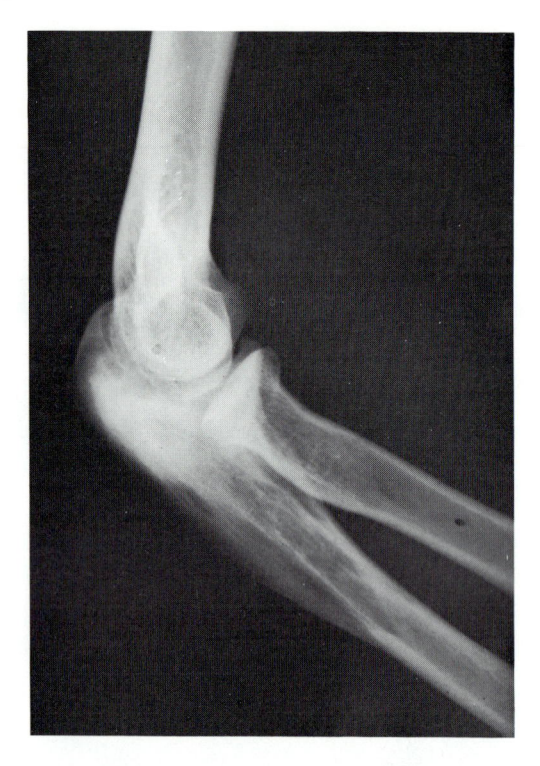

Fig. 11-2. Roentgenogram showing early (monostotic) Paget involvement in a proximal ulna. A film taken 4 months earlier showed a transverse pathologic fracture (now healed). Biopsy showed a richly vascular lesion of Paget's disease in an early resorptive phase.

is localized. When Paget's disease is complicated by osteogenic sarcoma, one may get fantastically high levels, exceeding those in any other condition.

The condition may develop in one, several, or many bones. While symptomatic lesions predilect the calvarium, the innominate bones, the vertebral column, and the long limb bones, one may occasionally find them in such sites as the sternum, clavicle, and hand and foot bones. Although there is wide variation in the extent and tempo of the disease, the usual history is one of slow progress over a period of many years. By the same token, the condition is compatible with long life, so that most patients die of natural causes rather than from bone sarcoma, cardiovascular disease, or other sequelae of Paget's disease. However, it should be emphasized that not all cases of Paget's disease show steady progression to an advanced stage, and the spontaneous healing tendency in the condition is well known.[4,10]

Treatment. Pain is often, though not necessarily, an early distressing symptom, especially in the lower back (Fig. 11-5) or in a bone of a lower extremity, particularly the tibia. Symptomatic relief has been noted,[4] though not consistently, after the administration of a variety of remedies, including androgen (to men) and estrogen (to women) in the same doses that one would use for osteoporosis.

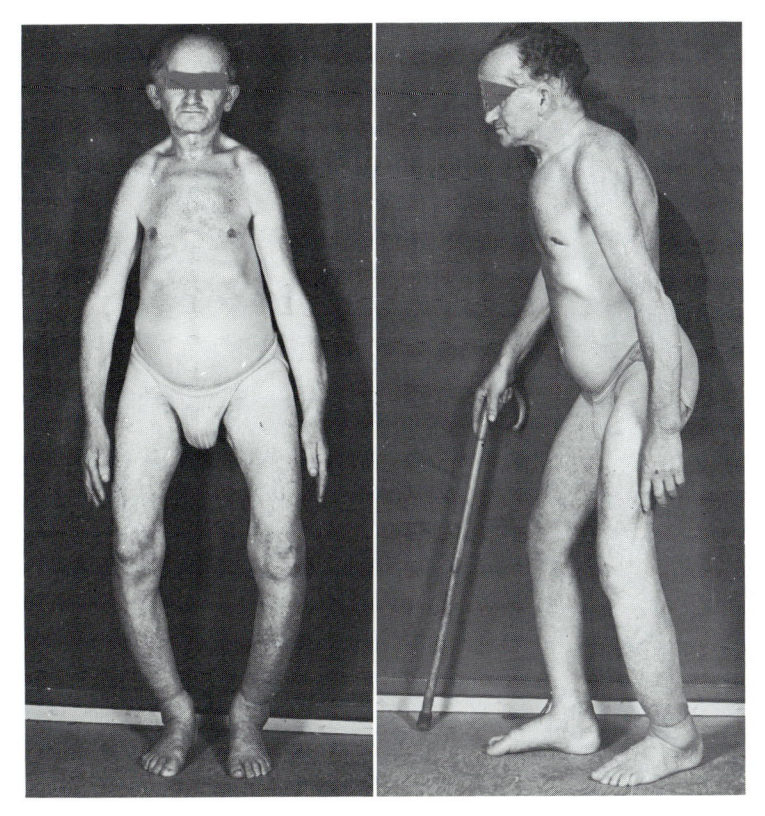

Fig. 11-3. Photographs of an elderly patient with widespread, advanced Paget's disease. Note the enlarged head, kyphosis with foreshortened barrel chest, bowing of the femora and tibiae, and marked widening and deformity of the tibiae, especially the left tibia.

These hormones also tend to reverse hypercalcuria, when present. For refractory pain not responding to any other measures, small fractional doses of x-ray irradiation may be effective, perhaps because it tends to reduce vascularity. Large dosage, however, is contraindicated and may induce a pathologic fracture that will not heal (see Fig. 13-3).

Many patients with Paget's disease are in negative calcium balance, and this can sometimes be corrected by treatment with sodium fluoride administered orally.[11]

Three new therapeutic anti-osteolytic agents have been introduced recently that are promising enough to deserve further clinical trial, although they apparently fall short of ideal treatment, namely, mithramycin, calcitonin, and diphosphonates. The antibiotic mithramycin is said to afford symptomatic relief and to suppress the activity of Paget's disease through inhibition of bone resorption, as determined by changes in the serum alkaline phosphatase and urinary hydroxyproline levels. It has been recommended[12] for patients with more severe active disease, coupled with the admonition that close supervision is re-

Diseases of bone and joints

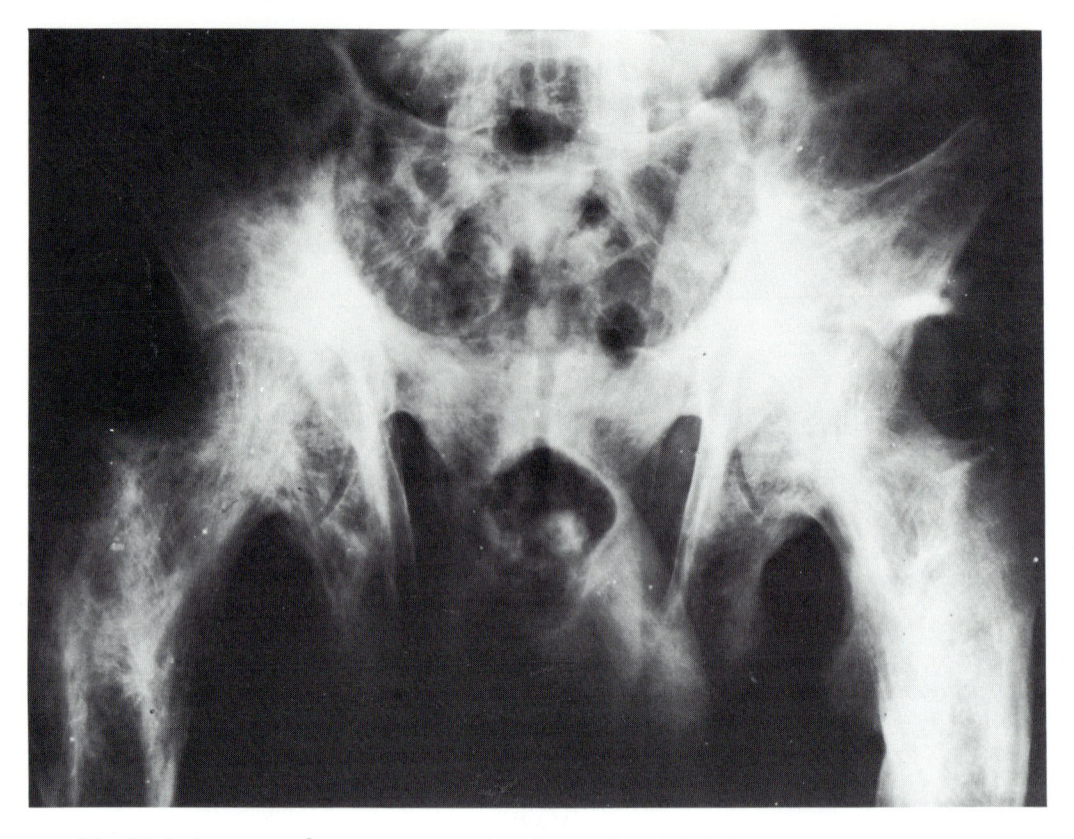

Fig. 11-4. An extraordinary instance of widespread and full-blown Paget's disease in a patient, aged 18.

quired to guard against its cytotoxic effect on platelets, as well as hepatic and renal function.

The possibility of long-term treatment of Paget's disease with synthetic calcitonin (of porcine or salmon[13] origin) has also been explored with encouraging results, but the potential hazard here is the development of hyperparathyroidism secondary to the hormone-induced hypocalcemia.

Diphosphonate compounds[14] administered orally are said to suppress excessive bone turnover (by building hydroxyapatite crystals), which would seem to be a prime objective, but experience with them is still limited.

Other manifestations that may require orthopedic or medical attention are bowing of the femur or tibia, infractions (particularly transverse fissure fractures on the convex side of bowed bones), urolithiasis (from hypercalcuria), and sometimes deafness, blindness, or proptosis from pronounced thickening of the skull. Because of the hazard of fractures and of hypercalcuria and stone formation, one should avoid immobilization, high calcium diet, and vitamin D. If immobilization is required temporarily, calcium should be limted and fluid intake kept high, to avoid potentially serious hypercalcemia.

Both multiple myeloma and hyperparathyroidism have been noted to occur in

Paget's disease of bone (osteitis deformans)

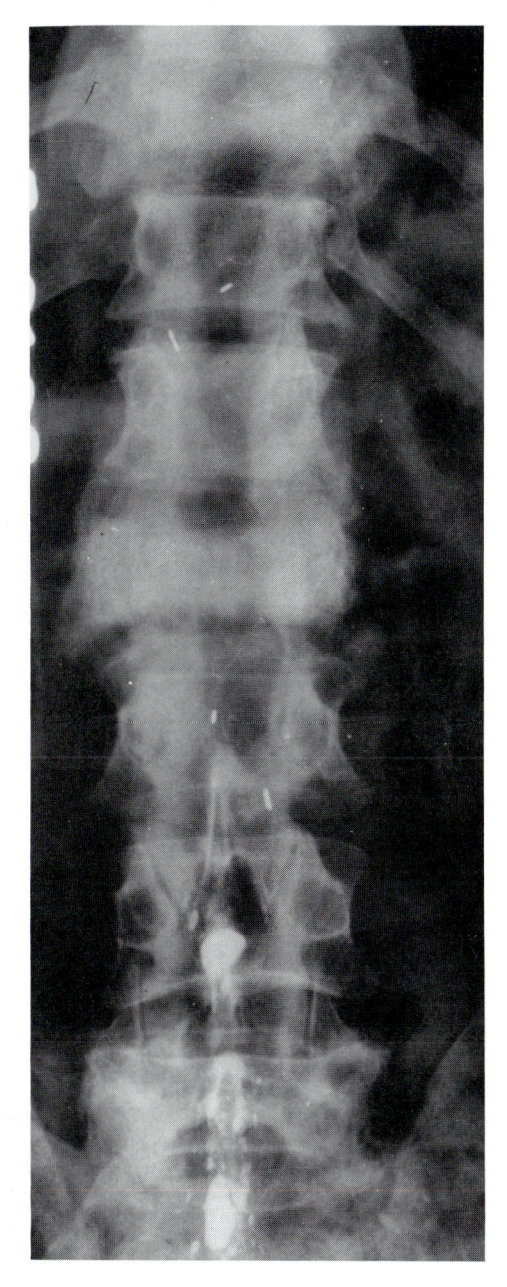

Fig. 11-5. Roentgenogram showing changes of Paget's disease in two separate vertebral bodies, D-11 and L-2. The lower one is distinctly broadened and compressed, and it produced symptoms of cord compression.

Diseases of bone and joints

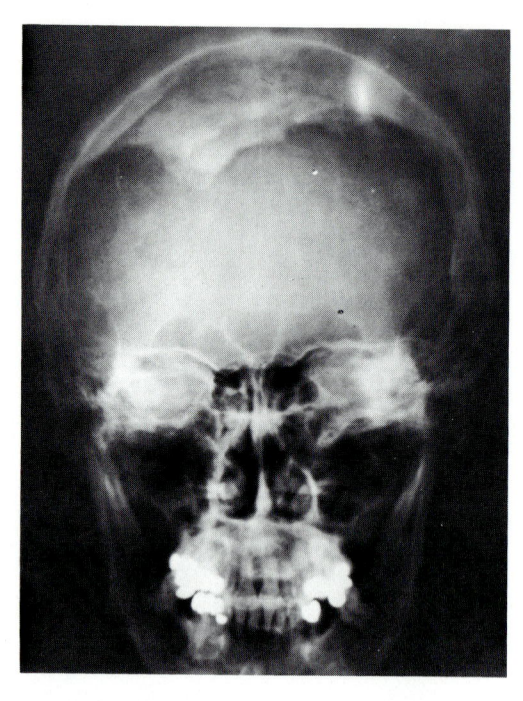

Fig. 11-6. Roentgenogram of a skull showing huge lucent areas of rarefaction reflecting the early resorptive phase of Paget's disease (so-called osteoporosis circumscripta cranii).

association with Paget's disease of bone, but this appears to be coincidental or fortuitous.

Pathologic changes. As indicated, sizable circumscribed rarefied skeletal defects reflect the early resorptive changes in Paget's disease. Their appearance and significance in the calvarium (Fig. 11-6) are well recognized (so-called osteoporosis circumscripta cranii).[15] Comparable defects may, of course, develop in other bones—an innominate bone, a tibia, or a humerus—as a forerunner of typical Paget transformation. When a tibia is involved, it is frequently the upper half of the shaft that is altered, although occasionally the lower end may display comparable changes (Fig. 11-7). While the rarefied defect often appears to terminate sharply, the process tends to progress along the shaft and is likely to be associated with some expansion of the bone and thinning of its cortex. Although there is not, as yet, any discernible coarse trabecular architecture, even at this stage of evolution, the microscopic changes observed in a biopsy specimen can be readily identified as those of Paget's disease (Fig. 11-8).

Whatever the site of early or initial resorption, it is apparently brought about by inordinate vascularity and, even more so, by intense osteoclastic activity (far exceeding that seen in hyperparathyroidism, for example). The resorbed bone is inevitably replaced by fibrous tissue, in which new bone is laid down by proliferating osteoblasts (Fig. 11-8). This, in turn, undergoes resorption. Thus the cycle goes on and on, until eventually the bone presents a peculiar complex pat-

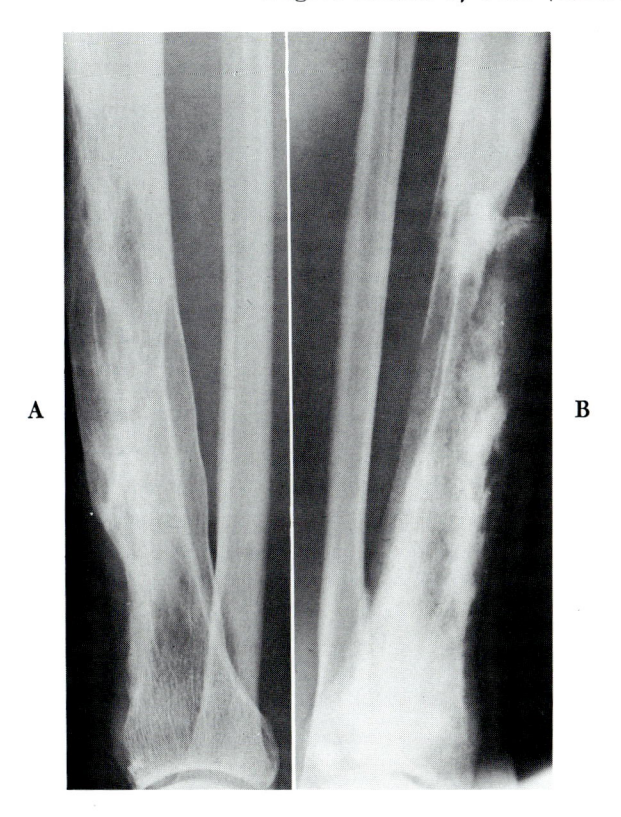

Fig. 11-7. **A,** Roentgenogram of a lesion of early Paget's disease in a lower tibia, which is still in a resorptive stage. Note the advancing cortical resorption at the proximal limit of the lesion. **B,** Roentgenogram of another lesion of relatively early (monostotic) Paget's disease in a distal tibia showing a pathologic fracture through its proximal end.

tern described by Schmorl as mosaic. It no longer has an orderly lamellar structure but instead is composed of irregular bits and pieces of bone, demarcated by unusually prominent cement lines (Fig. 11-9). It should be emphasized, however, that this jigsaw or mosaic architecture is a feature of advanced or late Paget transformation and, as such, is not a sine qua non for diagnosis in biopsy specimens, for example.

Grossly, transformed Paget bone presents a peculiar coarsened trabecular architecture, which is brought out particularly well in macerated preparations (Fig. 11-9, *D* and *E*) and, of course, is reflected roentgenographically (Fig. 11-10). The new bone is deposited endosteally and to some extent within the general medullary cavity and is also irregularly laid down by the periosteum, so that the surface of the affected bone appears rough and pumicelike. In the process there is an appreciable increase in the width of the bone (Fig. 11-11). Further, since this porous bone lacks customary structural strength and solidity, it is not only vulnerable to infraction but also yields under stress, so that the development of such deformities as tibial and femoral bowing, coxa vara, and kyphoscoliosis

Diseases of bone and joints

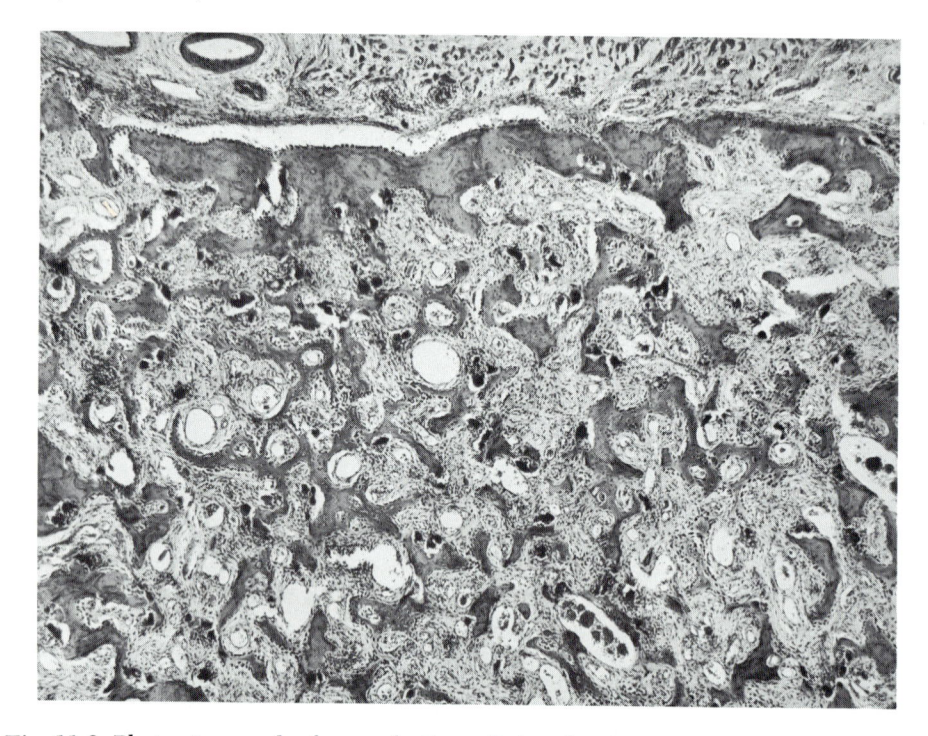

Fig. 11-8. Photomicrograph of an early Paget lesion showing extensive resorption of the cortical bone, replacement by vascular connective tissue, intense osteoclastic activity, and numerous small trabeculae of new bone rimmed by osteoblasts.

Fig. 11-9. **A**, Photomicrograph of a representative field from a biopsy of a tibial cortex showing a later stage of Paget's disease. In the bone at the lower left one sees the development of a mosaic pattern (numerous small irregular bits of bone outlined by conspicuous cement lines). This pattern can be accentuated by polarized light. On the cortical surface (top), there are layers of reconstructed new bone. **B**, Photomicrograph showing the changes of well-established Paget's disease is an active resorptive phase (though not the initial one). Note the striking number of osteoclasts and replacement of resorbed bone by young connective tissue. The bone area to left of center already shows the beginning of a mosaic pattern (heavy, irregular cement lines). **C**, Photomicrograph of another instance of Paget's disease showing a well-developed mosaic pattern. Note the numerous dark cement lines demarcating irregular bits and pieces of extensively reconstructed bone. Only occasional osteoclasts are in evidence, and the disease process in this area is apparently approaching its end stage. **D**, Macerated preparation (enlarged) of a portion of a lumbar vertebral body of a patient with Paget's disease showing the thickened and coarsened architecture of the cancellous bone (compare with Fig. 8-7). **E**, Photograph of a macerated specimen of a portion of the vertebral column of an older man with Paget's disease. Note the thickening of the spongy bone structure in all of the bodies. The holes reflect sites of resorption. (**D** and **E** From Schmorl, G., and Junghanns, H.: Die Gesunde und die Kranke Wirbelsäule in Rontgenbild und Klinik, ed. 4, Stuttgart, 1972, Georg Thieme Verlag.)

Continued.

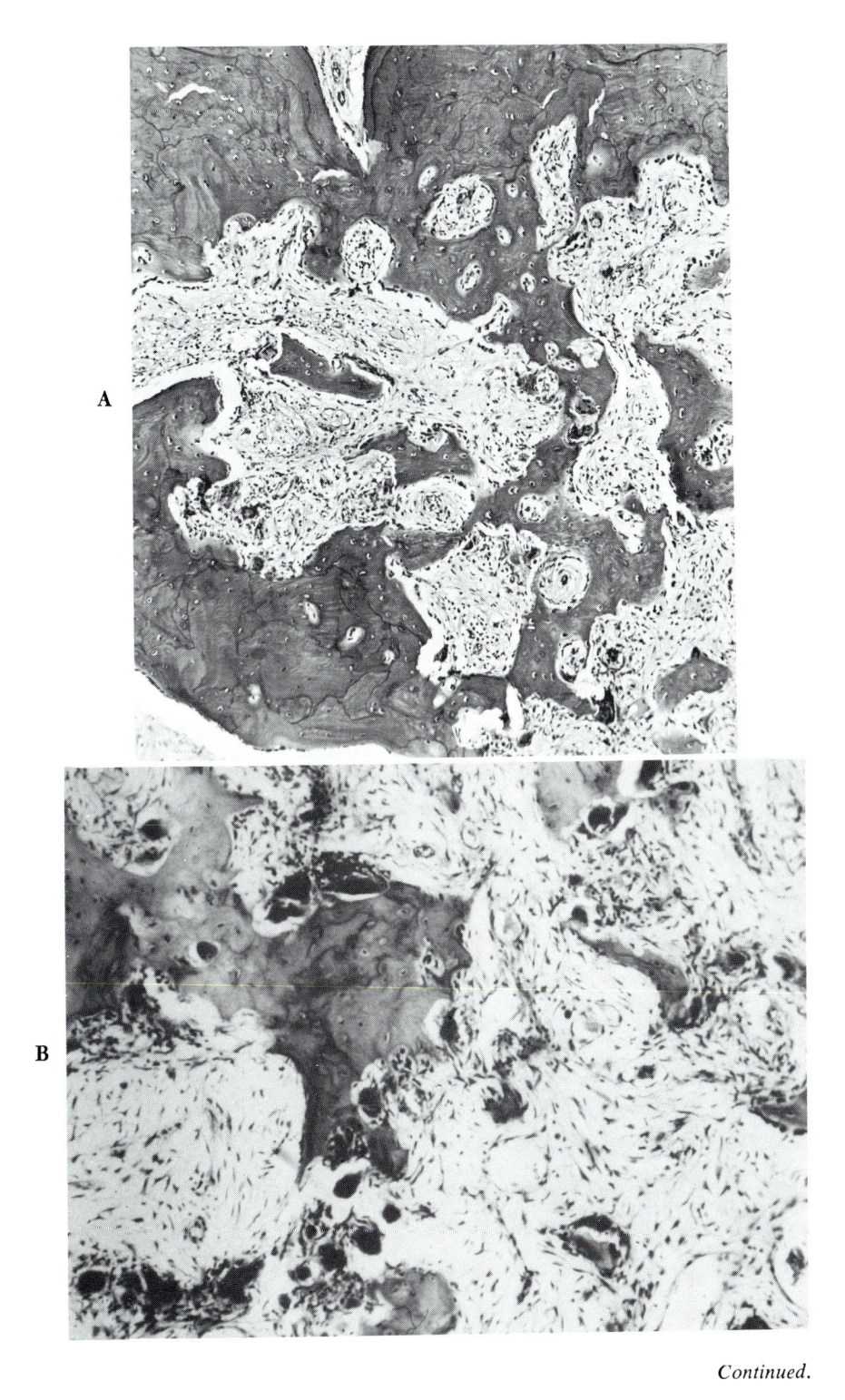

Fig. 11-9. For legend see opposite page.

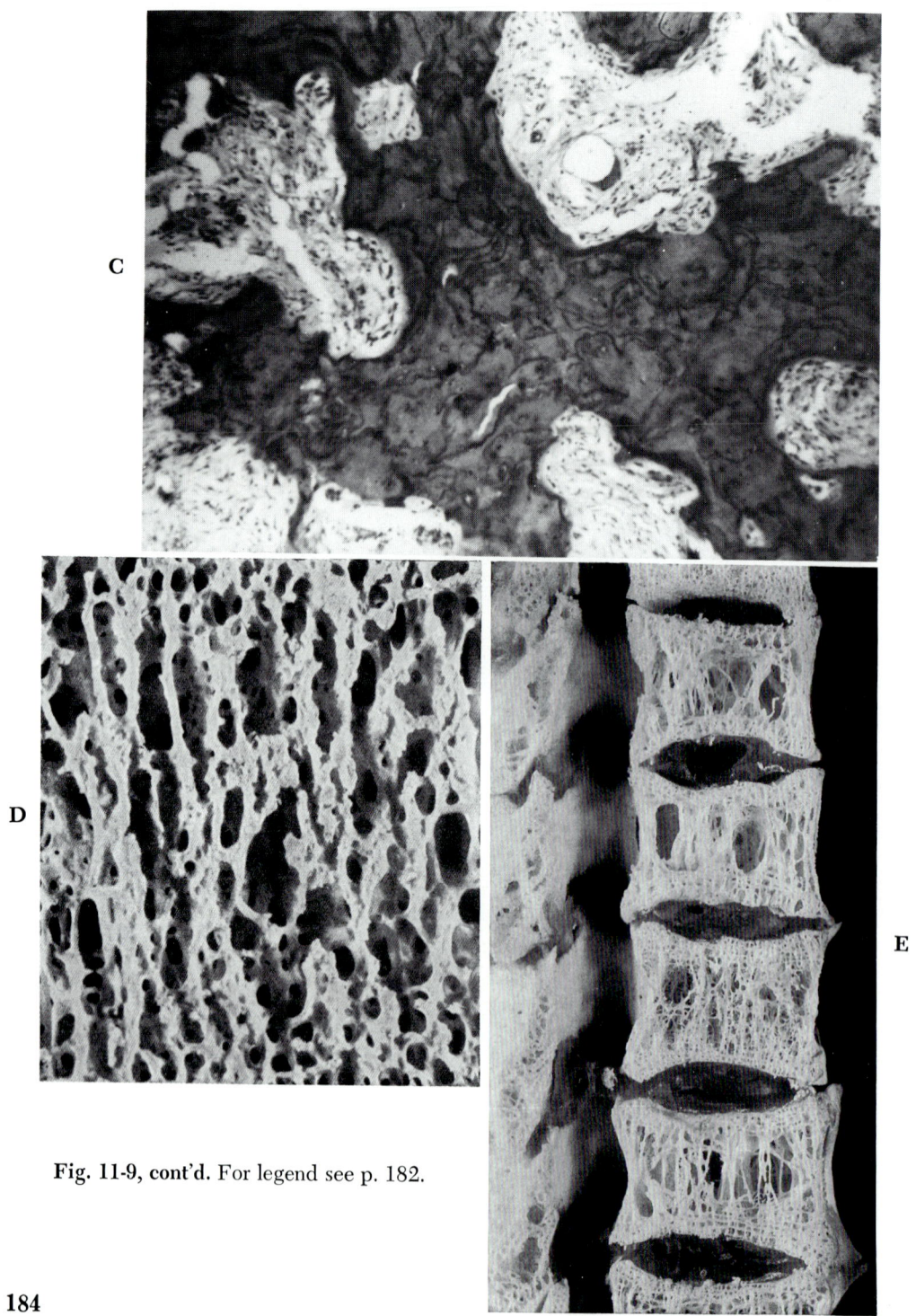

Diseases of bone and joints

C

D

E

Fig. 11-9, cont'd. For legend see p. 182.

Paget's disease of bone (osteitis deformans)

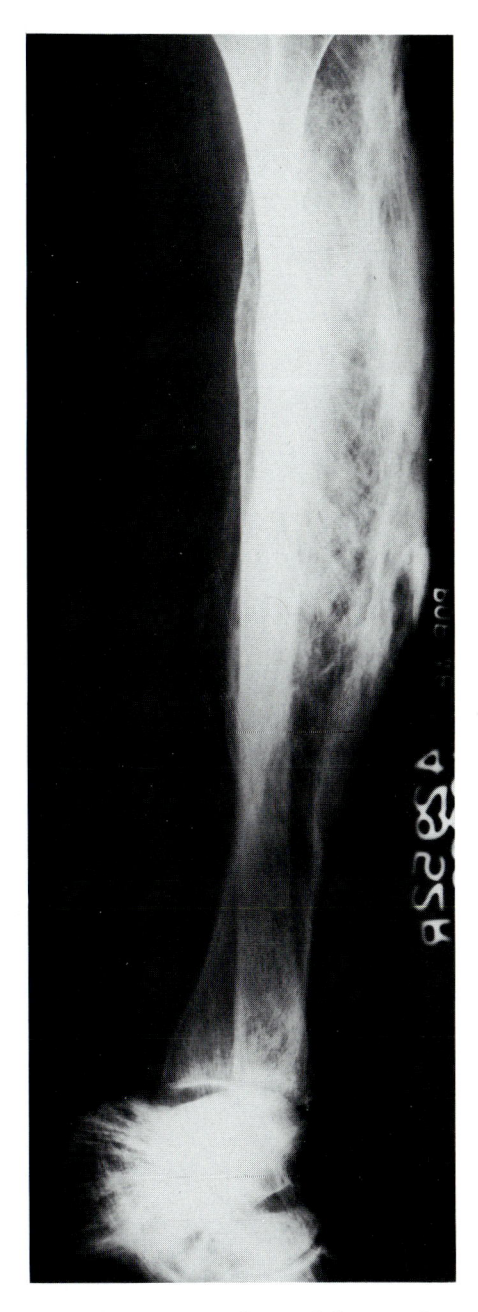

Fig. 11-10. Roentgenogram of a late or advanced lesion of Paget's disease in a tibia showing marked widening of the shaft and typical coarse trabecular architectural alteration. The latter is also evident in the calcaneus. Compare with Fig. 11-7, which shows an earlier stage in the evolution of the condition.

Diseases of bone and joints

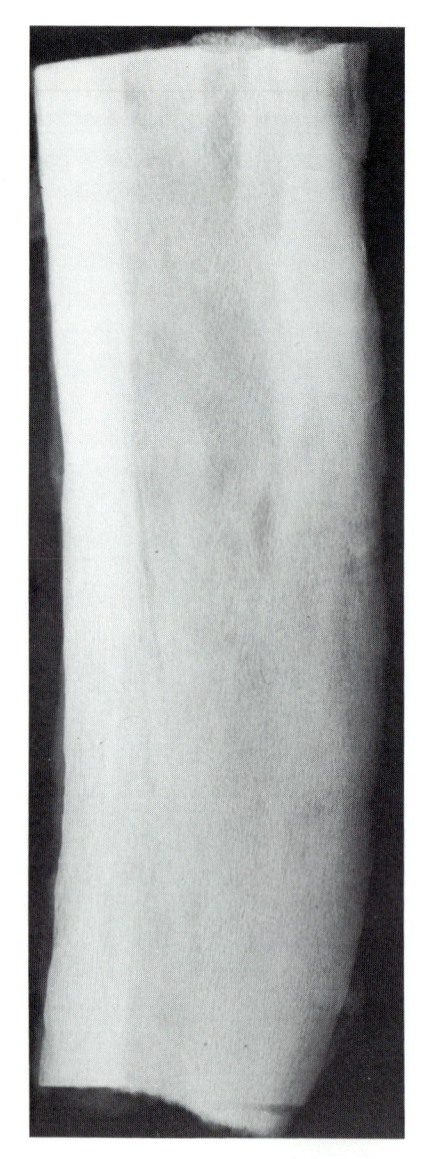

Fig. 11-11. Roentgenogram of a portion of the shaft of a tibia (obtained as an autopsy specimen) showing pronounced thickening and other changes of late Paget's disease.

(sometimes with cord compression) is quite understandable. In the skull, pronounced calvarial thickening as a late or end stage (Fig. 11-12) may lead to special problems (apart from headache) resulting from encroachment on the auditory canal, cochlea, or orbit. Also, in some instances a cosmetic problem is created by concomitant involvement of facial bones and maxillae (but not the mandible, as a rule).

For a meticulously detailed account of the pathologic anatomy of Paget bone, the natural tendency to healing, and the unusual development of osteosclerosis

Paget's disease of bone (osteitis deformans)

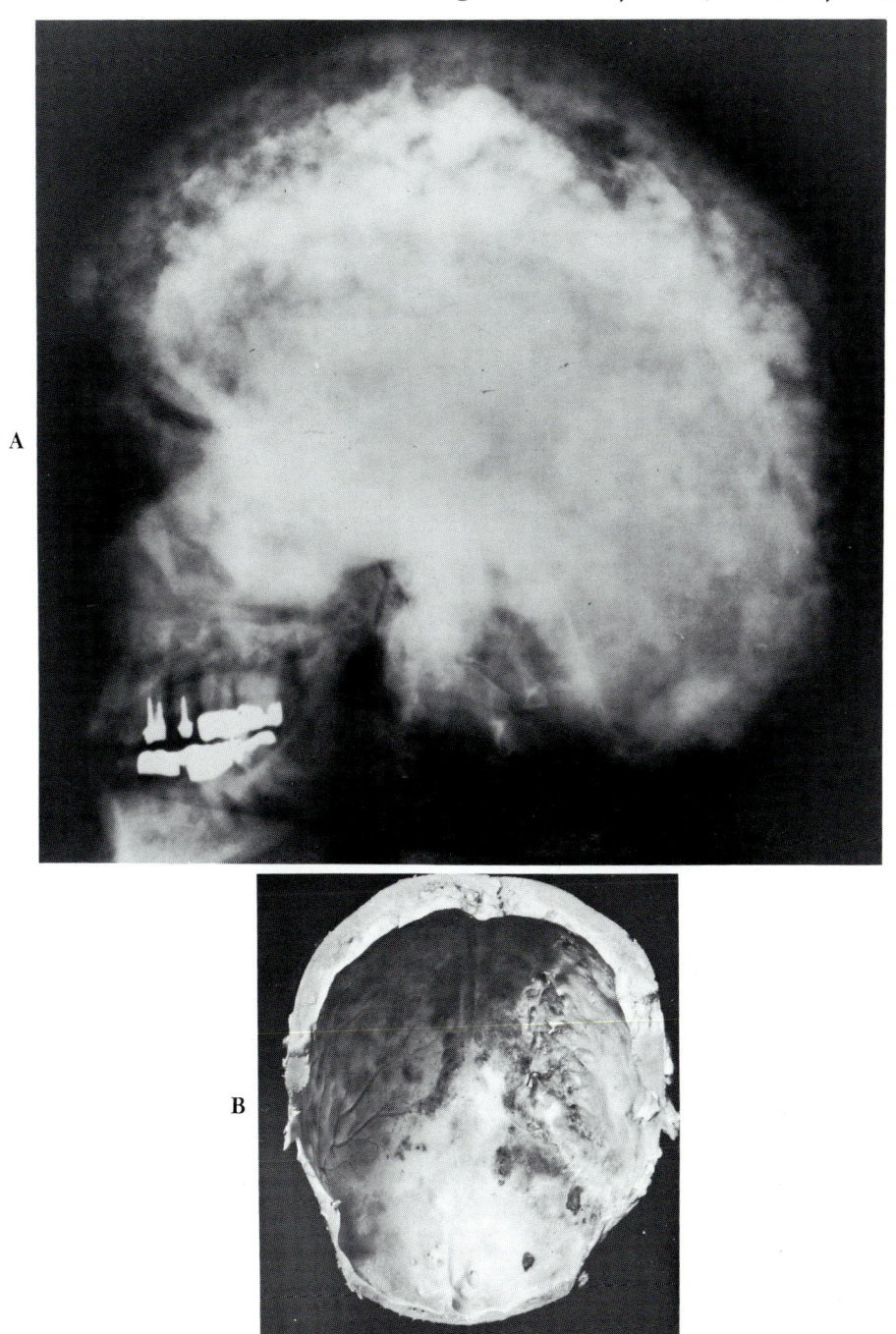

Fig. 11-12. **A,** Roentgenogram of a strikingly thickened and enlarged skull in a later stage of Paget's disease (so-called cotton-wool calvarium) showing transformation of its tables and relatively dense areas of new bone formation irregularly interspersed among more lucent areas of resorption. **B,** Frontal section through a calvarium showing pronounced thickening from Paget's disease in its posterior half (top of figure). The anterior half was uninvolved and serves as a normal control for comparison.

Diseases of bone and joints

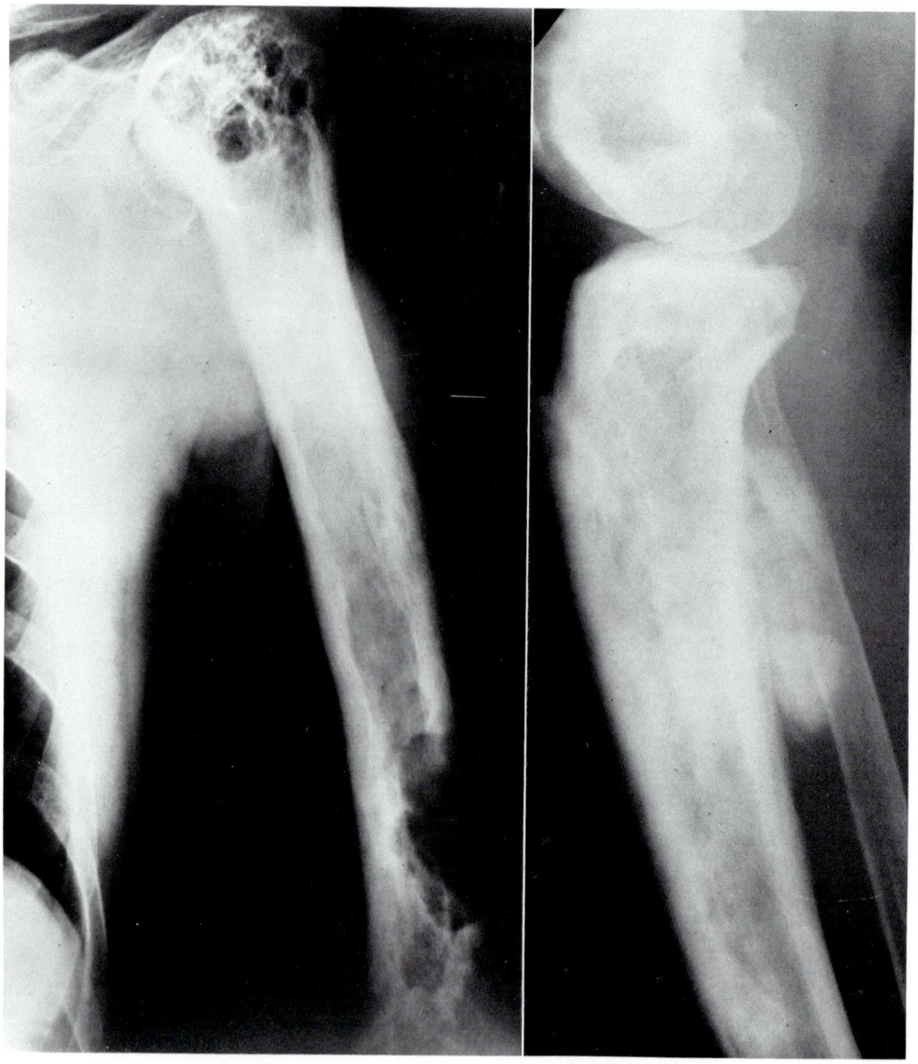

Fig. 11-13. **A,** Roentgenogram showing the development of two separate osteolytic foci of fibrosarcoma in Paget bone of a humerus, one in the upper end of the bone and the other in the lower shaft. The patient was a man in his sixties. **B,** Another Paget's sarcoma in a tibia of a woman, 77 years of age, that is clearly osteogenic in character. This patient also had changes of Paget's disease in the pelvis (not illustrated). **C,** Photomicrograph (low magnification) showing a moderately anaplastic fibrosarcoma developing in Paget bone (at the top). The latter is still undergoing active osteoclastic resorption.

Paget's disease of bone (osteitis deformans)

C

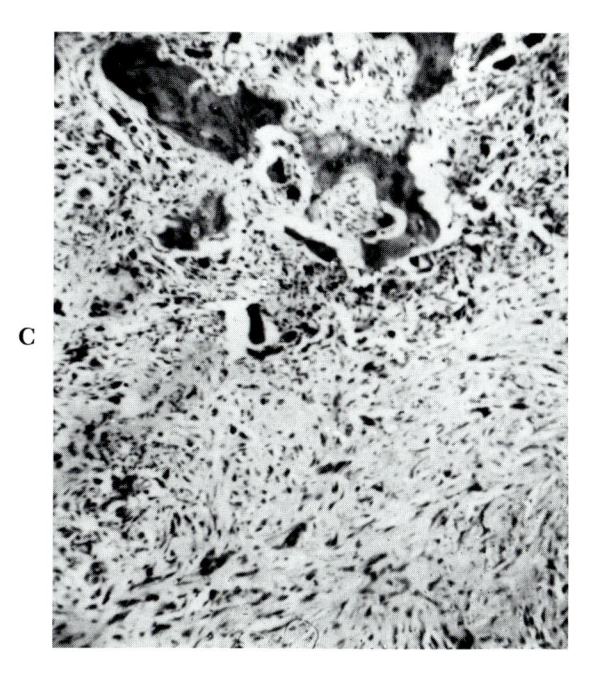

Fig. 11-13, cont'd. For legend see opposite page.

as an end stage in occasional instances, the reader may have profitable recourse to the articles of Jaffe[10,16] dating back to 1933. For highlights of some of the relevant clinical problems, as well as pathologic features, the richly illustrated paper of Goldenberg[4] is recommended.

Malignant change in Paget's disease. The problem of sarcoma developing in Paget's disease is an important one and has received considerable attention in recent years.[3] Sarcoma is usually observed in patients with fairly extensive Paget's disease of long standing, but it may occur even in monostotic Paget's disease. Commonly, it is some one bone that manifests malignant change. This is shown roentgenographically by the appearance of an ominous rarefied defect that had not been previously noted. However, it is not at all unusual to observe the development of two or more sarcomas simultaneously within bones transformed by Paget's disease, such as in the calvarium and in one or more of the large limb bones, particularly the femur, tibia, and humerus (Fig. 11-13).

The neoplasm that develops is most often an osteogenic sarcoma, but it need not be that. It may prove to be fibrosarcoma or an anaplastic tumor containing many multinuclear tumor cells, so as to simulate malignant giant cell tumor. The development of chondrosarcoma in Paget bone has also been observed,[4] although this is distinctly unusual. Whatever the type of sarcoma, it grows rapidly and metastasizes early, as a rule, so that the prognosis is distinctly bad. There are relatively few survivors beyond 1 year or less, even after well-conceived, prompt radical surgery.

189

Diseases of bone and joints

OTHER HYPEROSTOSES AFFECTING THE SKULL PARTICULARLY

There are many diverse conditions that may lead to localized thickening of the calvarium, facial bones, or jaw bones.

Hyperostosis frontalis interna, as its name clearly indicates, is characterized by irregular thickening of the inner table of the frontal bone just above the orbital plate, from knobby or bosselated excrescences of bone, which may be compact or cancellous, but is usually of mature lamellar type. The condition develops in certain women, especially obese women past menopause, who may also be hirsute and display other signs of virilism. These observations date back to Morgagni (1761) and were the subject of a monograph by Henschen[17] in 1949.

It is interesting that focal hyperostoses, or accretions of woven bone, may sometimes develop in the skull of women during pregnancy, only to disappear after childbirth. This manifestation, presumably an estrogen effect, is reminiscent

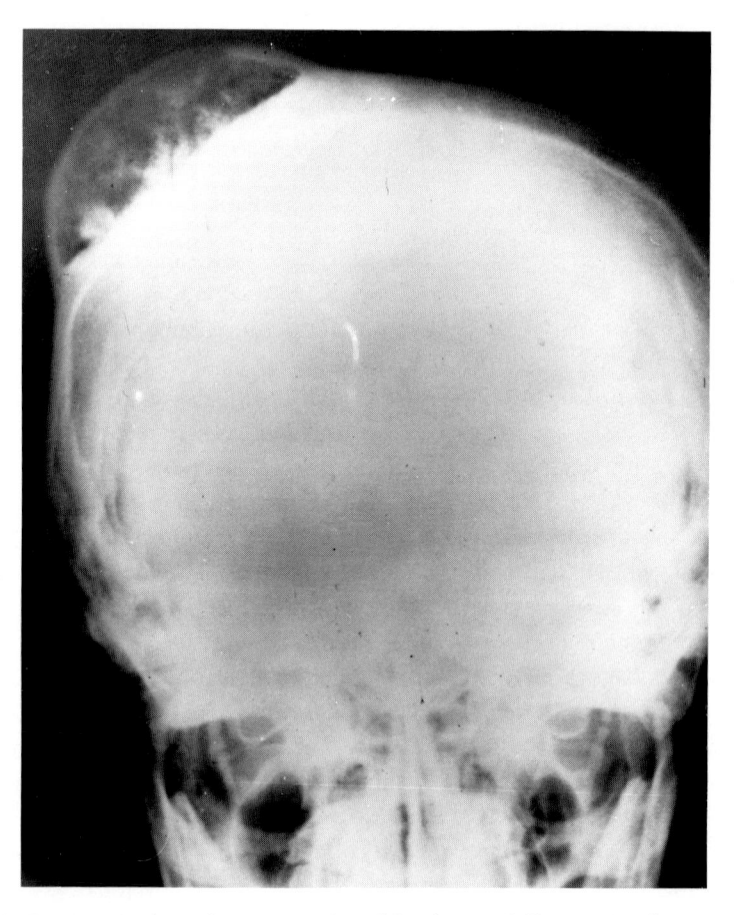

Fig. 11-14. Roentgenogram showing a blisterlike focus of fibrous dysplasia in a calvarium, where it has expanded the outer table. (The patient's chief complaint was that he could not keep his hat straight.)

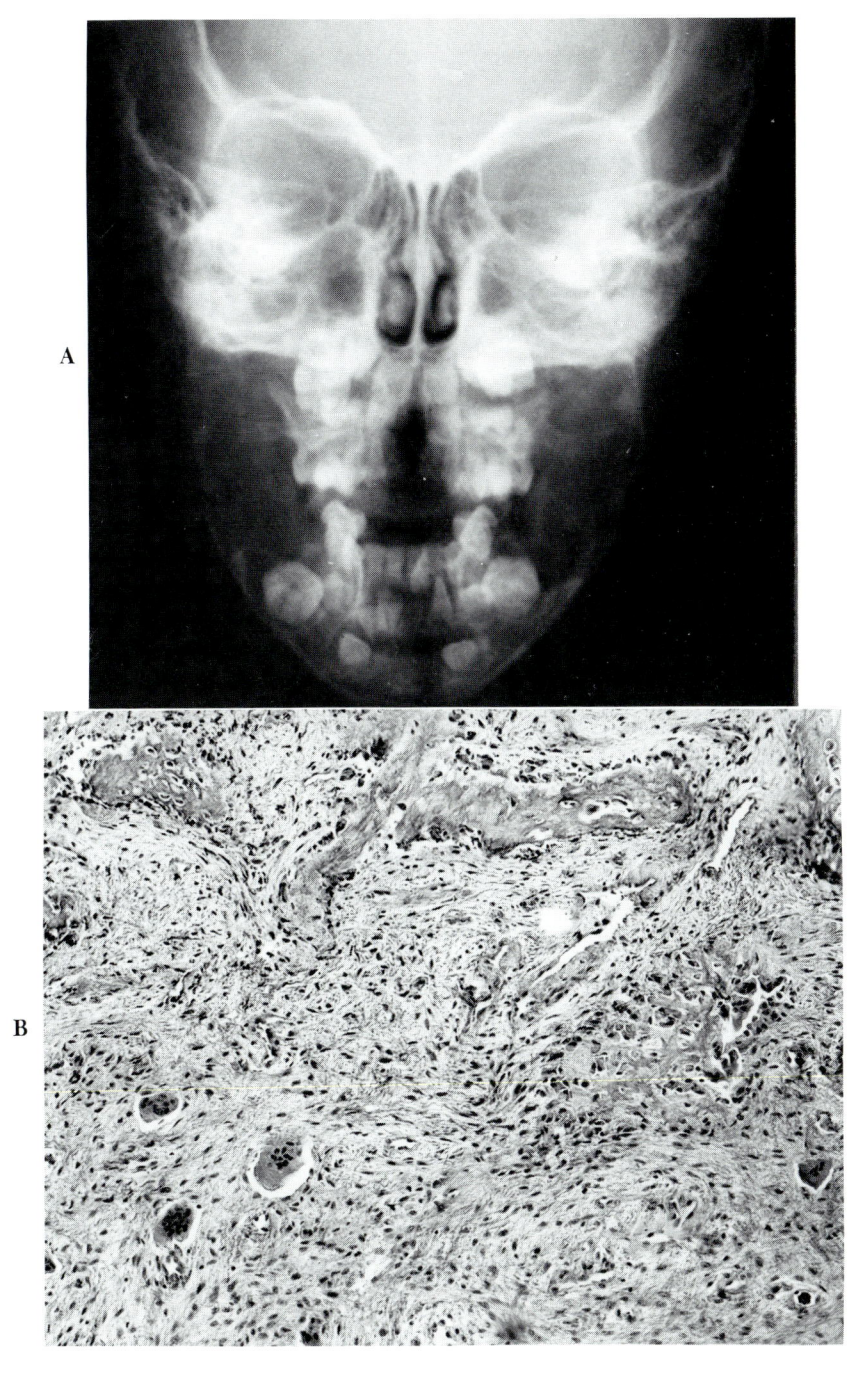

Fig. 11-15. **A,** Roentgenogram showing changes in the mandible of a child with cherubism. Note bilateral symmetrical expansion and marked thinning of the cortex. **B,** Photomicrograph of a representative field of the transformed mandible in the same child. The lesion apparently represents a peculiar fibro-osseous dysplasia different from fibrous dysplasia of bone. The osseous trabeculae were sparse and dispersed at random; elsewhere the lesion was more collagenous. The giant cells were obviously osteoclastlike macrophages found mainly within small vascular spaces. (×125.)

Diseases of bone and joints

of the rapid growth of temporary cancellous bone in the medullary cavity of the bones of egg-laying birds.

Osteomata may occasionally present on the outer surface of the calvarium as circumscribed, rounded, ivorylike exostoses, but more often they are found protruding into the orbit or one of the paranasal sinuses. If one examines such an osteoma before it is fully evolved, it is seen to be composed of prominent plaques and trabeculae of new bone within a benign osteoblastic connective tissue matrix.[3]

Localized gigantism, which may on rare occasions affect the skull and contiguous soft parts, is an example of a developmental anomaly producing asymmetrical enlargement and distortion.

Tumors, especially meningiomas, may also be responsible for localized hyperostosis of the calvarium. An appreciable number of meningiomas penetrate the dura and invade the overlying bone, and occasionally the reactive osteosclerosis that ensues may be sufficiently pronounced to produce a prominent, tumorlike protuberance (meningeom-hyperostose).[18] On the other hand, meningioma en plaque extensively invading the calvarium may sometimes have a striking lytic effect on the bone. I have seen a case in point in which, over a period of several years, virtually the entire anterior half of the calvarium disappeared radiographically. A focus of myeloma in the calvarium may sometimes produce not the customary rarefied defect but reactive osteosclerosis with perpendicular orientation of the new bone striae to the tables, so that the roentgenogram simulates that of reaction to a meningioma.

Fibrous dysplasia is still another condition that may bring about a sizable, localized, blisterlike expansion of the outer table of the calvarium (Fig. 11-14), although more often it induces thickening of the bones at the base of the skull. It may also manifest itself in deforming localized expansion of one or both of the jaw bones, especially in young patients (see Figs. 2-1, *B* and 2-4, *A*).

Symmetrical enlargement of the mandibles and distinctive eye changes may be observed in the peculiar localized developmental disorder known as *cherubism* (Fig. 11-5).

Congenital syphilis may sometimes result in pronounced skeletal hyperostoses. In these circumstances, parts of the skull and facial bones (as well as the limb bones) may become abnormally thick and dense. This unusual picture is said to be similar to that in certain cases of *goundou*.[19] The latter, a peculiar form of exostosis of the maxilla, is thought by Hackett[20] to be a manifestation of tertiary yaws.

In some instances of *Paget's disease*, the skull, facial bones, and maxillae alone are affected. (Such cases were at one time thought to represent leontiasis ossea.)

There may well be additional unusual causes of hyperostosis and transformation of one or another part of the skull, but the long list that has been presented will suffice to indicate that the problem in differential diagnosis can be quite complex.

Instances of slowly developing, more generalized thickening of the facial

Paget's disease of bone (osteitis deformans)

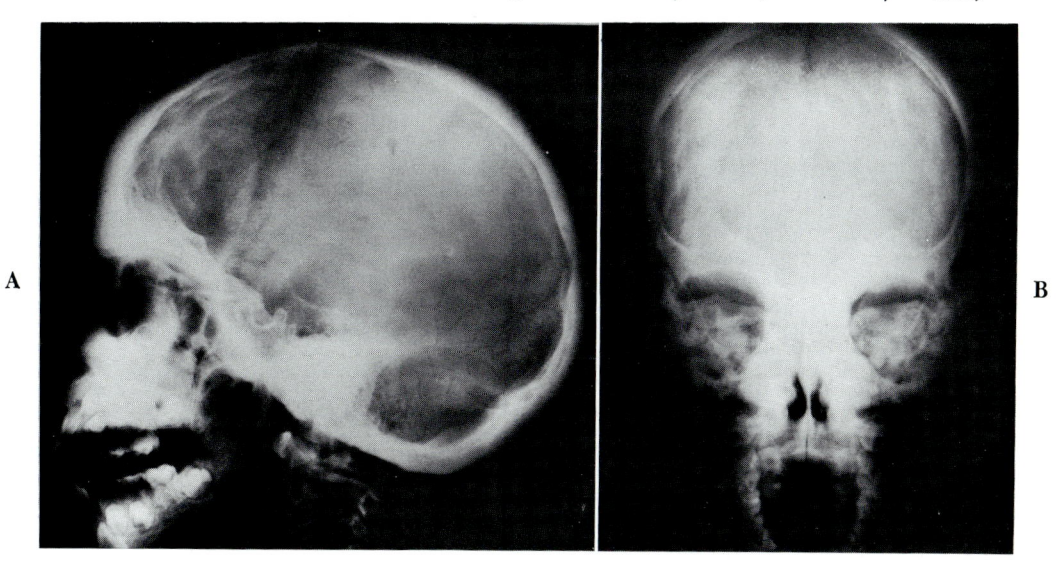

Fig. 11-16. Lateral and anteroposterior views showing the striking changes of familial hyperostosis of the skull and facial bones. Two other children in the family showed similar changes. (Courtesy Dr. E. C. H. Lehmann, Vancouver, British Columbia.)

bones, often associated with comparable changes in the lower jaw and cranium (not resulting from any of the specific conditions previously mentioned) have for a long time been designated as *leontiasis ossea*.[21-23] The swelling and deformity of these bones, depending on their extent, may or may not result in nasal obstruction, proptosis, or impairment of vision. Leontiasis ossea, however, is not a pathologic entity. It appears rather to represent a miscellaneous category, some components of which are not as well understood as they might be. Some instances in point apparently result from a spreading, sclerosing, inflammatory osteoperiostitis (thought possibly to be infectious, but actually of obscure nature). Others are associated with polyposis of the colon and soft tissue tumors and have a familial pattern,[24] apparently indicative of a peculiar developmental disorder predicated on a gene defect (Gardner's syndrome). In still others, the thickened bones are said to be rarefied rather than sclerotic, and there is apparently no significant inflammatory reaction (infection) in evidence. What the latter cases represent, no one knows.

That familial hyperostosis of the skull and facial bones can occur without associated intestinal polyposis or other apparent anomalies is evidenced by a case in point that I saw in consultation in 1955 for Dr. E. C. H. Lehmann of Vancouver, British Columbia.[25] In this family, three siblings presented unusual, diffuse thickening of the facial bones and of the skull, especially along its base (Fig. 11-16). Biopsy of the parietal bone of one of the children, then 6 years of age, showed great thickening of the bone without any significant alteration in its histologic pattern. Comparable involvement (seen roentgenographically) of the calvarium, facial bones, and mandible, as well as of other extracranial bones (ribs, clavicles, metacarpals, metatarsals, phalanges, and so forth) has been reported by van Buchem and his associates[26] under the title of "Hyperostosis Corticalis Generalisata." It is noteworthy that of their seven patients there was a set of twins and another pair of siblings. Subsequently, Fosmoe, Holm, and Hildreth[27] reported the roentgenographic findings in another case (in an adult) of even greater extent and severity under the heading of van Buchem's disease. Whether the cases presenting familial cranial hyperostosis exclusively and those presenting extracranial skeletal involvement as well are closely related would appear to be a moot point at this time.

Still another distinctive familial expression of dysplasia distorting the craniofacial bones, especially the mandible, but involving other parts of the skeleton as well, was described recently by Anderson and associates[28] under the title of "Familial Osteodysplasia." These authors also cite several other genetic disorders described in the literature that feature malformation of the facial bones. Altogether, it is apparent that the subject as a whole is quite complex and requires further clarification beyond anything possible at this time.

REFERENCES

1. Edholm, O. G., Howarth, S., and McMichael, J.: Heart failure and bone blood flow in osteitis deformans, Clin. Sci. **5:** 249, 1945.
2. Schmorl, G.: Über osteitis deformans Paget, Virch. Arch. Path. Anat. **283:**694, 1932.
3. Lichtenstein, L.: Bone tumors, ed. 4, St. Louis, 1972, The C. V. Mosby Co., p. 228.
4. Goldenberg, R. R.: The skeleton in Paget's disease, Bull. Hosp. Joint Dis. **12:** 229, 1951.
5. Hutter, R. V. P., Foote, F. W., Jr., Frazell, E. L., and Francis, K. C.: Giant cell tumors complicating Paget's disease of bone, Cancer **16:**1044, 1963.
6. Paget, J.: On a form of chronic inflammation of bones (osteitis deformans), Trans. R. Chir. Soc. London **60:**37, 1877.
7. Reifenstein, E. C., Jr., and Albright, F.: Paget's disease: a concept as to its pathologic physiology and the importance of this in the complication arising from fracture and immobilization, N. Engl. J. Med. **231:**525, 1944.
8. Wagner, M.: Report of case of Paget's disease in 18-year-old male, with review of literature, Wis. Med. J. **46:**1098, 1947.
9. Evens, R. G., and Bartter, F. C.: The hereditary aspects of Paget's disease (osteitis deformans), J.A.M.A. **205:**900, 1968.
10. Jaffe, H. L.: Paget's disease of bone, Arch. Pathol. **15:**83, 1933. (Contains a survey of pathologic alterations.)
11. Purves, M. J.: Some effects of administering sodium fluoride to patients with Paget's disease, Lancet **2:**1188, 1962.
12. Ryan, W. G., Schwartz, T. B., and Northrop, G.: Experiences in the treatment of Paget's disease of bone with mithramycin, J.A.M.A. **213:**1153, 1970.
13. Goldfield, E. B., Braiker, B. M., Prendergast, J., and Kolb, F. O.: Synthetic salmon calcitonin: treatment of Paget's disease and osteogenesis imperfecta, J.A.M.A. **221:**1127, 1972.
14. Smith, R., Russell, R. G. G., and Bishop, M.: Diphosphonates and Paget's disease of bone, Lancet **1:**945, 1971.
15. Erdheim, J.: Über die genese der Pagetschen Knochenerkrankung, Beitr. Path. Anat. Path. **96:**1, 1935.
16. Jaffe, H. L.: Atypical form of Paget's disease appearing as generalized osteosclerosis, Arch. Pathol. **16:**769, 1933.
17. Henschen, F.: Morgagni's syndrome: hyperostosis frontalis interna, virilismus, obesitas, Edinburgh, 1949, Oliver and Boyd, Ltd.
18. Oehlecker, F.: Eine ungewöhnliche Geschwülst des Schädeldaches (Meningeom-Hyperostose), Zbl. Chir. **34:**1433, 1952.
19. Hodges, P. C., Phemister, D. B., and Brunschwig, A.: The roentgen-ray diagnosis of diseases of the bones and joints, New York, 1938, Thomas Nelson & Sons, p. 44.

20. Hackett, C. J.: Bone lesions of yaws in Uganda, Oxford, 1951, Blackwell Scientific Publications, Ltd.
21. Evans, J.: Leontiasis ossea: a critical review with report of 4 original cases, J. Bone Joint Surg. 35-B:229, 1953.
22. Fairbanks, H. A. T.: An atlas of general affections of the skeleton, Edinburgh, 1951, E. & S. Livingstone Ltd., pp. 206-208.
23. Knaggs, R. L.: Leontiasis ossea, Br. J. Surg. 11:347, 1923.
24. Plenk, H. P., and Gardner, E. J.: Osteomatosis (leontiasis ossea): hereditary disease of membranous bone formation associated in one family with polyposis of the colon, Radiology 62:830, 1954.
25. Lehmann, E. C. H.: Familial hyperostosis of the skull and facial bones, J. Bone Joint Surg. 39-B:313, 1957.
26. Van Buchem, F. S., Hadders, H. N., Hansen, J. F., and Woldring, M. G.: Hyperostosis corticalis generalisata: report of seven cases, Am. J. Med. 33:387, 1962.
27. Fosmoe, R. J., Holm, R. S., and Hildreth, R. C.: Van Buchem's disease (hyperostosis corticalis generalisata familiaris), Radiology 90:771, 1968.
28. Anderson, L. G., Cook, A. J., Coccaro, P. J., Coro, C. J., and Bosma, J. F.: Familial osteodysplasia, J.A.M.A. 220:1687, 1972.

GENERAL REFERENCES

Barry, H. C.: Paget's disease of bone, Baltimore, 1970, The Williams & Wilkins Co.

Editorial: Newer therapies in Paget's disease of bone, J.A.M.A. 217:1383, 1971.

chapter 12

Histiocytosis X
(eosinophilic granuloma, Letterer-Siwe disease, and Schüller-Christian disease)

The integrated concept[1-5] of eosinophilic granuloma of bone, Letterer-Siwe disease, and Shüller-Christian disease as interrelated manifestations of a single nosologic entity has gained wide acceptance in recent years. The name "histiocytosis X," proposed by me[2] in 1953 as a provisional broad general designation for this malady, likewise appears to have taken hold. For an account of the historic development of this concept to which many American and European investigators have contributed, for the detailed pathologic evidence in its support, and for convenient clinical orientation including discussion of specific indications for rational therapy, the reader may have recourse to critical reviews on the subject published in 1953 and 1964, respectively.[2,5]

The interrelationship of the various clinical and pathologic manifestations is outlined in the following classification of histiocytosis X, first set forth[2] in 1953. The recognized types of clinical involvement can be grouped under the general heading and still be differentiated from one another, so that useful distinctions having a bearing on treatment and prognosis are maintained.

CLASSIFICATION OF HISTIOCYTOSIS X

Histiocytosis X, localized to bone (eosinophilic granuloma, solitary or multiple)
Histiocytosis X, disseminated, acute or subacute (Letterer-Siwe syndrome)
    With destructive skeletal lesions (eosinophilic granuloma)
    With transition to chronic phase (Schüller-Christian disease)
Histiocytosis X, disseminated, chronic (Schüller-Christian syndrome)
    With destructive skeletal lesions (eosinophilic granuloma)
    With early extraskeletal lesions (indicate sites) resembling eosinophilic granuloma
    With acute or subacute exacerbation (Letterer-Siwe disease)
    With involvement predominantly of bones, the lungs, pituitary gland, the brain, skin, and mucous membranes (oral, anal, genital), the liver or lymph nodes, and so on (in varying combinations, as the case may be)

There can no longer be any doubt that Letterer-Siwe disease and Schüller-Christian disease represent acute (or subacute) and chronic expressions, respectively, of the disseminated form of the malady. In this connection, it must be

Histiocytosis X

recognized that both these eponyms were adopted as convenient provisional designations for ostensibly finite clinical syndromes at a time when their intimate relationship could hardly be suspected. In other ways also, our concept of the conditions so designated has broadened in scope far beyond anything the authors concerned could ever envision.

As for the lesion of eosinophilic granuloma, it seems clear from pathologic evidence now available that it represents the pathologic expression of early, rapidly developing reaction to the etiologic agent, whatever it may ultimately prove to be. As such, it may appear not only within bone, where its presence was first recognized,[6] but also in many other sites, notably in lymph nodes, oral cavity (gingiva, palate, and so on), and anogenital region, as well as in the lungs, thymus, liver, kidneys, female genitalia, and possibly the eye and cranial nerves (in time, there will undoubtedly be other additions). Further, the lesion of eosinophilic granuloma may also appear in the lungs, liver, bones, and other sites as the pathologic expression of recrudescence in well-established, chronic, disseminated histiocytosis X, even of long standing (Fig. 12-1).

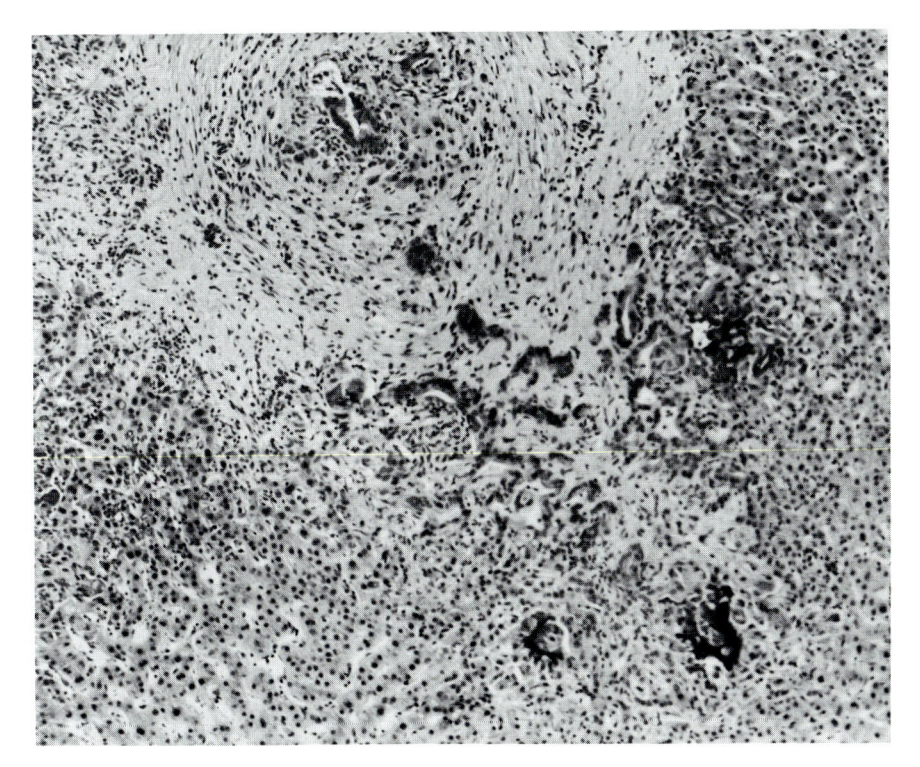

Fig. 12-1. Photomicrograph of a liver biopsy from an adult with long-standing chronic disseminated histiocytosis in recrudescence (he had had recurring osseous, buccal, and cutaneous lesions over a period of some 15 years). Note the small bile duct (at the top) surrounded by an involuting histiocytic nodule (containing some eosinophils) and enveloped by inflammatory scar tissue. In its vicinity one also sees proliferating bile ducts and markedly distended bile canaliculi (going on in the other areas to bile lakes). (×90.)

In regard to the etiology of histiocytosis X, I still favor infection, conceivably of viral nature, as a more plausible explanation than any alternative. Although no specific infectious agent has been identified, there are indirect clinical indications suggesting infection, notably the bouts of fever associated at times with the appearance of fresh lesions in bone and other sites; the fever, night sweats, and loss of weight associated with the onset of severe pulmonary involvement in some cases, so that the initial clinical impression is active tuberculosis; and the spread of lesions in skin and bone to regional lymph nodes.[5] Further, I have seen material from a case of eosinophilic granuloma in the skull of a teenage girl whose father also developed a focus of eosinophilic granuloma in the skull the following year. These are admittedly only straws in the wind, but they all seem to lean in the same direction.

The question of an infectious origin should undoubtedly be investigated further with modern techniques of virus culture, tissue culture, and electron microscopy. In recent years there has been some activity along these lines. A group of French investigators[7] has demonstrated cytoplasmic rod-shaped inclusion bodies in electron microscopic preparations from pulmonary and osseous lesions of histiocytosis X. This observation has been confirmed by DeMans,[8] but the significance of these bodies is still uncertain, since they have been found in Langerhans' cells in lymph nodes and skin in other conditions.[9]

The discussion that follows represents essentially a digest of the views expressed in previous articles on the subject by myself and my colleagues,[1-5] especially the reviews published in 1953[2] and 1964.[5] My observations since then have served to confirm the usefulness of these concepts as a basis for comprehensive orientation. I have not found it necessary to postulate atypical or transition forms of the disorder to explain the clinical and pathologic findings in any given case, as was the vogue some years ago. The extensive literature has further substantiated these views and broadened their scope.

EOSINOPHILIC GRANULOMA OF BONE
(histiocytosis X localized in bone)

The mildest and most favorable expression of the disease (histiocytosis X) is represented by cases presenting one, several, or occasionally many destructive foci within the skeleton, and otherwise showing neither apparent constitutional indications of illness nor any discernible evidence of cutaneous, pulmonary, hypophyseal, or other extraskeletal involvement. The pathologically descriptive name "eosinophilic granuloma of bone"[6] still seems to be an appropriate designation for such instances, which merit special consideration by virtue of their auspicious prognosis. I am inclined to regard this skeletal localization as an indication of successful confinement of the etiologic agent, which may well account for the favorable outcome. One can venture a good prognosis for recovery in such cases, even though an appreciable number of skeletal lesions are present and even though additional skeletal lesions subsequently make their appearance, as occasionally happens.

Histiocytosis X

In the matter of clinical diagnosis, it is worth emphasizing again that a focus of eosinophilic granuloma of bone is prone to develop so rapidly and to break through the cortex of the affected bone so readily that, prior to biopsy, it is often mistaken clinically for a primary malignant tumor, especially Ewing's sarcoma (Fig. 12-2). By the same token, comparable multiple foci appearing in the skeleton of a child, for example, may conceivably give rise to the initial impression of metastatic neuroblastoma. Despite their seemingly ominous behavior, however, it is well known that such lesions heal readily following curettement or roentgen therapy (in relatively small dosage). It has also been demonstrated[1] that they may even regress or disappear spontaneously.

It is also important to emphasize that, in actual practice, it is not always possible on initial examination, especially in a young child, to be certain that skeletal lesions pathologically identified as eosinophilic granuloma do not have

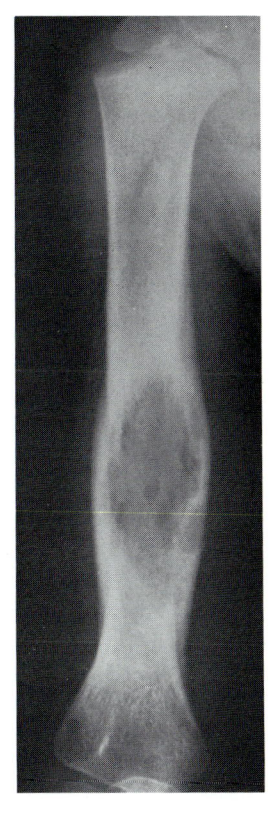

Fig. 12-2. Roentgenogram of a solitary focus of eosinophilic granuloma in the lower shaft of the humerus of a child, 2 years of age, who had restricted motion and some tenderness for about 2 months. The lesion was thought to be a tumor and the affected segment of the bone was resected. Good reconstruction was obtained by the use of a tibial graft reinforced by abundant cancellous bone from the iliac crest. Had the diagnosis been established by frozen section at the time of surgery, thorough curetment and packing would have sufficed for cure.

Diseases of bone and joints

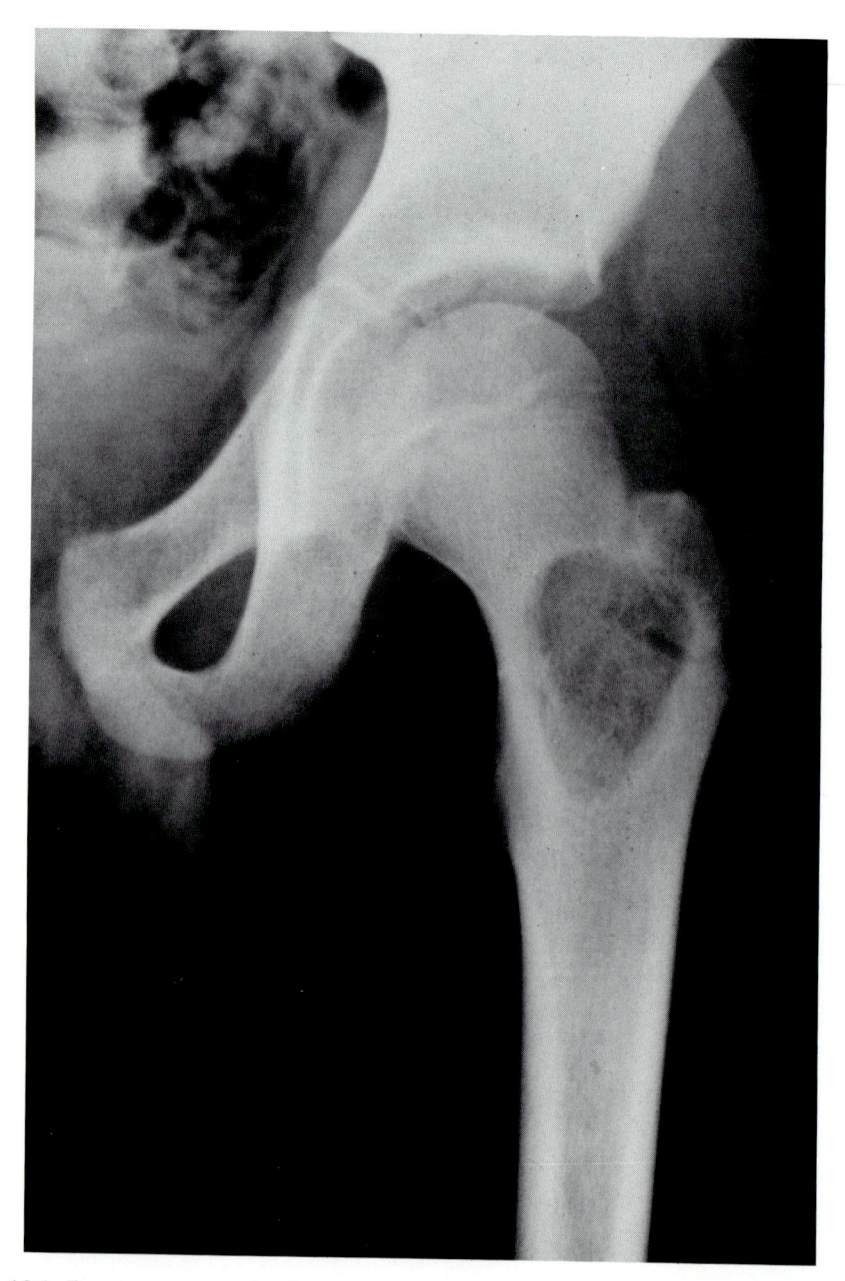

Fig. 12-3. Roentgenogram of a lesion of eosinophilic granuloma in the intertrochanteric region of a femur in a child, which was thought to be a bone cyst before surgery. Cure was obtained by thorough curetment and packing with bone chips. No additional foci were found on skeletal survey.

Histiocytosis X

their histiocytic counterpart elsewhere, or that extraskeletal lesions will not manifest themselves subsequently, even though at the time roentgenographic examination of the chest is negative and physical examination fails to reveal involvement of the skin, mucous membranes, or hemopoietic organs. To be more explicit, inasmuch as the pathologic lesion of eosinophilic granuloma of bone represents the expression of acute skeletal involvement in the disease as a whole (histiocytosis X), whether this be localized or disseminated, it follows that from the roentgenogram of such a lesion, or even from a biopsy of it alone, one cannot make any reliable forecast as to prognosis, since this depends largely upon whether there is associated visceral involvement and more particularly upon the distribution, extent, and severity of these visceral lesions. In certain instances, it may be necessary to reserve judgment and to follow the patient closely for a number of months or even for several years. In particular, the clinician must be on the alert for such indications as fatigability, chronic malnutrition, loss of weight, slight fever, predisposition to secondary infections, and the frequent appearance of new skeletal defects as harbingers of systemic involvement of potentially serious import.

Today experienced radiologists are very likely to consider the possibility of

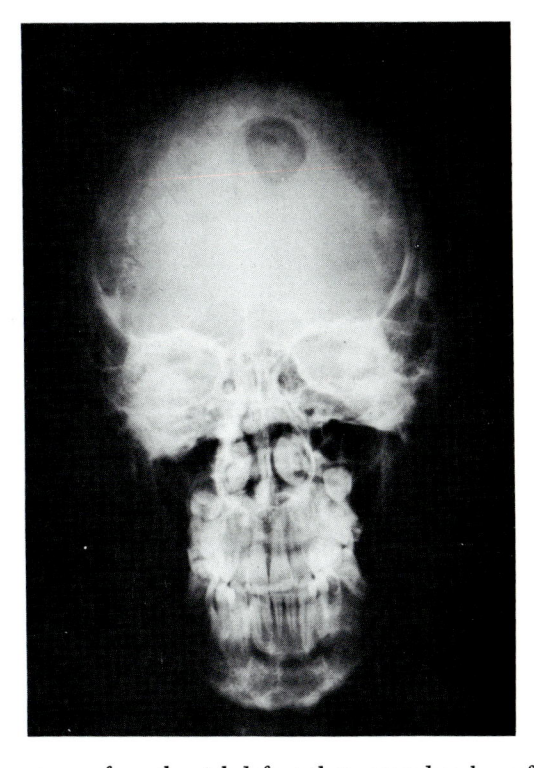

Fig. 12-4. Roentgenogram of a calvarial defect that proved to be a focus of eosinophilic granuloma. This is a common site of localization. To venture any opinion as to prognosis, one would have to know whether the disease was disseminated or confined to bone.

Diseases of bone and joints

eosinophilic granuloma in the differential diagnosis of rapidly developing, destructive lesions of bone (Figs. 12-2 to 12-4). Recognition of the lesion by pathologists in most instances occasions little difficulty, even when the histologic picture is altered by extensive hemorrhage and necrosis with giant cell reaction. When the diagnosis is missed or is not clear at the onset, it is generally for one of two reasons. First, prolonged acid treatment of the surgical specimen for decalcification interferes with the staining of the eosinophilic granules within leukocytes—whenever possible, bits of soft tissue not requiring decalcification should be processed separately. Second, lesions that are removed relatively late may be extensively modified by pathologic fracture, cortical perforation, scarring, and periosteal new bone reaction. In these circumstances, one may have to scrutinize all available tissue fragments closely for telltale foci of eosinophilic granuloma featuring proliferating histiocytes admixed with clumps of eosinophils (Figs. 12-6 and 12-7, A).

With reference to age incidence, eosinophilic granuloma of bone may occasionally affect infants as well as older children and adults. In older adults, a lesion of eosinophilic granuloma (in a rib, for example) may be asymptomatic.

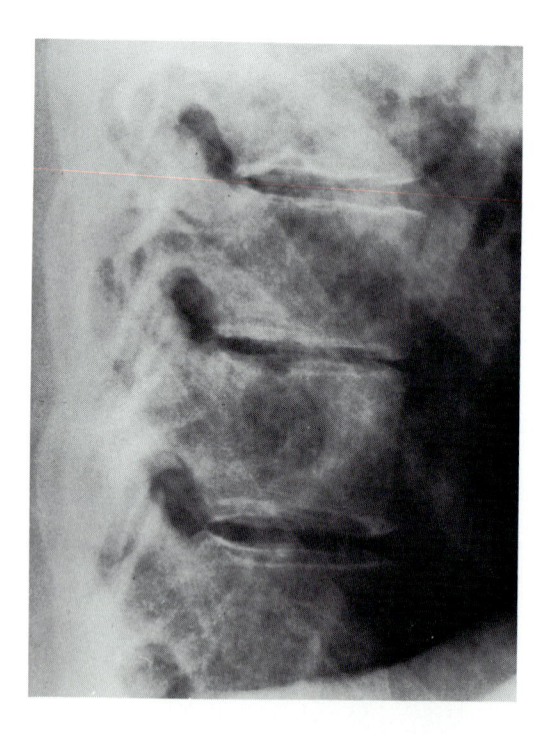

Fig. 12-5. Roentgenogram of a rarefied lesion of eosinophilic granuloma in the body of the tenth thoracic vertebra of an adult, who also presented additional foci in several other bones as well as diffuse bilateral pulmonary infiltration indicative of chronic disseminated histiocytosis X. (The importance of a chest film and of thorough physical examination in such patients must be emphasized.) The skeletal lesions were effectively controlled by roentgen therapy in comparatively small dosage.

The most common sites of localization are the limb bones, skull, vertebral column, and innominate bone (Figs. 12-2 to 12-5), but the lesion may be encountered elsewhere.

When eosinophilic granuloma localizes in a vertebral body, it may lead to compression fracture with pronounced flattening and, sometimes, to spinal cord or nerve root impingement. In children, this may develop insidiously without early detection. Vertebra plana (Calvé's disease), long thought to result from avascular necrosis, is commonly a sequel of eosinophilic granuloma.

ACUTE (OR SUBACUTE) DISSEMINATED HISTIOCYTOSIS X
(Letterer-Siwe syndrome)

Before instituting treatment or venturing an opinion as to prognosis, one should be certain of the diagnosis on pathologic as well as clinical grounds. It must be borne in mind that the German pediatrician Siwe described only a clinical syndrome rather than a pathologic entity. It so happens that the same combination of clinical manifestations may be caused not only by acute disseminated histiocytosis X but also by neoplastic reticulosis (or reticuloendotheliosis) with or without associated leukemia. Although the necessity for making a sharp distinction between the two conditions seems clear enough, there

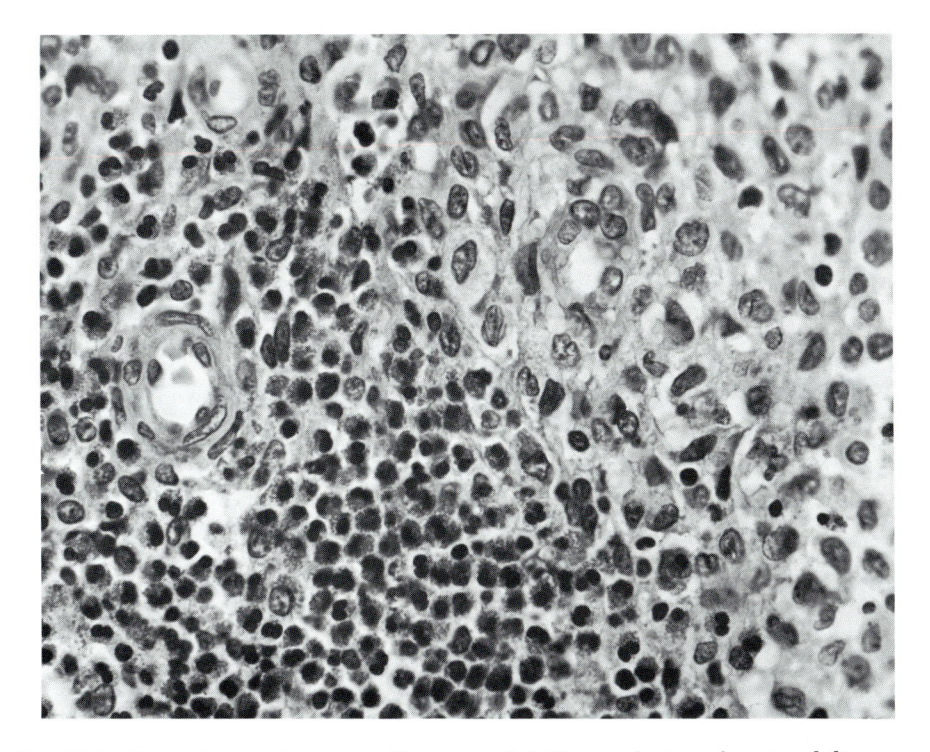

Fig. 12-6. Photomicrograph of a well-preserved field in a lesion of eosinophilic granuloma of bone. The leukocytes massed on the left are all eosinophils, many of them young forms. The large pale cells to the right are of histiocytic nature. (×450.)

Diseases of bone and joints

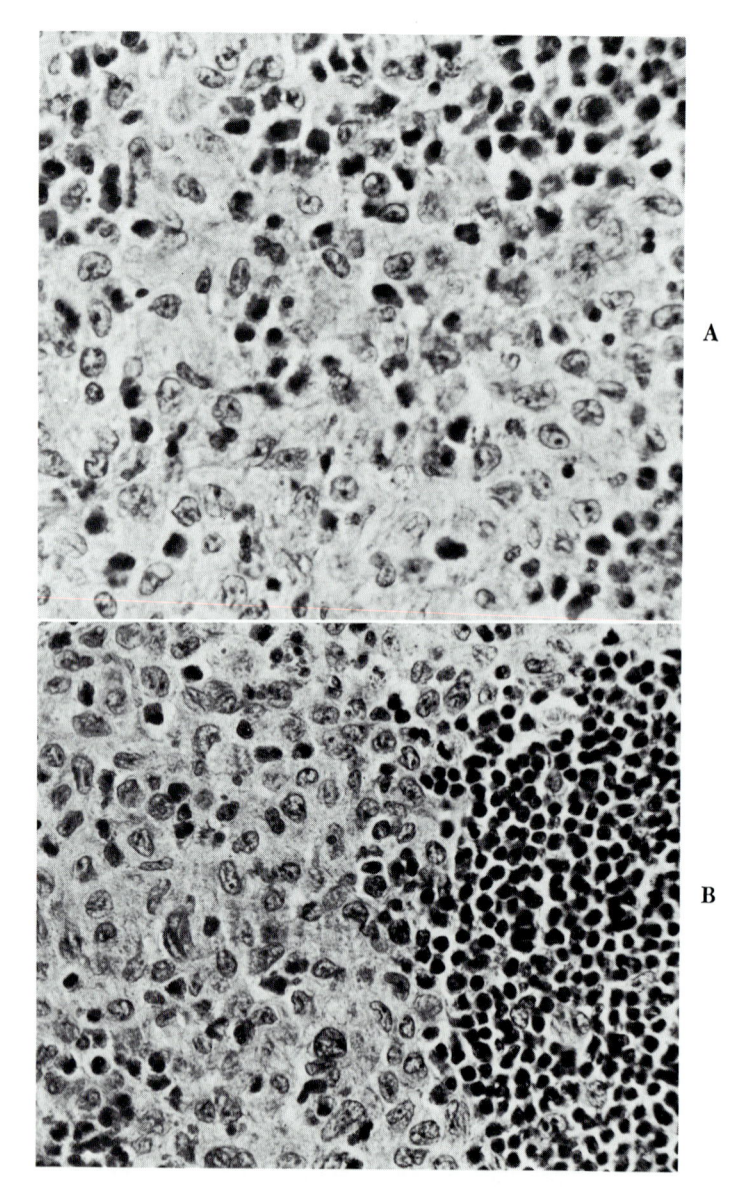

Fig. 12-7. **A,** Section of an eosinophilic granuloma in the frontal bone of a 15-year-old boy. The dark-staining cells interspersed among the histiocytes are eosinophilic leukocytes. (×470.) **B,** From an enlarged cervical lymph node in the case illustrated in **A,** showing the picture of eosinophilic granuloma on the left and residual lymphoid tissue on the right, for contrast.

Histiocytosis X

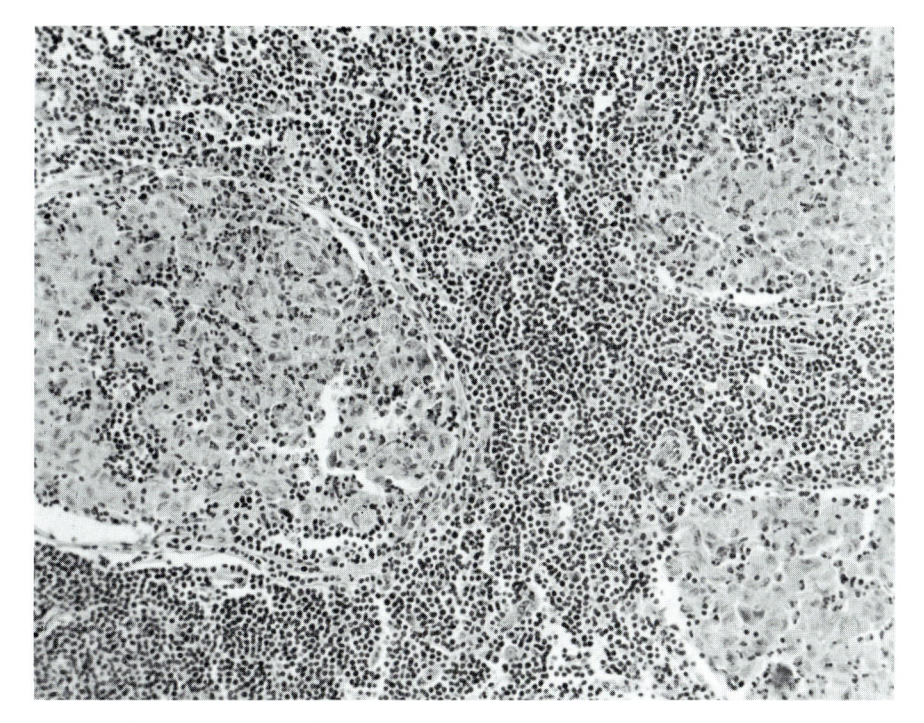

Fig. 12-8. Photomicrograph (low magnification) of a lymph node involved by eosinophilic granuloma. Note the focal nodular aggregates of histiocytes; the small dark cells within these nodules are eosinophils.

are still some cancer therapy groups[10,11] that apparently fail to recognize it. I suspect they have been treating systemic neoplastic disease in children and calling it "Letterer-Siwe disease" and, conversely, treating some children with acute disseminated histiocytosis X with cytotoxic agents as though they had leukemia, probably with unfortunate results. This problem in differential diagnosis has been highlighted in an excellent recent paper by Henderson and Sage,[12] "Malignant Histiocytosis with Eosinophilia," in which they advocate that the use of the eponym "Letterer-Siwe disease" be discontinued altogether because of the confusion it may create.

One must resort to biopsy whenever possible to distinguish the two. Thus a young child with a destructive focus of eosinophilic granuloma in bone (Fig. 12-6), mucocutaneous lesions showing histiocytic proliferation (with or without associated eosinophil reaction), enlarged lymph nodes showing focal nodular histiocytosis (Fig. 12-8), and bone marrow that fails to show any neoplastic growth can, with assurance, be said to be suffering from acute (or subacute) disseminated histiocytosis X, rather than from something akin to acute leukemia. Adequate steroid therapy for such a child may well be lifesaving if the disease is not fulminant, whereas the use of marrow-damaging cytotoxic agents, like nitrogen mustard, or of radioactive elements might well have serious consequences.

Diseases of bone and joints

Some lingering misconceptions still need to be dispelled. Acute (or subacute) disseminated histiocytosis X may be observed occasionally in adults as well as young children. The condition, although serious, is not necessarily fatal, as was once thought. With improved therapy, an appreciable number of patients have remissions of significant duration and presumably go into the chronic phase of the disease (Schüller-Christian). Attention should be directed particularly to the use of selected antibiotics to control secondary bacterial infections and to the value of steroid therapy in critical situations. Autopsy experience indicates that when the outcome is fatal despite well-conceived therapy, it is usually because the disease is fulminant or because of unresponsive secondary infection, extensive pulmonary involvement, or serious hepatic damage leading to cirrhosis.

CHRONIC DISSEMINATED HISTIOCYTOSIS X
(Schüller-Christian disease)

The following concepts concerning the chronic form of histiocytosis X may be reemphasized[5] here in list form for the sake of brevity.

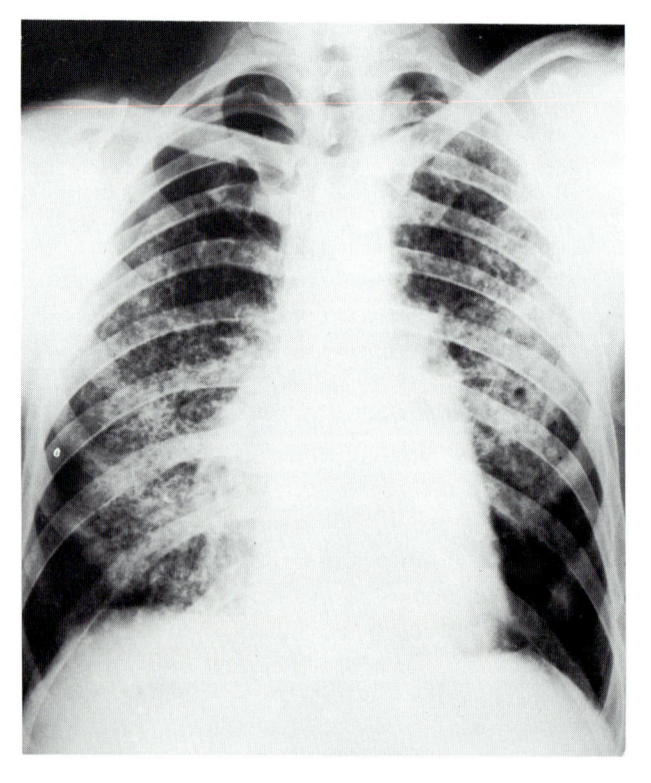

Fig. 12-9. Roentgenogram showing old dense infiltration of both lung fields in a man of 29, who had also had symptoms of diabetes insipidus for about 4 years and then developed a lesion of eosinophilic granuloma in the calvarium. (From Lichtenstein, L.: Histiocytosis X, Arch. Path. **56**:84, 1953.)

Histiocytosis X

1. The old belief that chronic histiocytosis X represents a primary disorder of lipid metabolism (or a functional disturbance of the reticuloendothelial system) should be discarded as no longer having any justification.
2. Only a minority of patients, perhaps no more than one in ten, manifests the complete Christian triad—calvarial defects, exophthalmos, and diabetes insipidus.
3. Skeletal lesions should no longer be considered to be a sine qua non for the diagnosis, since they may be absent or, if they do appear, they may not become manifest until lesions in extraskeletal sites (such as the lungs or pituitary gland) are already well established (Fig. 12-9).
4. Although the clinical picture may vary considerably from case to case, all manifestations fit within a unified framework of reference as clinical expressions of chronic disseminated histiocytosis X, of which the tempo, severity, and localization may vary within wide limits. The major types of involvement are skeletal, pulmonary, cutaneous, and hypophyseal (or cerebral).

When the condition proves fatal, as it may in adults as well as children, it is usually for one of the following reasons: acute exacerbation,

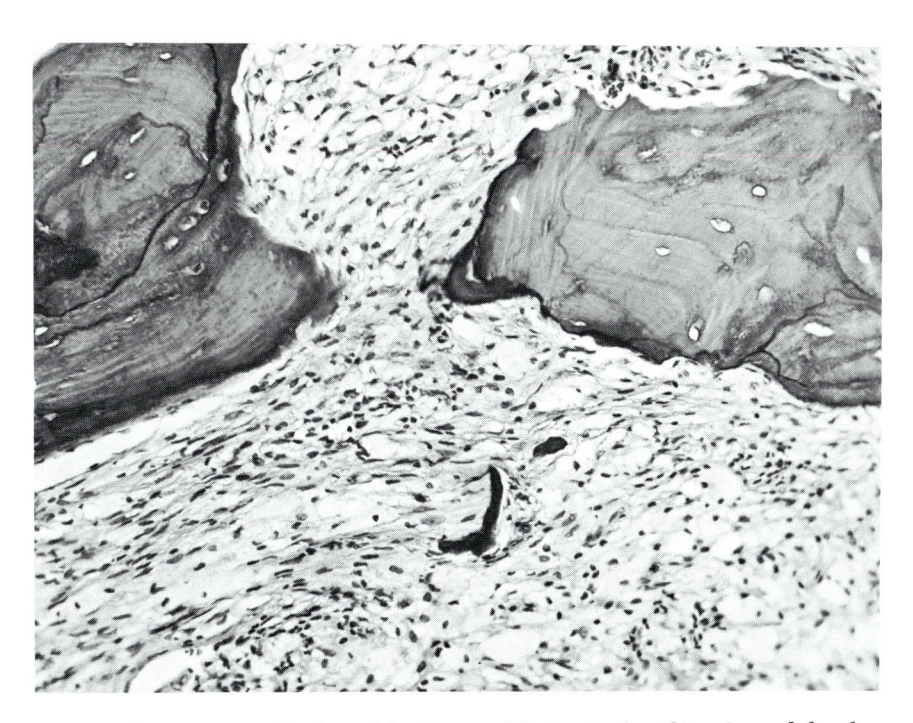

Fig. 12-10. Photomicrograph of an old sclerotized lesion in the tibia of an adult who presented no clinical manifestations of extraskeletal involvement (burned out or healed end stage of Schüller-Christian disease). Note the presence of numerous lipophages and collagen-forming fibroblasts in the tissue between the sclerotic trabeculae of spongy bone. This is the picture once referred to as "lipoid granulomatosis." (From Lichtenstein, L.: Histiocytosis X, Arch. Path. **56**:84, 1953.)

Diseases of bone and joints

extensive pituitary damage (in cases manifesting diabetes insipidus), progressive pulmonary disease leading to honeycomb lungs and resulting cor pulmonale, or hepatic involvement resulting in intrahepatic obstructive jaundice[4] and eventually cirrhosis (if the patient survives long enough).

5. The initial pathologic picture is essentially that of an inflammatory histiocytosis that may or may not be accompanied by intense eosinophil reaction. Fibrosis and conversion of histiocytes to lipophages are secondary, if not late, changes (Fig. 12-10).

6. Finally—and this of prime importance—early, rapidly developing lesions as seen in biopsy specimens commonly have the characteristics of eosinophilic granuloma. This is true not only in bone but also in skin, oral cavity (gingiva, palate, or tongue), anogenital region, lungs, lymph nodes, liver, kidney, and other sites.

Of particular interest are the observations showing that the early disseminated nodular lesions in the lungs resemble eosinophilic granuloma. This is apparently an important portal of entry of the etiologic agent (Fig. 12-11). Similarly, the early lesions in the liver around portal radicles likewise have the character of eosinophilic granuloma and may lead rather rapidly to serious intrahepatic ob-

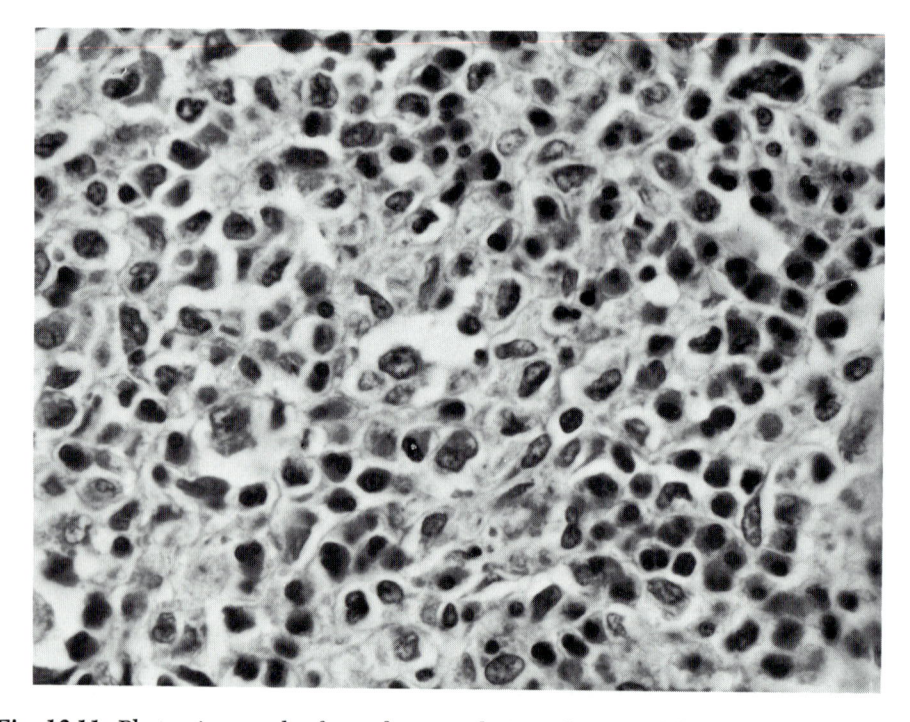

Fig. 12-11. Photomicrograph of a pulmonary lesion of eosinophilic granuloma showing replacement of pulmonary parenchyma by histiocytes interspersed with eosinophilic leukocytes. (The smaller dark cells are young eosinophils, many of them uninuclear or bilobed.)

structive jaundice[4] (Fig. 12-1). Also noteworthy are the observations[5] indicating that lesions of eosinophilic granuloma in bone, as well as in the cutis, may extend to regional lymph nodes (Fig. 12-7, *B*).

In the matter of treatment, one may stress the established value of roentgen irradiation (in limited dosage) in the control of osseous and mucocutaneous lesions, particularly; adequate therapy for the control of diabetes insipidus (when present); and the usefulness of steroids for pulmonary involvement, especially in its early stage and for critical exacerbation in general.

REFERENCES

1. Jaffe, H. L., and Lichtenstein, L.: Eosinophilic granuloma of bone: a condition affecting one, several or many bones, but apparently limited to the skeleton, and representing the mildest clinical expression of the peculiar inflammatory histiocytosis also underlying Letterer-Siwe disease and Schüller-Christian disease, Arch. Pathol. **37**:99, 1944.
2. Lichtenstein, L.: Histiocytosis X: integration of eosinophilic granuloma of bone, "Letterer-Siwe disease" and "Schüller-Christian disease" as related manifestations of a single nosologic entity, Arch. Pathol. **56**:84, 1953.
3. Lichtenstein, L.: Medical progress, pathology: diseases of bone, N. Engl. J. Med. **255**:427, 1956.
4. Parker, J. W., and Lichtenstein, L.: Severe hepatic involvement in chronic disseminated histiocytosis X, Am. J. Clin. Pathol. **40**:624, 1963.
5. Lichtenstein, L.: Histiocytosis X (eosinophilic granuloma of bone, Letterer-Siwe disease, and Schüller-Christian disease): further observations of pathological and clinical importance, J. Bone Joint Surg. **46-A**:76, 1964.
6. Lichtenstein, L., and Jaffe, H. L.: Eosinophilic granuloma of bone, Am. J. Pathol. **16**:595, 1940.
7. Basset, F., Nézelof, M. C., and Turiaf, M. J.: Présence en microscopie electronique de structures filamenteuses originales dans les lésions pulmonaires et osseuses de l'histiocytosis X, Bull. Soc. Med. Hôp. Paris. **117**:413, 1966.
8. DeMan, J. C. H.: Rod-like tubular structures in the cytoplasm of histiocytes in histiocytosis X, J. Pathol. **95**:123, 1968.
9. Shamoto, M., Kaplan, C., and Katoh, A, K.: Langerhans cell granules in human hyperplastic lymph nodes, Arch. Pathol. **92**:46, 1971.
10. Lieberman, P. H., Jones, C. R., Dargeon, H. W. K., and Begg, C. F.: A reappraisal of eosinophilic granuloma of bone, Hand-Schüller-Christian syndrome and Letterer-Siwe syndrome, Medicine **48**:375, 1969.
11. Brough, A. J., and Yang, S. S.: Histiocytosis X—fact or fancy? Abstract, Scientific proceedings, The Pediatric Pathology Club, March 6, 1971, p. 14a.
12. Henderson, D. W., and Sage, R. E.: Malignant histiocytosis with eosinophilia, Cancer, **32**:1421, 1973.

chapter 13

Chemical and radiation effects on bone

CHEMICAL EFFECTS ON BONE

With reference to chemical damage, apart from benzol poisoning (which can cause aplastic anemia), we are concerned here mainly with the pathologic effects of certain chemical elements, some of which have been well documented in the past as important industrial hazards. This concise survey will deal only with the manifestations in bone. For discussion of the other noxious systemic effects of these chemical agents, the reader may have recourse to standard reference texts on toxicology and internal medicine.

Lead. In chronic lead poisoning (plumbism, saturnism), the heavy metal is stored in bone or in other depots (brain, kidneys, and liver). In the skeleton, it is deposited mainly in newly formed bone and in cancellous bone, rather than cortex. In limb bones specifically, it tends to be concentrated in the ends of the bone. In affected adults (painters, pottery workers, white-lead workers, and others), this deposition does not cause any apparent untoward effects except for anemia and a bluish line along the gums adjacent to the teeth. In children (who ingest lead-containing paint on their cribs or even the walls), one characteristically sees a transverse radiopaque line or band on the metaphyseal side of the growth plates of the long limb bones (Fig. 13-1). The width of this dense zone radiographically indicates the duration of exposure to lead. Its appearance apparently reflects abnormally condensed, calcified cartilage and newly formed bone, rather than the presence of lead itself.[1] That the hazard to children of plumbism and its untoward sequelae is not negligible has been demonstrated once again in a recent screening study[2] of preschool children in an impoverished section of Boston (based on analysis of lead in hair), which showed 98 of 705 children (14%) to have a significantly increased lead burden.

Bismuth. After the administration of bismuth to babies (or experimental young animals[3]), one also sees transverse dense bands in the juxtaepiphyseal regions of long bones, although this observation is only of historic interest now

Chemical and radiation effects on bone

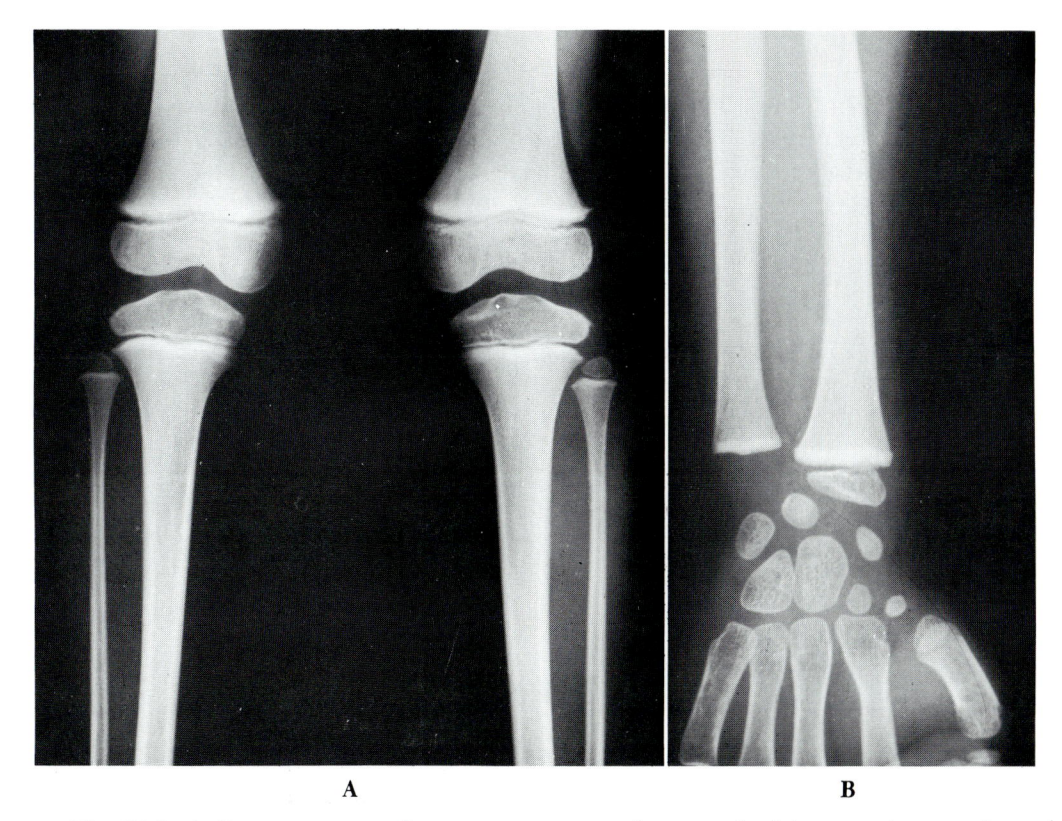

Fig. 13-1. A, Roentgenogram showing transverse radiopaque lead lines at the growth plates of a child (who had ingested lead paint from his crib). **B,** Comparable changes in the distal radius and ulna.

that penicillin has replaced bismuth in the treatment of congenital syphilis. As in the case of comparable lead lines, the radiopaque zones contain abundant compacted calcified cartilage, reflecting interference with orderly endochondral ossification. As these zones later move away from the growth plate and undergo reconstruction, they remain relatively dense for some time.

Phosphorus. Still another chemical agent that may produce radiopaque bands in or adjacent to the growth zones of long bones in babies or children is phosphorus, which was once used (as yellow phosphorus or phosphorized cod liver oil) in the treatment of rickets.[4] As an industrial poison, yellow phosphorus (in workers in match factories, particularly) was once responsible for more or less extensive necrosis of the jaw bones and refractory osteomyelitis, sometimes leading to massive sequestration and involucrum ("phossy jaw").

Fluoride. Fluoride intake in small amounts may have beneficial effects. That the addition of fluoride to the water supply in minute concentration reduces the incidence of dental caries in children now appears to be established by well-controlled statistical surveys. Those who still object to this public health measure may be reminded that fluorine is ordinarily present in very small amounts in almost all human tissues, including bone, and that in such amounts it has no known pathologic effects. Fluoride tends to accumulate in bone, where it is compounded in the hydroxyapatite crystalline system of bone mineral and held there in relatively stable form. For this reason, it has been used therapeutically by some (as sodium fluoride) in certain malacic diseases of bone (for example, osteoporosis), with a view to strengthening the bone and retarding its resorption. As might be anticipated, it is incorporated more readily into active areas of bone growth, and the uptake is higher in young individuals.

Fluoride intake in large doses, on the other hand, has certain undesirable or deleterious effects. Excessive fluoride content in water in endemic areas where fluorosis is prevalent, such as parts of Texas and Oklahoma, may lead to mottling of the enamel of permanent teeth in children, after exposure during the first 8 years of life. In these circumstances, the fluorine interferes with enamel development and with the activity of ameloblasts (dental fluorosis[5-7]).

Chronic fluoride poisoning is a well-known industrial hazard in cryolite and certain phosphate rock miners. Huge quantities of fluorine-containing minerals are also used in the chemical, fertilizer, glass, and aluminum industries. The fluorine may be inhaled as a pollutant or ingested as a dust in the vicinity, or even in fluoride-contaminated crops. Fluoride absorbed into the blood stream is disposed of quickly—part is excreted by the kidneys and the remainder is deposited in bone.

In individuals subjected to relatively heavy industrial pollution particularly, there may be distressing symptoms of fluoride intoxication. These are migraine-like headaches, visual changes, serious gastrointestinal disturbances, and such orthopedic manifestations as pain and stiffness in the lumbar and cervical spine, with restricted motion, "arthritis" in other joints, myalgias and paresthesia in arms, legs, and shoulders, and impaired muscle power of hands and legs. In such patients, biopsy will show high fluoride content in bone and soft tissues, long before skeletal alterations become manifest radiologically.

The characteristic skeletal changes develop only after long-term fluoride intake, as a rule, and then only in some exposed individuals (chronic skeletal fluorosis). They feature uniform diffuse osteosclerosis[8] (Fig. 13-2), especially of the spine and pelvis; ossification of ligaments,[9] particularly the sacrotuberous and sacrospinatous ligaments, but also others; and in some instances, remarkable, sometimes massive, multiple periosteal hyperostoses (pseudotumor, periostitis deformans) on limb bones, hand bones, and others. It is interesting that the latter changes are reversible after cessation of fluoride intake.[10] Continuing, osteophytes may extend into tendon insertions, as well as ligaments, and in the vertebral column can give rise to a crippling rigidity, simulating that of ankylosing spondylitis. In the long bones, the massive periosteal exostoses, often taking the form of an involucrumlike sleeve, overlie the original cortex, which has undergone extensive resorption (as in osteoporosis). There may also be wide osteoid borders microscopically (as in osteomalacia), indicating interference in the mineralization process. As Collins[5] emphasized, the pathologic process, as a

Chemical and radiation effects on bone

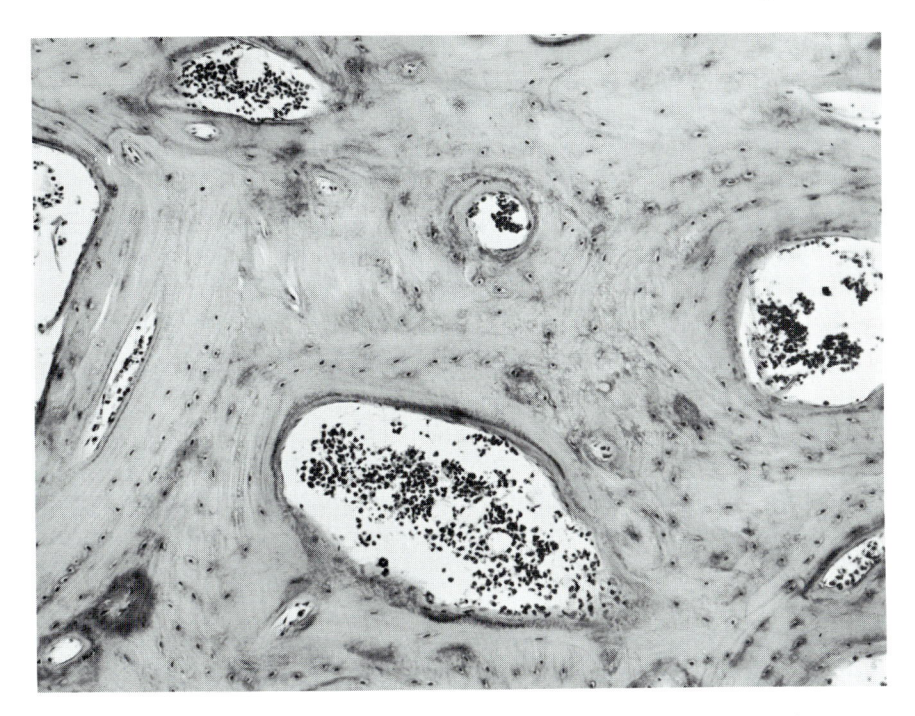

Fig. 13-2. Photomicrograph showing abnormally dense bone (osteosclerosis), as seen in chronic fluoride poisoning of long duration in an adult dying of other natural causes.

whole, is actually complex, featuring osteoclastic resorption, extensive bone regeneration, and abnormalities of osteoid calcification.

Cadmium. Cadmium poisoning, which has been recognized in Japan particularly as an industrial hazard in certain zinc-refining workers, is said to cause marked fragility of the bones, as well as renal damage and excruciating abdominal pain.

Mercury. Mercury poisoning is far less common than it was when mercurial drugs and ointments were used in the treatment of syphilis. It is still seen as an industrial disease or, very occasionally, following attempts at suicide with mercuric bichloride. (Today, people intent on suicide jump off the Golden Gate Bridge instead.) The only skeletal effect, if it can be called that, is loosening of the teeth.

Beryllium. Beryllium poisoning, observed in workers in beryllium ore extraction, the making of fluorescent light tubes, and the preparation of beryllium-copper alloys, produces histiocytic granulomas in the lungs, lymph nodes, and skin, but apparently not in bone.

It may be mentioned here that beryllium, when implanted in bone experimentally or administered intravenously,[11,12] provokes reactive osteosclerosis leading to the development of osteogenic sarcoma in 8 to 18 months. Such tumors may be multiple. This observation is of greater academic interest than practical moment.

Diseases of bone and joints

Lathyrism. In human lathyrism resulting from excessive consumption of peas (in time of famine), the clinical manifestations are neurologic rather than skeletal. However, experimental lathyrism[13] induced in rats by a diet of sweet pea seeds, leads to profound disturbance of the skeleton, as well as alterations in connective tissue elsewhere. Succinctly stated, the bone changes include fractures, focal resorption of cortices, formation of osteophytes, kyphoscoliosis, proliferation of fibrous tissue, and interference with the growth of cartilage and its ossification. These are all held to be manifestations of injury to connective tissue matrix, especially its mucopolysaccharide component, by β-aminopropionitrile, the active chemical agent.

RADIATION EFFECTS ON BONE

Occasional exposure to small doses of *roentgen rays* (delivered by well-calibrated and supervised equipment) in the course of diagnostic procedures is not held to be harmful. Repeated exposure over a long period of time, even when the usual safeguards are observed, may be a hazard—radiologists are more prone to develop leukemia than are other physicians. The possibility of the insidious induction of gene mutations in these circumstances has also been raised by concerned biologists and geneticists, although this still appears to be a moot point.

Roentgen irradiation in heavy doses employed in therapy[14] (for the destruction or control of neoplasms particularly) regularly induces certain well-recognized pathologic changes in tissues within the beam of irradiation, including bone. The major effects are the following: calcification (Fig. 13-3), narrowing or obliteration of blood vessels, necrosis or necrobiosis, scarring and hyalinization, and, in the reparative phase, the appearance of abnormal fibroblasts with large swollen nuclei. Still larger or massive doses may, of course, be followed by obvious gross changes as well, including destruction and ulceration of the skin, necrosis of soft tissues (including muscle) in the irradiated field, and partial necrosis in the bone itself.

Another important consideration is the occasional development of sarcoma in bone (or soft tissues) following therapeutic irradiation[15] after a latent interval that may be as short as 3 years or as long as 20 to 30 years or more. The mean is about 5 to 6 years. When postirradiation sarcoma develops in bone, it is most often an osteogenic sarcoma, but it may be fibrosarcoma or even chondrosarcoma. As a rule, the hazard is directly proportional to the dosage employed, although there are undoubtedly exceptions. With increasing recognition of such cases, there has been a growing feeling, first, that nonneoplastic lesions in bone or in joints should be treated by irradiation only when there is a clear, specific indication for it, and second, that when irradiation is employed, whatever the reason may be (and this applies also to tumors), one should use the smallest dose calculated to be effective.

Brief comment is in order here on the nature of injury to bone from *external radiation* in less dramatic circumstances. Although bone is near the bottom of

Chemical and radiation effects on bone

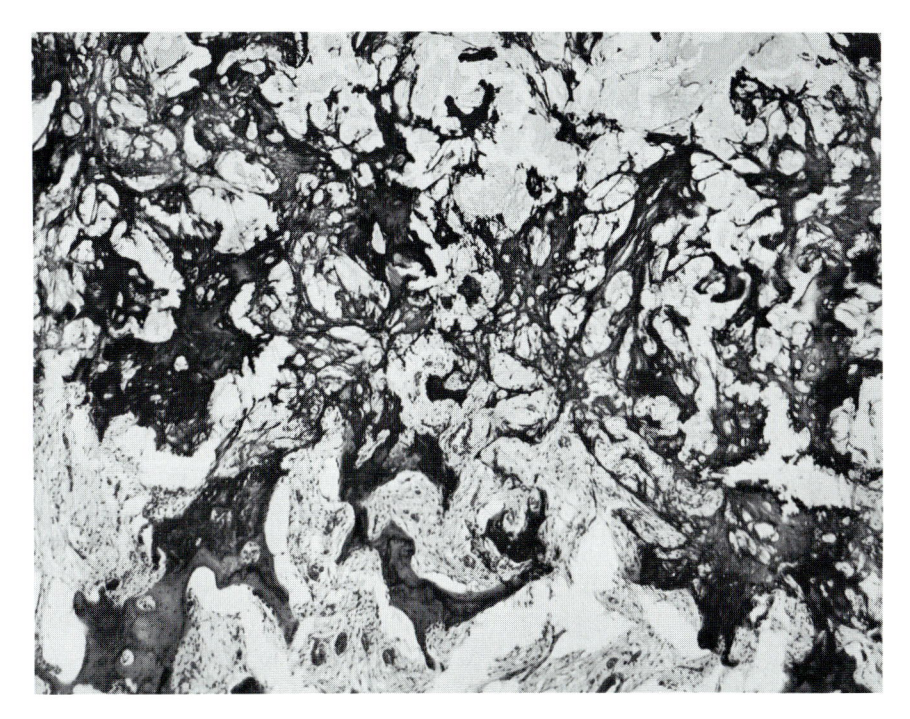

Fig. 13-3. Photomicrograph of a representative field of a lesion of Paget's disease in a tibia, which had been heavily irradiated on the mistaken premise that it represented a malignant tumor (pathologic fracture and nonunion developed, and the leg was eventually amputated). The intense calcification of Paget bone and the necrobiosis in places are postirradiation changes.

the list of tissues arranged in order of relative radiosensitivity, it will sustain damage if the total dose to bone is sufficiently large. The injurious effects of radiation on bone itself may be summarized as necrosis, inflammation, interference with or distortion of growth, and sometimes tumor induction. Naturally, the effect on the sensitive hemopoietic cells in the marrow is more pronounced. In so-called radiation osteitis, induced by external radiation, the significant histologic changes are destruction of osteoblasts; damage to blood vessels with necrosis of bone, as noted; abnormal resorption; and proliferation of abnormal osteogenic connective tissue (with or without the development of sarcoma). As is well known, such devitalized bones (for example, in the jaw), are more prone to develop osteomyelitis. Also, their weakened structure may at times lead to pathologic fracture. These changes are reflected roentgenographically by coarsening of trabecular pattern, localized areas of bone resorption, patchy sclerosis, and areas of avascular necrosis.[16]

In children, following irradiation (usually of tumors) a number of undesirable skeletal changes have been noted.[17,18] These depend on dosage and the field of irradiation, and may include distortion of vertebral bodies, scoliosis, hypoplasia of the iliac bone and rib cage, osteocartilaginous exostoses, and, in the extremities, damage to growth plates and epiphyseal ossification centers, with growth arrest, discrepancy of limb length, and deformity. Also, when one irradiates growing bone, not only is there the possibility of disturbing normal growth, but the hazard of postirradiation sarcoma is greater than it is in adults.

With reference to *internal radiation,* or emanation from a radioactive source within the tissues of the body, we know that bone can hold many radioactive elements in its hydroxyapatite crystals, concentrated in "hot" spots as visualized by microradiographic and autoradiographic techniques.[19] These are found particularly in metabolically active areas, such as endosteal and periosteal surfaces where new bone apposition is taking place, or in haversian systems that are undergoing new construction and mineralization. Moreover, such foci may become buried or locked in by the further accumulation of new bone lamellae,[20] so that they are not eradicated readily.

It is now well established that osteogenic sarcoma can be induced in experimental rats and mice by the administration of radium,[21] plutonium, and strontium 90.

As for tumor induction in man, apart from sporadic mishaps in nuclear energy plants or in above-ground atomic testing, there have been two documented major catastrophic experiences, with long-term followup, that may serve as models of what happens when significant amounts of radium are taken up. For the past 20 years or more, a study of over 400 persons bearing a detectable body burden of ^{226}Ra has been underway at the Argonne National Laboratory and the Argonne Cancer Research Hospital.[16] Many of them received radium chloride intravenously or orally as a medicament between 1920 and 1933, appalling as that may seem today. A substantial number of bone sarcomas subsequently developed in these individuals (and I have seen material from several of them), but if any precise analysis of tumor incidence and other ill effects in the group as a whole has ever been published, I am not aware of it. The other large group is made up of former radium (and mesothorium) watch-dial painters during the period 1920 to 1940; some 219 have had roentgenographic surveys and radium body determinations on at least one occasion,[16] demonstrating their long-term radium burden. Gary and his associates,[22] also following up the pioneer study by Martland,[23] observed a 10% incidence (as of 1964) of osteogenic sarcoma in persons who had had symptomatic radium poisoning. Other significant long-term sequelae were focal necrosis and eventual loss of teeth, radiographically mottled areas of radiation necrosis and "osteitis" that are prone to fracture, osteomyelitis (of the jaw bones, particularly), and, in a few instances, carcinoma of the paranasal sinuses or mastoid.

These investigators pointed out again that radium and mesothorium are deposited in bone in an irregular pattern, with "hot" spots in metabolically active areas[20] that contain a hundred times the concentration of radioactivity found in adjacent areas of bone. Inasmuch as these deposits, small as they may be, set up a never-ending alpha particle bombardment over a long period of time, one may have justifiable concern about the long-term effects of radioactive fallout, especially that of the bone-seeking radioactive elements, such as plutonium or strontium 90. It is quite conceivable that we may yet witness a significant rise in the incidence of osteogenic sarcoma, as well as of leukemia, in populations subjected to radioactive fallout, and that we may perforce have to revise our present estimates of what constitutes a "safe" concentration.

REFERENCES

1. Caffey, J.: Clinical and experimental lead poisoning: some roentgenologic and anatomic changes in growing bones, Radiology **17:**957, 1931.
2. Pueschel, S. M., Kopito, L., and Schwachman, H.: Children with an increased lead burden: a screening and follow-up study, J.A.M.A. **222:**462, 1972.
3. Caffey, J.: Changes in growing skeleton after administration of bismuth, Am. J. Dis. Child. **53:**56, 1937.
4. Phemister, D. B., Miller, E. M., and Bonar, P. E.: Effects of phosphorus in rickets, J.A.M.A. **70:**850, 1921.
5. Collins, D. H.: Pathology of bone, London, 1966, Butterworth & Co. (Publishers) Ltd.
6. Bosworth, T. J.: Discussion of fluorosis in man and animals, Proc. R. Soc. Med. **34:**391, 1940.
7. Sutro, C. J.: Changes in teeth and bone in chronic fluoride poisoning, Arch. Pathol. **19:**159, 1935.
8. Stevenson, C. A., and Watson, A. R.: Fluoride osteosclerosis, Am. J. Roentgen. **78:**13, 1957.
9. Møller, P. F., and Gudjonsson, S. V.: Massive fluorosis of bones and ligaments, Acta Radiol. **13:**269, 1932.
10. Soriano, M.: Periostitis deformans, Rev. Clin. Esp. **97:**373, 1965.
11. Kelly, P. J., Janes, J. M., and Peterson, L. F. A.: The effect of beryllium on bone, J. Bone Joint Surg. **43-A:**829, 1961.
12. Barnes, J. M., Duz, F. A., and Sissons, H. A.: Beryllium bone sarcomata in rabbits, Br. J. Cancer **4:**212, 1950.
13. Angevine, D. M.: Injury to connective tissue. In Collins, D. H., editor: Modern trends in pathology, London, 1959, Butterworth & Co. (Publishers) Ltd., p. 45.
14. Rubin, P., and Casarett, G. W.: Clinical radiation pathology, Philadelphia, 1968, W. B. Saunders Co.
15. Hatcher, C. H.: Development of sarcoma in bone subjected to roentgen or radium irradiation, J. Bone Joint Surg. **27:**179, 1945.
16. Hasterlik, R. J., Miller, C. E., and Finkel, A. J.: Radiographic development of skeletal lesions in man many years after acquisition of radium burden, Radiology **93:**599, 1969.
17. Katzman, H., Waugh, T., and Berdon, W.: Skeletal changes following irradiation of childhood tumors, J. Bone Joint Surg. **51-A:**825, 1969.
18. Neuhauser, E. B. J., Wittenborg, M. H., Berman, C. Z., and Cohen, J.: Irradiation effects of roentgen therapy on the growing spine, Radiology **59:**637, 1952.
19. Looney, W. B., and Woodruff, L. A.: Investigation of radium deposits in human skeletons by gross and detailed autoradiography, Arch. Pathol. **56:**1, 1953.
20. Marshall, J. H.: Radioactive hot spots, bone growth and bone cancer: self-burial of calcium-like hot spots. In McLean, F. C., Lacroix, P., and Budy, A., editors: Radioisotopes in bone, Oxford, 1962, Blackwell Scientific Publications, Ltd., p. 35.
21. Dunlap, C. E., Aub, J. C., Evans, R. D., and Harris, R. S.: Transplantable osteogenic sarcomas induced in rats by feeding radium, Am. J. Path. **20:**1, 1944.
22. Gary, G. E., Clark, S. D., and Evans, R. D.: Radium and mesothorium poisoning in human beings: report of over 375 cases, presented at American Medical Association meeting, San Francisco, June, 1964.
23. Martland, H. S.: Occurrence of malignancy in radioactive persons: a general review of data gathered in the study of the radium dial painters, with special reference to the occurrence of osteogenic sarcoma and the inter-relationship of certain blood diseases, Am. J. Cancer **15:**2435, 1931.

GENERAL REFERENCE

Baserga, R. R., Lisco, H., and Cater, D. B.: The delayed effects of external gamma irradiation of the bones of rats, Am. J. Pathol. **39:**455, 1961.

chapter 14

Pathology of some common and unusual orthopedic conditions

This chapter will deal concisely with some thirty miscellaneous, more or less common orthopedic conditions not considered in preceding chapters. It is concerned mainly with "bread and butter" orthopedic pathology and puts together, for convenient reference, observations that may not be readily available elsewhere, although they are generally well known. It is intended primarily to aid general surgical pathologists, who, by force of circumstances, often have limited experience in the field of skeletal disease. Orthopedic surgeons who are well grounded in basic pathology will not find much with which they are unfamiliar, although they may find some of the illustrations rewarding.

PATHOLOGY OF MENISCI OF THE KNEE

Lacerated meniscus. Though commonly referred to as "cartilages," the menisci are actually composed of dense collagenous connective tissue. As sports buffs are well aware, they are often torn following injury to the knee and must then be removed before damage to other articular structures ensues. Because of their limited blood supply, spontaneous repair or healing of menisci following laceration is apt to be so slight as to be negligible. Extensive injury may lead to complete bucket-handle tear (Fig. 14-1, *A*), but less extensive types of laceration are also commonly observed (Fig. 14-1, *B* and *C*). When a meniscus "regenerates" following removal, it takes the form usually of a fibrous cord. Calcification of meniscal connective tissue is seen only infrequently.

Sections for microscopic examination are best taken in a vertical plane at right angles to the site of apparent or suspected laceration. As a rule, they show nothing more striking than degeneration and fraying or fibrillization of the connective tissue and, sometimes, slight focal capillary vascularization as well. It is essential for the examining pathologist to distinguish clearly the irregularly

Pathology of some common and unusual orthopedic conditions

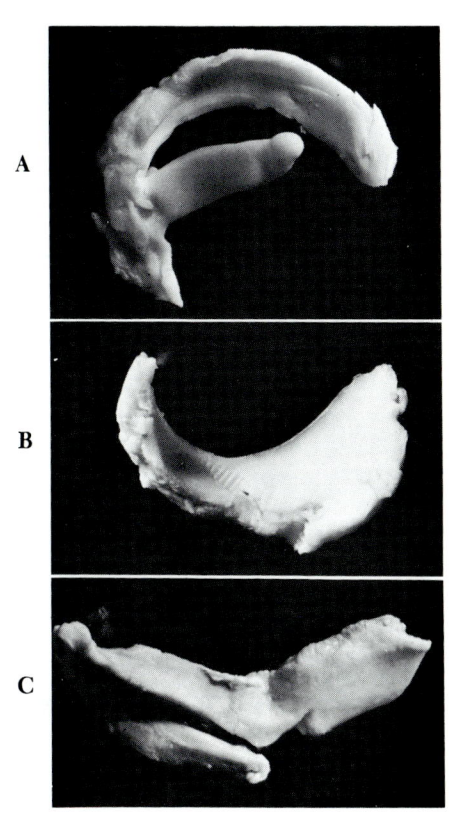

Fig. 14-1. **A**, Photograph of a lacerated meniscus of a knee showing a bucket-handle tear. **B** and **C**, Other examples of torn menisci.

roughened, modified tract of a tear from the clear, sharp, inadvertent cut of the surgeon's scalpel.

Discoid meniscus. Discoid meniscus manifesting an anomalous broadened structure (as its name implies) is of practical moment in that it is peculiarly vulnerable to horizontal splitting (Fig. 14-2), as well as degeneration.

Meniscal or parameniscal cysts. Meniscal cysts result from focal myxoid degeneration and cystic softening of meniscal collagenous connective tissue, usually toward the meniscocapsular junction. In many ways, their formation is reminiscent of the way in which a ganglion develops (Fig. 14-5). There is a tendency for the multifocal cystic areas to coalesce (Fig. 14-3), and occasionally a sizable, clinically evident mass may be formed. I have seen a specimen of a cyst of a lateral meniscus of a knee, containing colorless viscid fluid, that had attained the size of a fist.

CHRONIC BURSITIS

Chronically irritated bursal sacs develop with great frequency in many paraskeletal sites, particularly where there has been friction between apposing glid-

Diseases of bone and joints

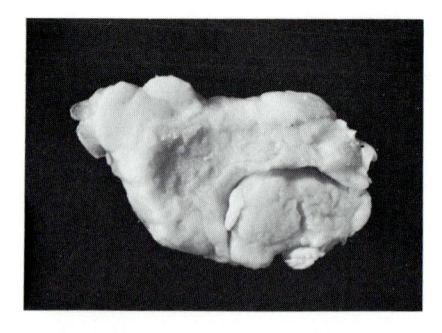

Fig. 14-2. Photograph of a surgically removed broadened discoid meniscus of a knee.

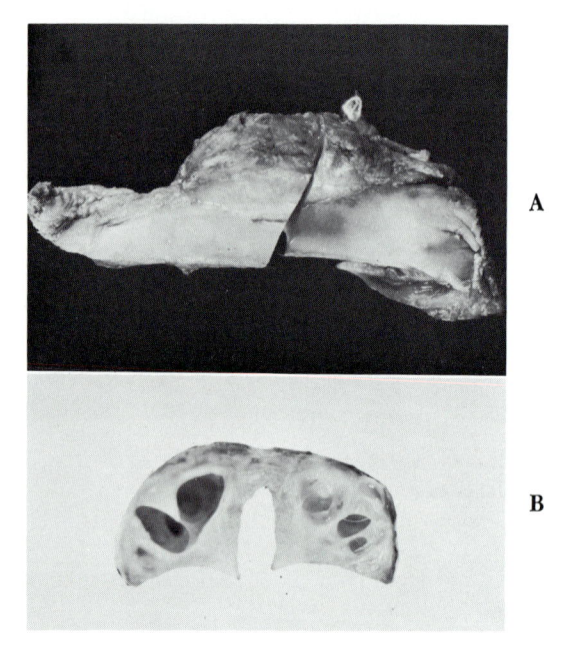

Fig. 14-3. **A,** Photograph of a cyst of a medial meniscus (external view). **B,** Section of the specimen illustrated in **A.**

ing surfaces or over bony prominences (housemaid's knee and philosopher's elbow, for example, have become colloquialisms). Bursal sacs are commonly operated on because of swelling or painful motion. At such sites, the connective tissue undergoes appreciable thickening and encompasses a cystlike space containing mucinous fluid.

The lining of the sac may come to resemble synovium, but this is not necessarily so. In any event, the lining usually presents irregular ridges and small nodular excrescences, often discolored yellow-brown by hemosiderin pigment. There may also be deposits of fibrinoid material on or within the lining surface, and its organization often leads to fibrous strands or cords traversing the lumen of the bursal sac (Fig. 14-4, A). It is not uncommon also to find fibrin rice

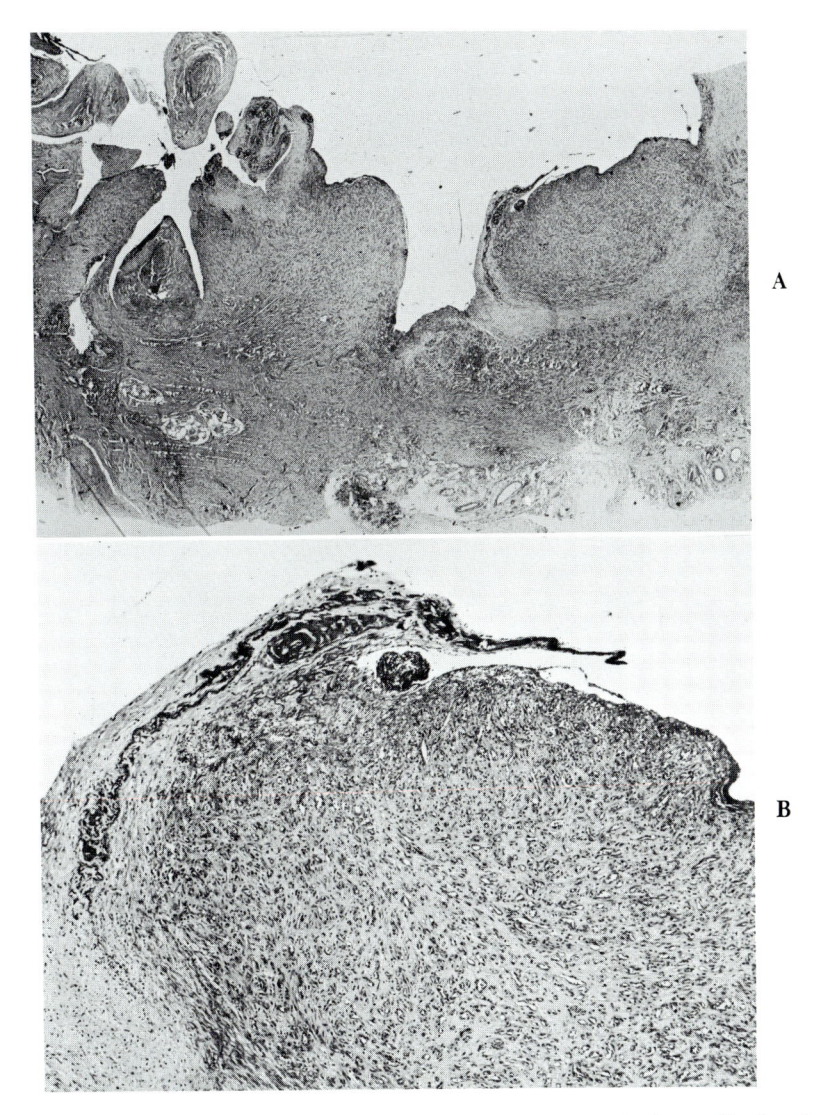

Pathology of some common and unusual orthopedic conditions

Fig. 14-4. **A,** Low-power photomicrograph of a section through the wall of a bursal sac. Note the vascularized collagenous wall and the papillary excrescences on the lining, some of which are organizing fibrin deposits. **B,** Higher magnification of an area of the lining of the bursal sac illustrated in **A,** showing intense capillary vascularization as well as organizing fibrin on its surface. This reaction to chronic irritation should not be interpreted as showing hemangioma formation.

bodies attached to the lining or lying free within the sac. Very occasionally, calcified chondral bodies resembling joint mice are encountered.

These features are evident in microscopic sections, which, in addition, show more or less intense vascularization of the lining by innumerable sprouting capillaries (Fig. 14-4, *B*). Despite the common designation of bursitis, there is usually no inflammatory exudative reaction.

Diseases of bone and joints

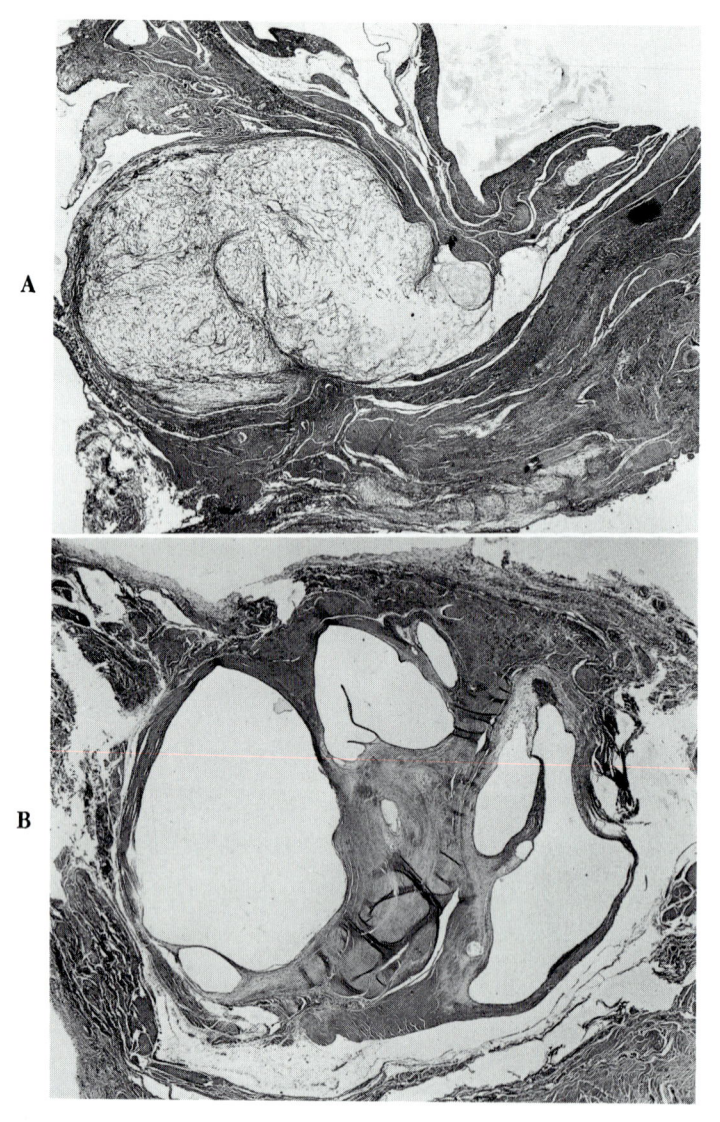

Fig. 14-5. **A**, Low-power photomicrograph showing ganglion formation through myxoid change and cystic softening of the collagenous connective tissue of a joint capsule (in the wrist region). (×8.) **B**, Photomicrograph of another ganglion showing its multilocular structure. The spaces contained colorless, viscid fluid in the gross. (×9.)

GANGLION FORMATION

The common ganglion is a thin-walled, fibrous cystic structure containing a small amount of colorless mucous fluid (rich in hyaluronic acid). It is found most often on the hand or in the wrist, but may be encountered in many other joint regions and occasionally in unusual sites.[1] A ganglion develops through myxoid degeneration and cystic softening of the collagenous connective tissue of a joint capsule or tendon sheath. As such, it constitutes a "tumor" only in the limited clinical sense of a swelling (Fig. 14-5, A). As in comparable multilocular cyst formation within parameniscal connective tissue of the knee joint, it enlarges and ramifies through coalescence of areas of cystic change (Fig. 14-5, B). Obviously, crushing of a ganglion alone will not prevent its reappearance, since it does not remove the connective tissue implicated in its formation.

Intraosseous ganglion ("synovial cyst"). On occasion one may encounter a cystic lesion *in bone* that contains viscid, mucoid, or gelatinous fluid (rich in hyaluronic acid) and that, microscopically also, is reminiscent of the common (extraosseous) ganglion. Since the paper by Hicks[2] in 1956 directing attention to it, a number of additional reports[1,3] have described instances in point in limb bones (especially the proximal tibia), as well as in the innominate, carpal, and tarsal bones.

In my teaching files, I have reports of two such lesions in the proximal tibia and a third in the distal radius, which I had interpreted provisionally as intraosseous ganglia. In one of the tibial cases, there was also a parosteal ganglion and an eroded aperture in the cortical bone between it and the intraosseous lesion, clearly suggesting communication. In the instance in the distal radius, a cystlike rarefaction was discernible radiographically, which had enlarged perceptibly over a 7-year period of observation. At surgery, the lesion was found to contain yellowish, gelatinous fluid and to have a whitish lining, which was curetted. Sections showed connective tissue cells with oval or spindle-shaped, nuclei containing secretory vacuoles, clustered loosely within a ground substance that showed a tendency to disintegration and cystic softening. The stromal connective tissue cells looked more mesenchymal than fibroblastic. The delicate lining of the cyst was vascularized and slightly papillary, but its resemblance otherwise to synovium was only superficial.

It has been postulated[1] that lesions such as these represent the degenerative and cystic late stage of an antecedent growth of connective tissue cells, which produce hyaluronic acid. Incidentally, much the same sequence of events has been noted in the development of so-called "cutaneous myxoid cysts."[4]

HERNIATED INTERVERTEBRAL DISC TISSUE

Rupture of intervertebral discs with herniation and prolapse, and its clinical consequences, have been the subject of active investigation and discussion for more than 40 years.[5] Surgery for ostensibly herniated intervertebral disc tissue has become a major stock in trade for neurosurgeons and some orthopedists, although there are many who feel that it is undertaken too often on inconclusive evidence. In any event, the surgical pathologist, even in a smaller general hospital, has ample opportunity to learn to identify bits of intervertebral disc tissue (Fig. 14-6, A) and to distinguish them from fragments of hyaline cartilage, the concentric fibrous laminae of the annulus fibrosus, and the elastica-containing ligamentum flavum.

In the structure of intervertebral discs, the nucleus pulposus, which lies within the tough ligamentous annulus fibrosus, represents the adult remnant

Diseases of bone and joints

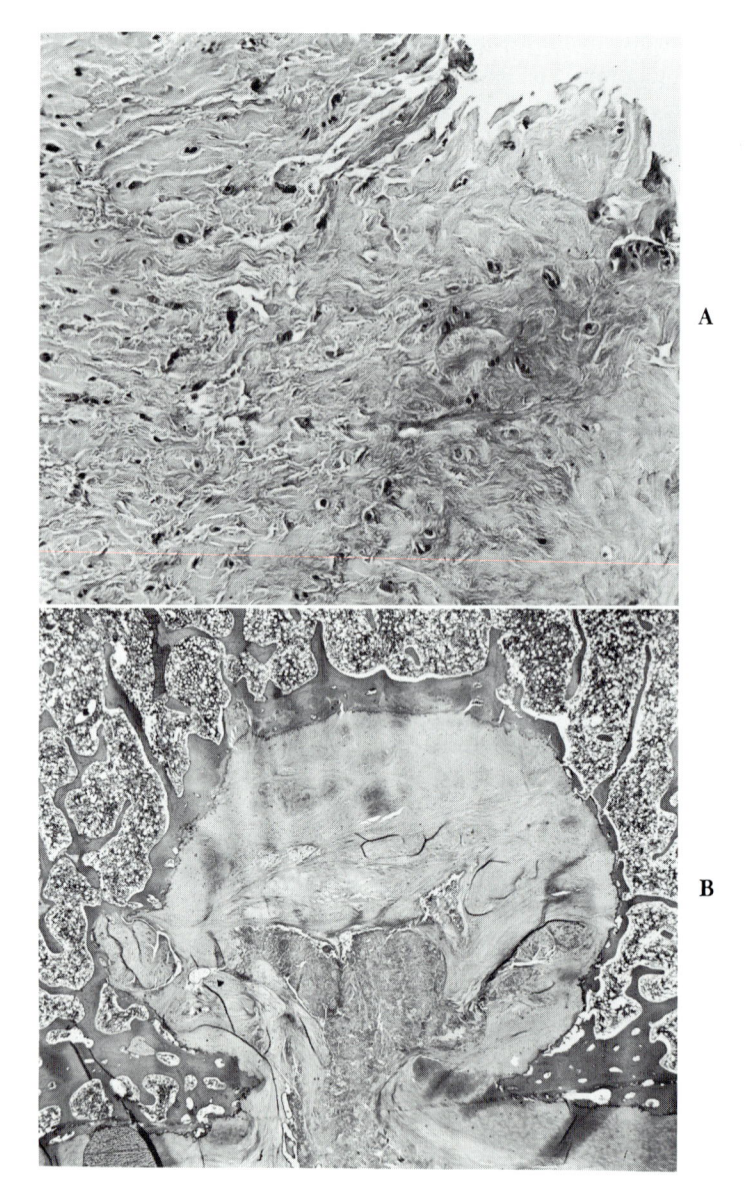

Fig. 14-6. A, Photomicrograph of a bit of (herniated) intervertebral disc tissue removed surgically. The resemblance of the nuclei to those of cartilage cells is only superficial. (Actually, the cells of the nucleus pulposus are of notochordal derivation.) **B,** Photomicrograph showing protrusion of disc tissue through a hiatus into a vertebral body and its walling-off by a thin plate of bone (Schmorl's node).

of the embryonic notochord, the primitive anlage of the vertebral column. It is turgid and hydrophilic, and histochemical stains show it to contain abundant mucopolysaccharides. With aging, it loses some of its aqueous content and is subject to fissuring and, sometimes, calcification. The annulus fibrosus, too, undergoes degenerative changes, with impaired tensile strength.

In describing intervertebral disc tissue fragments microscopically, the pathologist is not justified in stating that they were necessarily herniated, since the validity of this observation depends essentially on what was seen at the operating table. Nor is he justified ordinarily in stating that the intervertebral disc tissue submitted shows evidence of injury, unless there is reparative vascularization, or that it shows significant degenerative changes. The latter inference would require elaborate controls with reference to age, occupation, body build, previous history, and other relevant factors that are not readily available. In most instances, all one can say with any assurance is that bits of intervertebral disc tissue were actually removed at surgery, if that is the case.

As Schmorl, the distinguished German bone pathologist, demonstrated many years ago in a survey of thousands of whole vertebral columns, herniation of intervertebral disc tissue into adjacent vertebral bodies is often seen on examination of the vertebral column at autopsy, although it is asymptomatic and apparently of no practical consequence. Fig. 14-6, B shows a so-called Schmorl's node that has become walled off by a thin plate of bone, as is usually the case.

One occasionally observes herniation of the intervertebral disk ventrally or anteriorly. This, too, is apparently asymptomatic, although it tends to provoke reactive new bone formation leading to a conspicuous radiopaque beaklike protrusion of bone, which may appear curious and puzzling to those unfamiliar with it.

Any detailed consideration here of the pathogenesis of degenerative disc disease and its sequelae of lumbar and cervical disc protrusion and prolapse, adolescent kyphosis, senile kyphosis, the common spondylosis deformans (vertebral osteophytosis), and other disorders of the vertebral column is beyond the scope of this chapter. For this, the reader may have recourse to such sources as the superbly illustrated atlas of Schmorl and Junghanns[6] on the vertebral column, the lucid discussions by Collins[7] and Gardner,[8] and the monograph of DePalma and Rothman[9] on the intervertebral discs, among others. For a brief comprehensive review of cervical and lumbar disc disease, the article by Golub, Rovit, and Mankin[10] is recommended.

PATHOLOGIC CHANGES IN TENDONS AND THEIR SHEATHS

Many of the conditions that affect synovial joints have their counterpart in tendon sheaths (as well as bursae mucosae); the pathologic reaction is similar, whatever the localization. Thus one may encounter tenosynovial tuberculosis, chronic nonspecific inflammation (at the wrists, for example), rheumatoid inflammation, and, on occasion, even sarcoid. With reference to the last, I have

Diseases of bone and joints

observed a remarkable instance of sarcoid that involved primarily the tendon sheaths, rather than the usual sites (skin, lymph nodes, and bone, among others). Continuing the analogy, chondromatosis of tendon sheaths also occurs, as does, commonly, pigmented nodular tenosynovitis (formerly designated "giant cell tumor" of the tendon sheath). These lesions will be considered further on in relation to the pathology of synovial joints (see Chapter 15).

There are several noteworthy conditions affecting the collagenous connective tissue of tendons. Chief among them is *calcification*. This is seen most often in the supraspinatous tendon (and frequently in the subdeltoid bursa, as well), but on occasion it may also involve other tendons, such as the patellar, gluteus, peroneus and flexor carpi ulnaris. The pathogenesis of this calcium deposition is still uncertain, although there has been much speculation about it. Examination of surgical specimens from cases in point may show some degeneration of collagenous connective tissue or even focal necrobiosis, but I have not seen significant necrosis that might plausibly account for calcification as a sequel (Fig. 14-7).

In the shoulder region particularly, calcification is often painful and may require aspiration, cortisone injection, x-ray therapy, or other modalities for relief. As a rule, it is self-limited, but occasionally the problem may become a persistent one. In general, it may be observed that the paraskeletal collagenous connective tissue structures (and this applies to joint capsules and ligaments as well as

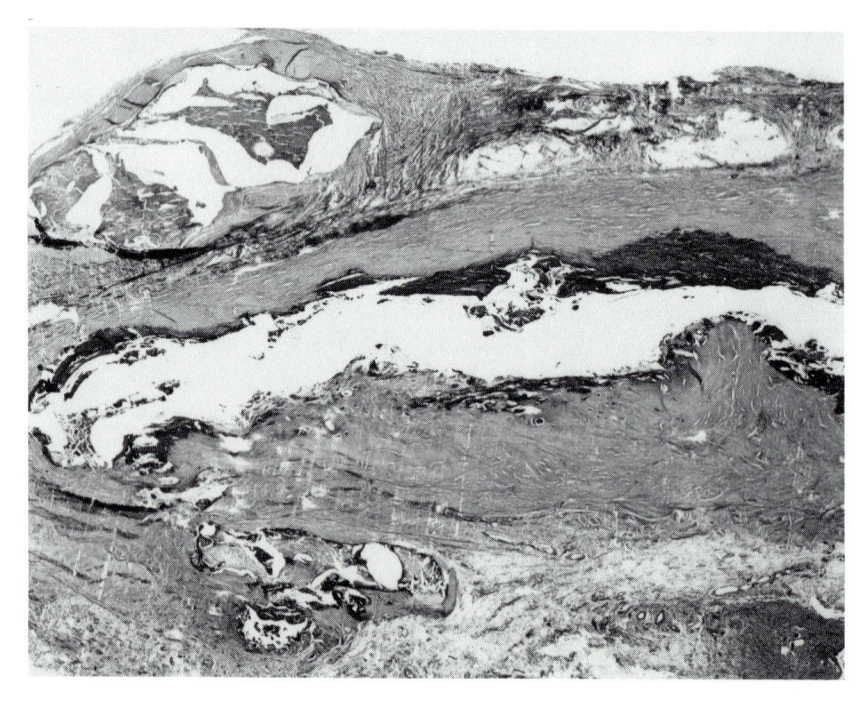

Fig. 14-7. Photomicrograph (low magnification) showing calcification in a patellar tendon. The dark-staining material represents calcium deposit; the cracks and spaces, artefact sustained in cutting the specimen. (×25.)

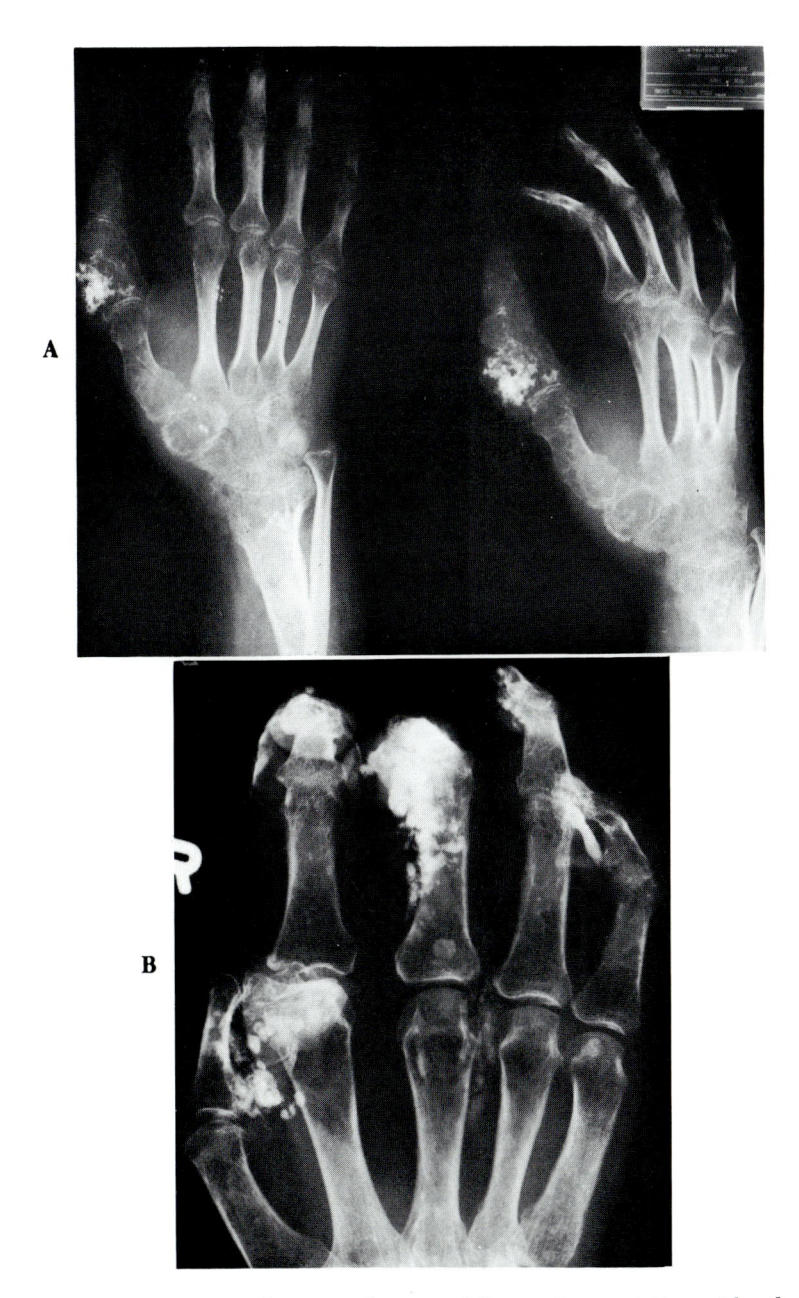

Fig. 14-8. Roentgenograms showing calcinosis of fingers in association with scleroderma.

Diseases of bone and joints

tendons) have a meager blood supply and thus usually require 3, 4, or even 6 months for an injury to heal and for concomitant relief of symptoms, regardless of what is done by way of treatment.

Localized calcification in soft parts—of the fingers, for example—may occur quite apart from calcification in tendons. Interestingly enough, such calcinosis may occur in association with scleroderma (Fig. 14-8), but it may be encountered

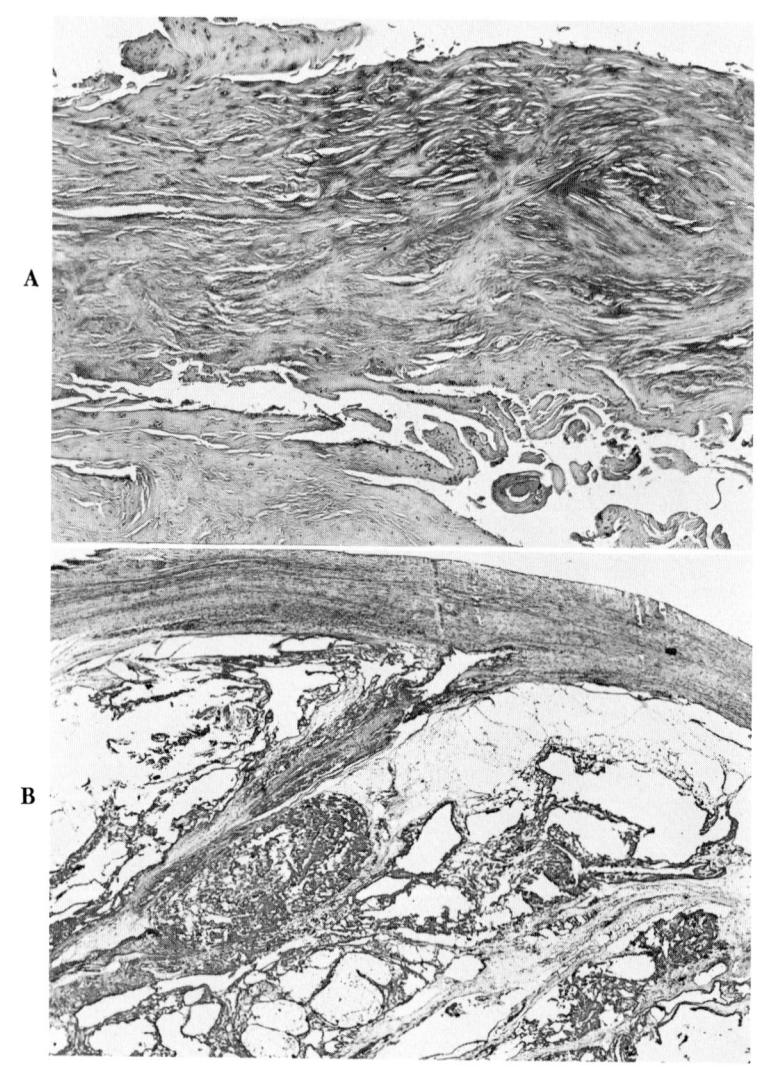

Fig. 14-9. **A**, Photomicrograph showing degeneration of collagenous connective tissue in a tendon. **B**, Myxoid degeneration and cystic softening of tendinous connective tissue, as a forerunner of spontaneous rupture (in an Achilles tendon). **C**, Photomicrograph of a section through the site of focal nodular thickening of a tendon sheath in a patient with stenosing tenovaginitis, or so-called trigger finger. Note the hyalinization of the connective tissue and its chondroid, or fibrocartilagenous, transformation. (×125.)

Pathology of some common and unusual orthopedic conditions

occasionally as an idiopathic manifestation. In the Burnett, or milk-alkali, syndrome[11] (seen in peptic ulcer patients), calcium deposits may also be laid down in skeletal structures, subcutaneous tissues, and the eye (band keratopathy); however, this is reversible.

Traumatic rupture of tendons is well known, especially in football players who may sever their heel cords or plantaris or patellar tendons, for example. Tendons, particularly the Achilles tendon, may also undergo significant *degenerative change* (Fig. 14-9, A). When the process develops relatively slowly over a period of years and allows for irregular scarring, a swelling or pseudotumor may be the result. More often, there is peculiar myxoid degeneration and cystic softening, for no apparent reason, predisposing to spontaneous rupture (Fig. 14-9, B).

Another condition that is noteworthy is *stenosing tenovaginitis*, particularly of a tendon sheath of a finger (so-called trigger finger). In this condition there is a block to the free movement of the tendon caused by a focal, nodular, fibrocartilagenous thickening of the tendon sheath, which must be excised to correct the condition (Fig. 14-9, C).

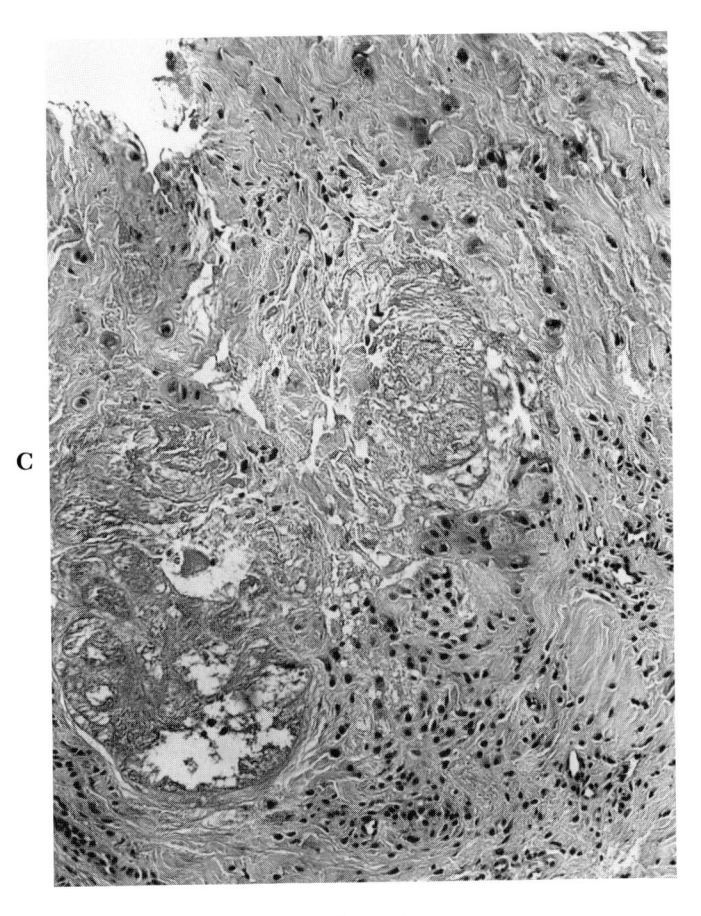

Fig. 14-9, cont'd. For legend see opposite page.

Diseases of bone and joints

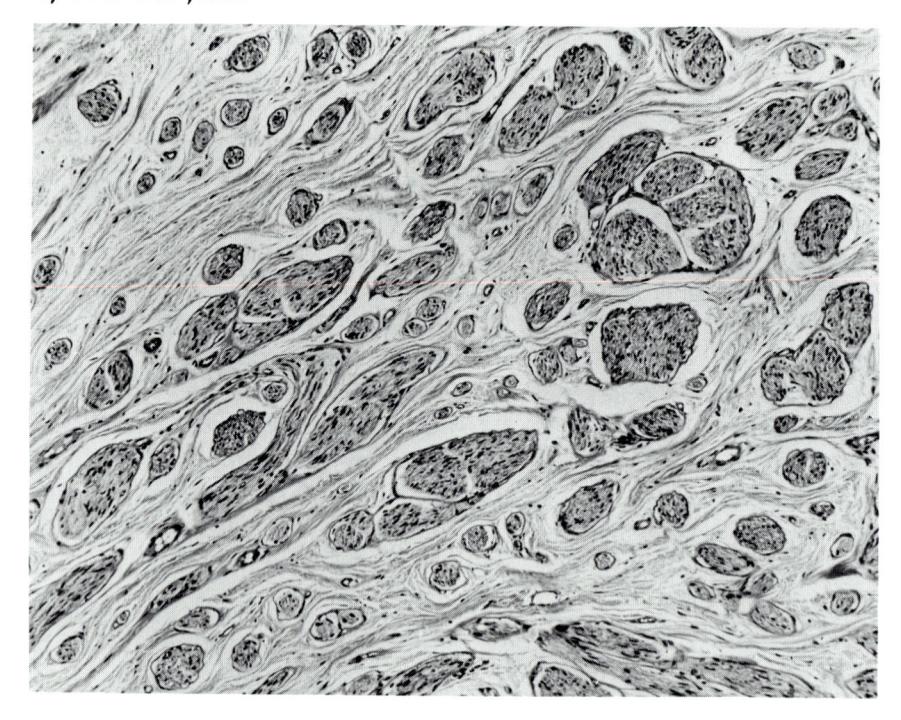

Fig. 14-10. Photomicrograph of a section taken through a bulbous amputation neuroma.

AMPUTATION NEUROMA

Amputation neuroma is a common cause of painful amputation stump, although it is also seen after the severance of peripheral nerves that are not repaired promptly and effectively for whatever reason. When explored, an amputation neuroma presents as a focal bulbous swelling at the site of severance. On microscopic examination one sees smaller and larger proliferating nerve bundles enveloped in scar tissue; these presumably fail to join their counterparts (Fig. 14-10).

VOLKMANN'S CONTRACTURE

Volkmann's contracture is the common orthopedic designation for contracture of muscle tissue following a deep laceration in which nutrient blood vessels are severed–for example, in the forearm, after the hand is thrust through a plateglass window. What happens pathologically is that, as a sequel of muscle necrosis, tracts of fibrous tissue grow into the muscle by way of attempted repair (Fig. 14-11). Whatever deformity ensues is the result of contraction of this scar tissue.

DUPUYTREN'S CONTRACTURE

Dupuytren's contracture is a fairly common surgical condition resulting from fibroplasia (or fibromatosis) of the palmar fascia–one of many sites of fibroplasia that may be encountered throughout the body. Continued interest in the subject

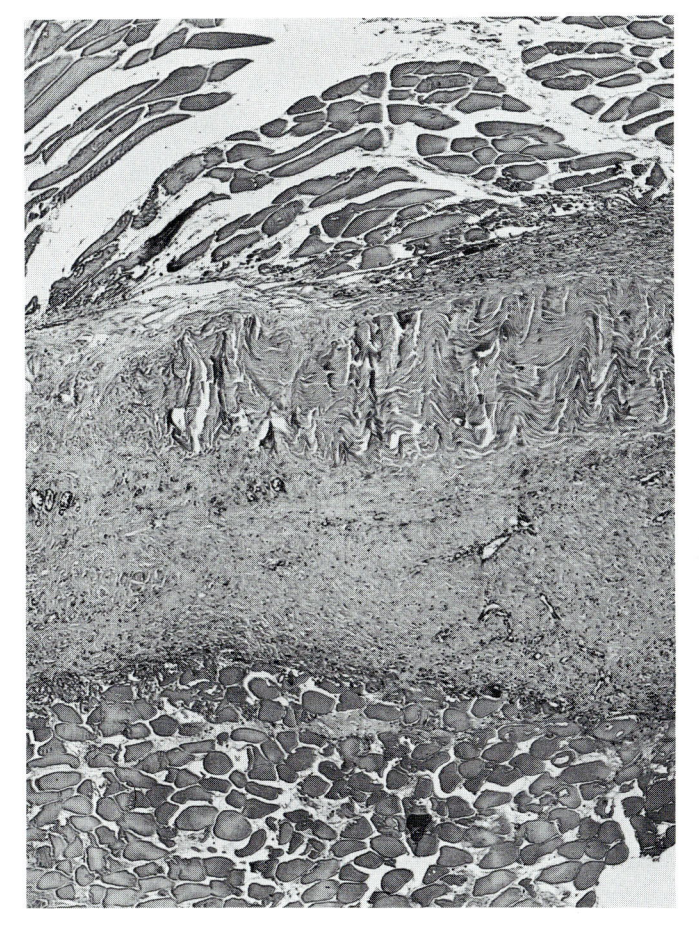

Pathology of some common and unusual orthopedic conditions

Fig. 14-11. Photomicrograph illustrating the changes found in Volkmann's contracture. Note the tract of scar tissue within the field of necrotic muscle. Deformity results from contraction of this scar tissue.

is evidenced by the recent publication of several monographs,[12,13] largely clinical in scope.

When the examining pathologist sections one or more of the gristly nodules in a relevant surgical specimen, he finds active spindle cell proliferation (Fig. 14-12), which may at times cause some concern over the possibility of fibrosarcoma. From examination by electron microscopy, it has been suggested[14] that these spindle cells are fibroblasts that have modulated into contractile cells (myofibroblasts), which play a role in the pathogenesis of the contracture observed clinically. The older quiescent areas show only more or less thickened fascia (not illustrated).

Actually, the process is self-limited; I have seen hundreds of cases in point and have no knowledge of a single instance of malignant change. What happens is that these cellular foci subside and collagen is formed, which contributes to

Diseases of bone and joints

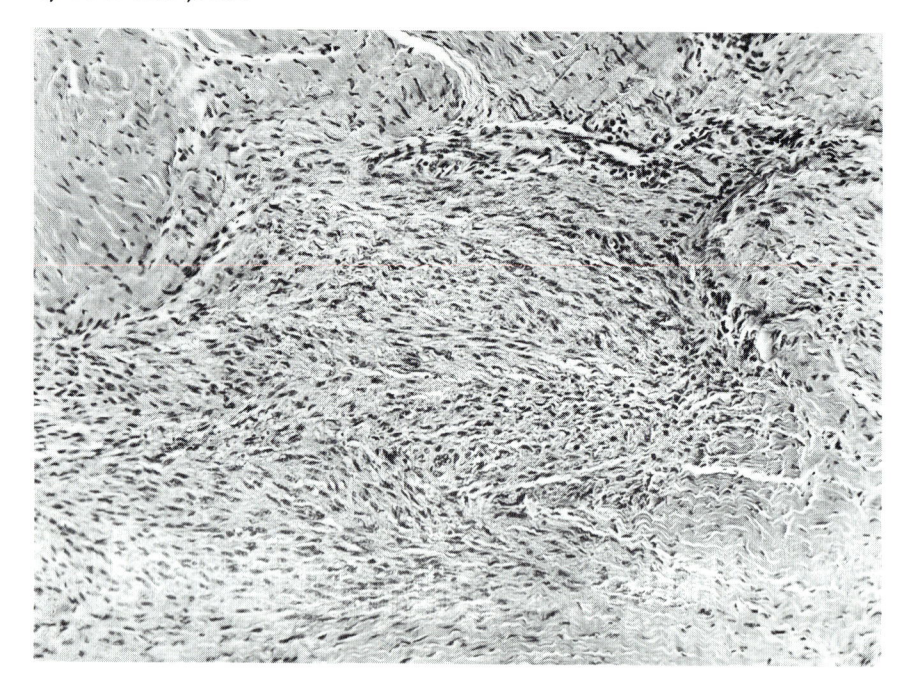

Fig. 14-12. Photomicrograph (low magnification) showing a focus of active fibroplasia in the palmar fascia of a patient with Dupuytren's contracture.

the thickening of the palmar fascia. Foci of active fibroplasia may, however, appear subsequently in other sites, accounting for the chronicity of the condition. This should not be construed as recurrence in pathologic terms. The collagen deposited tends to contract, and when this occurs in the fascial slips that extend into the flexor surface of the fingers, the latter are drawn into the palm of the hand, producing the characteristic deformity that Dupuytren described.

Essentially the same process is encountered at times in the plantar fascia of one or both feet.[15,16] Focal nodular fibroplasia in this site, however, seldom leads to contracture, as it does in the hand. Complete excision of the plantar fascia may be required for the relief of tender or painful nodes and to prevent "recurrence."

It may be noted also that fibroplasia or fibromatosis may develop in the connective tissue of muscle as well as in fascia, such as in the abdominal wall ("desmoid"), thigh, and sternocleidomastoid muscle of both newborn and older children. If the condition does not regress spontaneously in the last site listed, contracture of scar tissue may lead to the development of wryneck (*congenital torticollis, fibromatosis colli*).

BAKER'S CYST

The term "Baker's cyst" has come to be applied rather loosely to any cystlike structure in the popliteal space. Sometimes the cyst results from a herniation of the posterior capsule of the knee joint, although communication with the joint cannot always be demonstrated. In these circumstances, the sac may have a thin

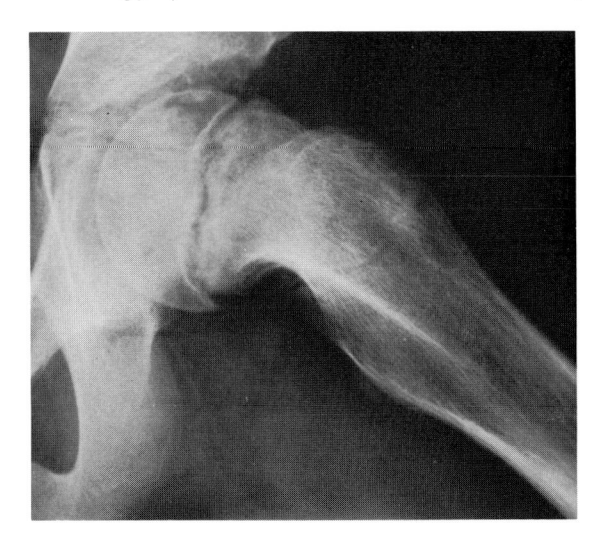

Pathology of some common and unusual orthopedic conditions

Fig. 14-13. Roentgenogram showing slipped capital femoral epiphysis (coxa anteverta). The patient was an obese adolescent.

wall, mucinous contents, and a delicate lining resembling synovium. Fibrous-walled bursal sacs in the popliteal area are also designated by some as Baker's cyst, although I do not follow this practice, preferring to avoid the eponym altogether as being unnecessarily confusing.

SLIPPED CAPITAL FEMORAL EPIPHYSIS

Slipped capital femoral epiphysis (adolescent coxa vara, coxa anteverta) is occasionally encountered as a spontaneous painful development in adolescents who tend to be overweight. Its pathogenesis has been the subject of much speculation for 30 years or more (Fig. 14-13). Adequate pathologic specimens are not readily available, inasmuch as the condition, if discovered early, may be corrected by closed manipulation. However, in the cases in which open surgery was done relatively early and sufficient bone was removed for pathologic examination, we had the distinct impression that the essential lesion was a shearing of the epiphyseal cartilage plate,[17] without necrosis, degeneration, or any other predisposing change, except perhaps for increased vascularity at the plate associated with a spurt of active growth at this period, as Trueta has emphasized. It is true that Lacroix and Verbrugge,[18] from their examination of a large specimen, postulated a fibrous transformation at the plate as the basic change. However, the condition in this case had been present for 3 years before a reconstructive procedure was done, and the changes they described may well have been secondary in nature.

CONGENITAL PSEUDOARTHROSIS OF TIBIA

Because it may be noted at birth or during childhood, this particular manifestation of pseudoarthrosis is held to be congenital. It is characterized clinically

Diseases of bone and joints

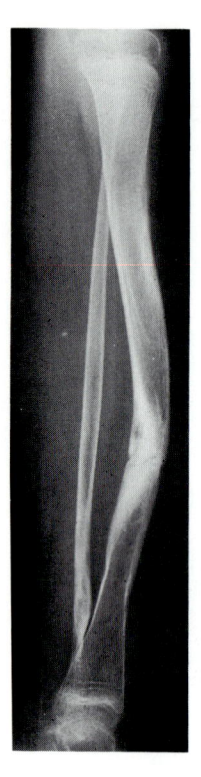

Fig. 14-14. Roentgenogram showing congenital pseudoarthrosis of the tibia in a child.

by thinning of the tibial cortex, predisposing to fracture through the shaft, and by a tendency to persistent fibrous union and pseudarthrosis, which is difficult to overcome surgically (Fig. 14-14). From the literature, it would appear that in about half of the cases reported there were cutaneous and other manifestation of von Recklinghausen's disease.

In the specimens of connective tissue and bone obtained in the course of corrective surgical procedures that we have had an opportunity to examine, we made it a point to search for indications of neurofibromatosis as a possible explanation for failure of bony union, but with no success. In line with this experience is a recent study[19] of the ultrastructure of the site of congenital pseudoarthrosis in three children with stigmata of neurofibromatosis, in which it was concluded that the connective tissue cells were fibroblasts, and not Schwann cells.

INFARCTS IN BONE *(avascular necrosis)*

Inasmuch as the long limb bones are supplied by nutrient arteries with limited collateral circulation, it is not surprising that infarcts, particularly at the bone ends, are found in a variety of predisposing circumstances, although they are not nearly as common as infarcts in certain viscera (heart, spleen, and kidneys, for example).

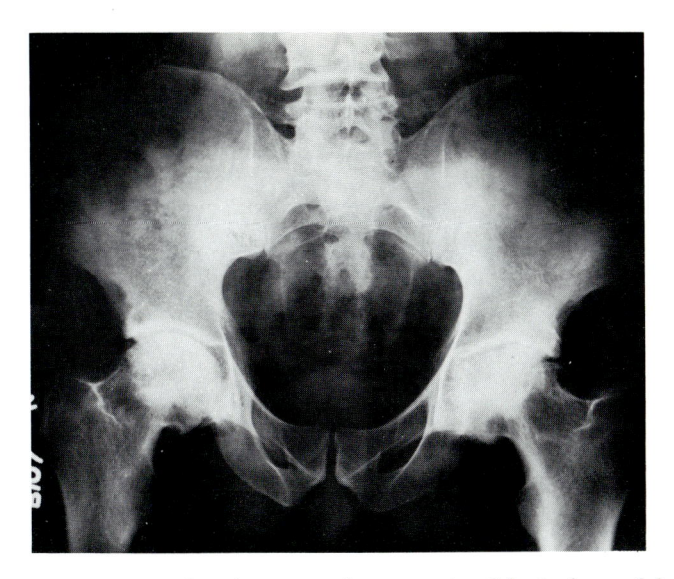

Fig. 14-15. Roentgenogram showing avascular necrosis of both femoral heads in caisson disease.

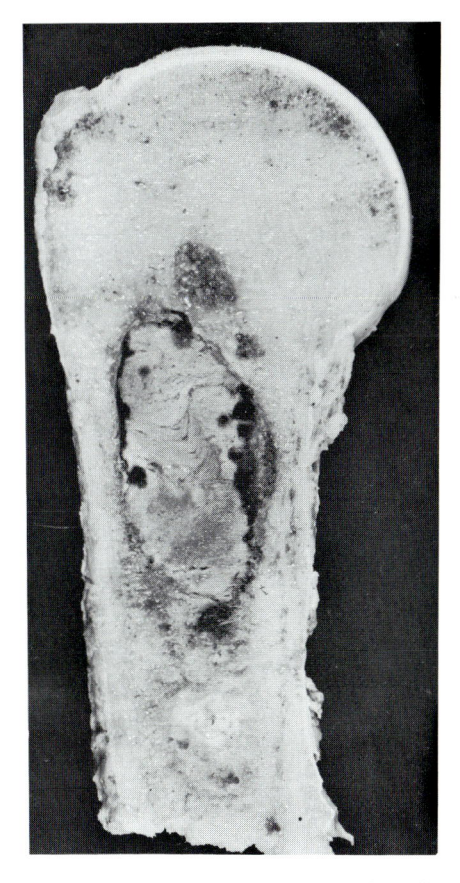

Fig. 14-16. Photograph showing an old infarct of bone found at autopsy in the upper femur of a 70-year-old man with heart block. Microscopically there was extensive secondary cholesterol deposition within the area of necrosis.

Diseases of bone and joints

Perhaps the most common cause of necrosis is loss of adequate blood supply following certain fractures, such as in the femoral head after fracture of the neck. Apart from this, bone infarcts, notably in one or both femoral heads, are seen in caisson workers (sandhogs) and occasionally in high altitude military flyers, presumably as a result of air (gas) embolism (Fig. 14-15). They are observed also in blacks with sickle cell anemia, apparently as a sequel of vascular occlusion. In patients with collagen disease, particularly disseminated lupus erythematosus, who have been on massive steroid therapy, infarcts of the femoral head have been noted too frequently for this to be fortuitous, although pathologic evidence (of endarteritis) is hard to come by.

Embolism in cardiac patients (Fig. 14-16), especially those with rheumatic heart disease and auricular fibrillation, is still another cause of infarcts in bone. I have observed an unusual instance in which a collapsed vertebra (T11) caus-

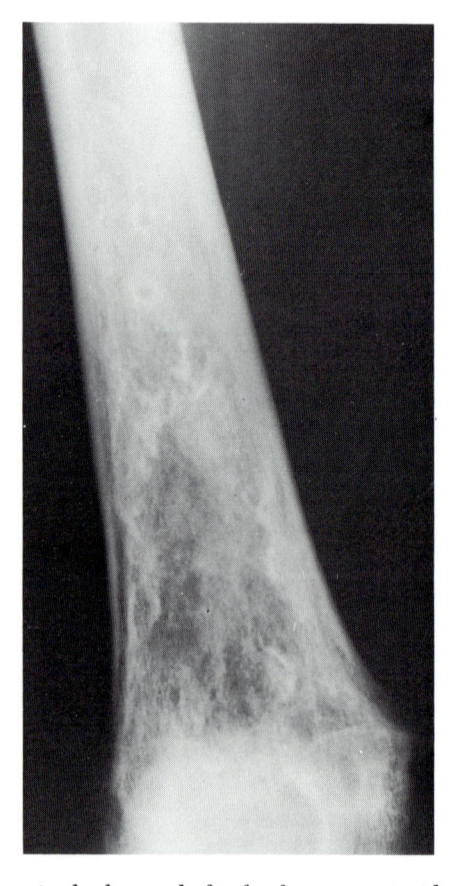

Fig. 14-17. An old infarct in the lower shaft of a femur—an incidental finding in an adult with an eosinophilic granuloma of a rib. There was a comparable symmetrical infarct in the opposite femur and similar smaller ones in both upper tibiae.

Pathology of some common and unusual orthopedic conditions

ing cord compression in a man, aged 66, who was recovering from an episode of congestive heart failure, showed a recent bone infarct on biopsy. As previously noted (see Fig. 6-2), deposition of abnormal lipid in bone, especially the femora in Gaucher's disease, may predispose to necrosis and collapse of the femoral head. Occasionally, infarction in the upper femur may be observed after injudicious forceful manipulation. From time to time, one may also observe old infarcts in bone that were clinically silent and for which there is no apparent cause (Fig. 14-17).

Whatever the cause of an infarct in bone, the involved area is, as a rule, readily recognizable in the gross as a well-demarcated, yellowish zone. In the femoral head, this often takes the form of a subchondral triangular wedge of varying size. A recent infarct (in the femoral head, for example) stands out radiographically as a relatively radiopaque area (Fig. 14-15). This may reflect the fact that the area of avascular necrosis retains its original density, whereas the surrounding bone undergoes resorption, making for appreciable contrast. An older infarct (in a femoral shaft, for example) may have variable density; it stands out because of the irregular calcification within it (Fig. 14-17). It should be pointed out, however, that intramedullary calcification may also outline a calcified enchondroma. At times, the differentiation may be difficult without tissue examination (Fig. 14-18).

Microscopically, there are two cardinal features that characterize an infarct in bone:

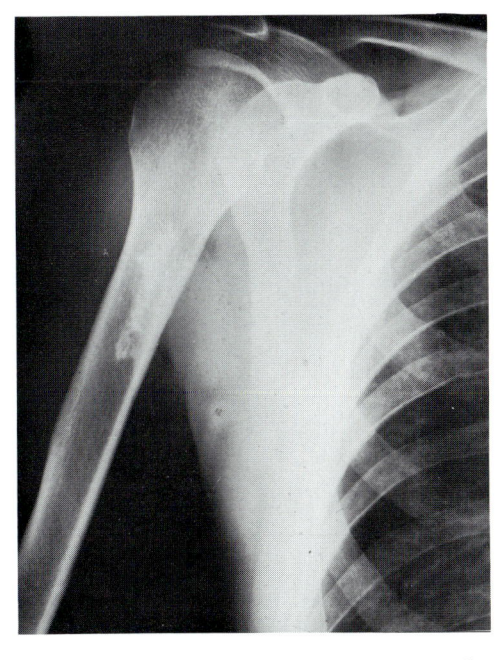

Fig. 14-18. Roentgenogram showing linear calcification within the upper shaft of a humerus, which may reflect either an old infarct or a calcified enchondroma.

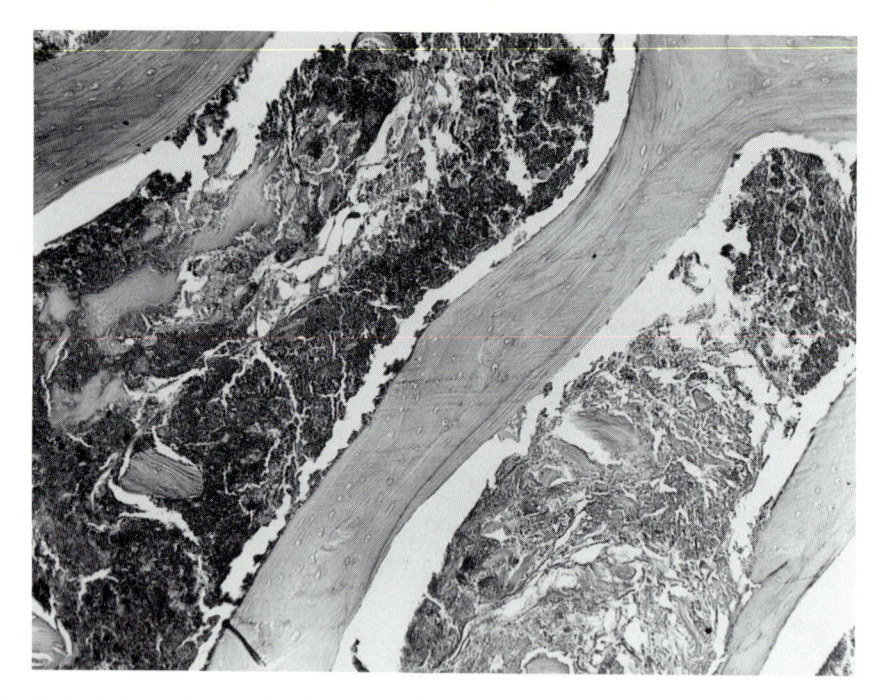

Fig. 14-19. Photomicrograph of an area of infarction in a femoral head showing necrosis of the bone and of the marrow as well. There was no creeping replacement or substitution of the dead bone in this field.

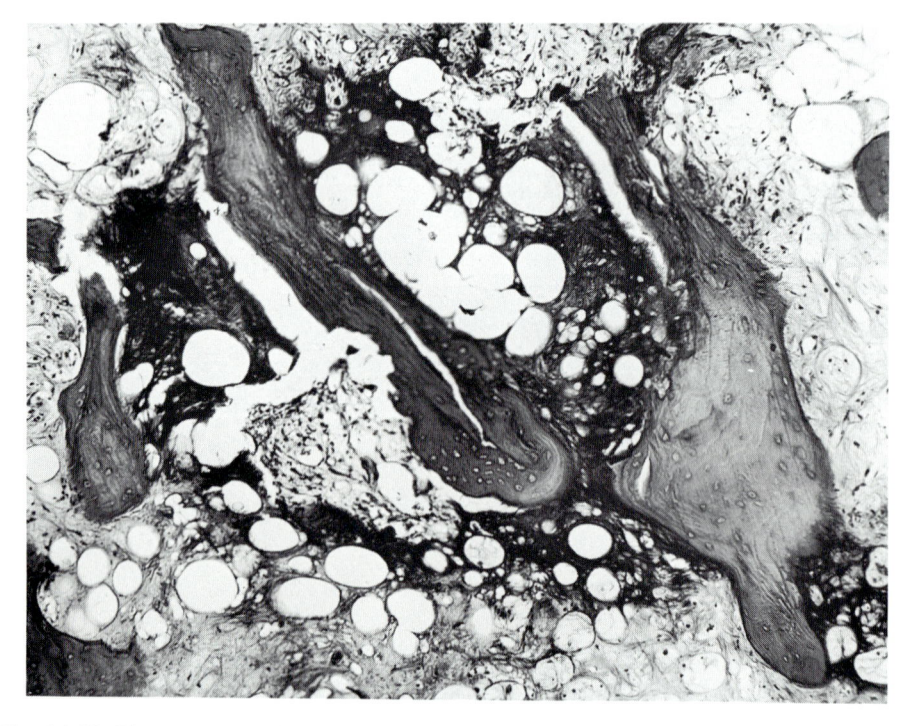

Fig. 14-20. Photomicrograph of an older area of infarction in which there has been appreciable calcification (black zones in the print) and organization of the necrotic fatty marrow.

1. Necrosis of the bone, as evidenced by the finding of empty lacunae devoid of osteocytes. This finding in itself is not sufficient, since it may follow a fracture.
2. The presence of necrotic detritus within the marrow spaces (Figs. 14-19 and 14-20).

An infarct in time tends to undergo certain secondary changes, namely scarring of the marrow, irregular calcification of dead bone and marrow, cholesterol deposition, and sometimes cystic softening (Fig. 14-20). With reference to the last, I have seen a specimen in point of a femoral head and neck in which there were cystic spaces up to 2 cm. in diameter containing clear viscid fluid. Reconstruction of the dead bone takes place, as previously noted (Chapter 1), by creeping replacement or substitution. Thin strips or tiers of new bone are deposited on top of the necrotic bone by osteoblasts accompanying vascular connective tissue that is able to penetrate the area of infarction. While this process is fairly rapid in a child (with Perthes' disease, for example), it is likely to be painfully slow in an adult, and many years may be required for any meaningful reconstruction of an infarct.

AVASCULAR NECROSIS OF BONE IN "JUVENILE OSTEOCHONDRITIS"

Infarcts of bone in so-called juvenile osteochondritis (epiphyseal osteochondritis of growth centers, osteochondritis deformans juvenilis, osteochondrosis, localized osteochondritis) comprise a special category about which reams have been written, much of it speculative. The nomenclature is obviously misleading in that inflammation is not a feature of the process. To make the subject more confusing, a dozen or more eponyms have been employed over the years to denote essentially the same pathologic lesion in various locations. Some of the better-known ones, in which significant pathologic data are available, are Legg-Perthe's disease (femoral head), Köhler's disease (tarsal navicular), Freiberg-Köhler's disease (metatarsal head), and Kienböck's disease (lunate). For a detailed discussion of the clinical and roentgenographic features of these disorders, as well as their pathogenesis, the reader may have profitable recourse to Chapter 19 in Jaffe's monograph.[20]

Irrespective of which primary or secondary epiphysis is affected, or whether a small circumscribed area or an entire epiphysis is involved, it seems clear from pathologic evidence that the essential change is that of avascular necrosis or infarction. In some instances, for example, Kienböck's disease of the lunate, there may be indications of fracture, as well as necrosis.

If one examines sections of an "osteochondritis dissecans" body from a knee joint, for example (Fig. 14-21)—and these are readily available as surgical specimens (either semidetached or as free joint bodies)—one finds necrosis of the subchondral bone and of the marrow as well (Fig. 14-22, A). The same is true of bone samples of the capital femoral epiphysis in Legg-Perthes' disease (Fig. 14-22, B). The cause of the infarct is presumed to be interference with or

Diseases of bone and joints

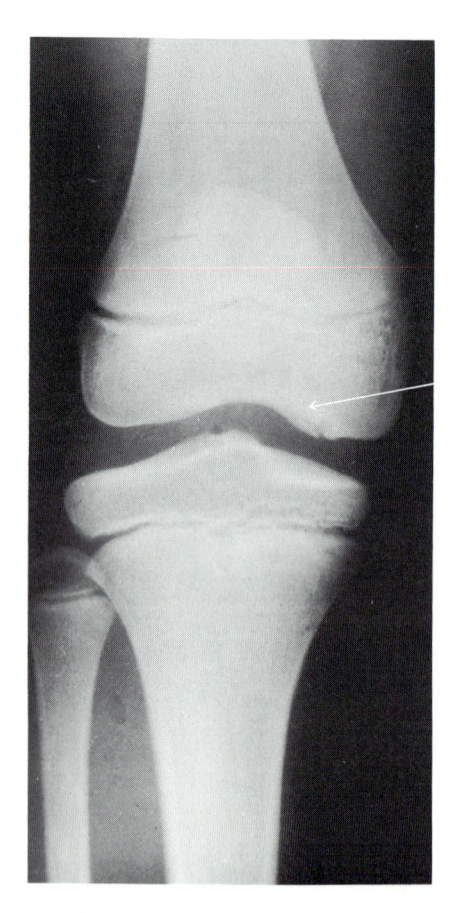

Fig. 14-21. Roentgenogram showing a small focus of osteochondritis dissecans in the medial femoral condyle of a child.

Fig. 14-22. **A**, Photomicrograph of a representative field of an osteochondritis dissecans body that was removed from a knee joint. The articular cartilage (above the dense horizontal cement line near the top) is viable. The subchondral bone, however, is substantially dead, and the marrow spaces within it contain dark-staining necrotic detritus. **B**, Photomicrograph of a section through the capital femoral epiphysis of a child with Perthe's disease (obtained by surgical-wedge biopsy). At top right is a bit of the articular cartilage of the femoral head. At bottom left is a bit of the epiphyseal cartilage plate. In the epiphysis, in between the two, one sees avascular necrosis of the bone (the lacunae were completely empty) and conspicuous (dark-staining) necrotic detritus in the marrow spaces. Together, these are clear indications of infarction. Compare with similar changes in osteochondritis dissecans, **A**. (×25.)

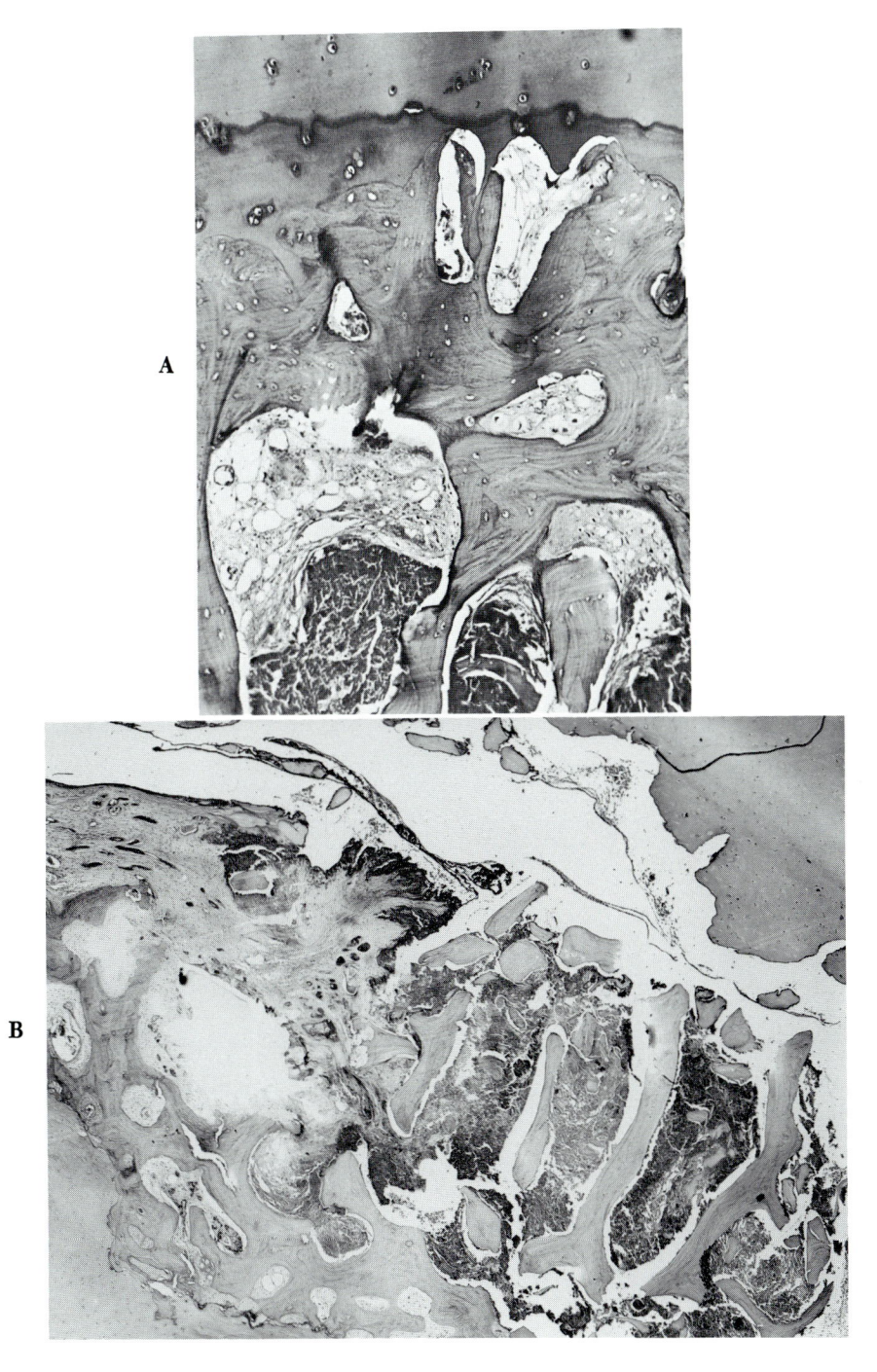

Pathology of some common and unusual orthopedic conditions

Fig. 14-22. For legend see opposite page.

Diseases of bone and joints

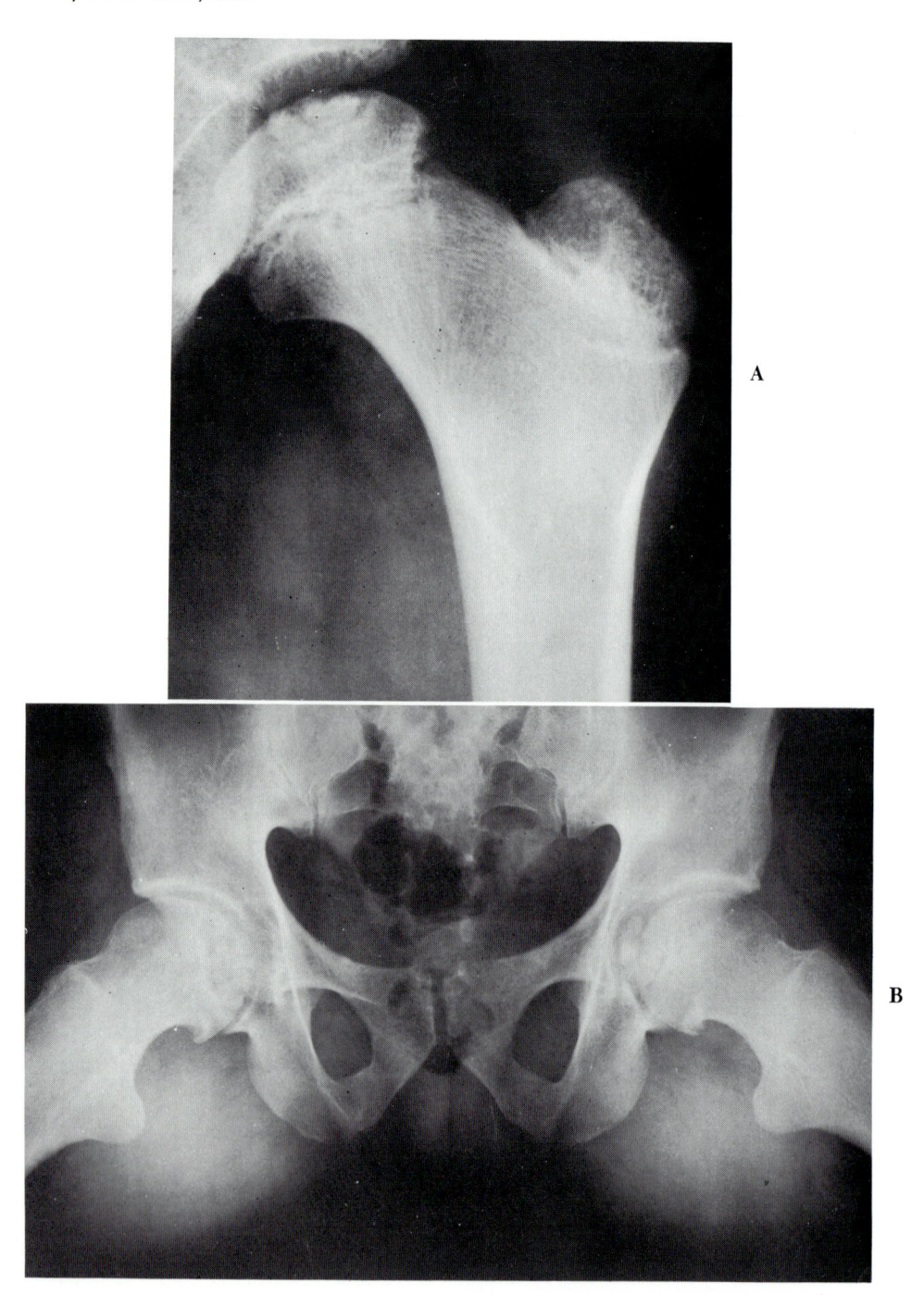

Fig. 14-23. **A,** Roentgenogram of a circumscribed focus of osteochondritis dissecans on the articular surface of a femoral head. **B,** Comparable lesions of osteochondritis dissecans in both femoral heads. It is noteworthy that at least two other members of this family had the same condition (familial occurrence of osteochondritis dissecans is well known).

Pathology of some common and unusual orthopedic conditions

loss of essential blood supply. This is a logical inference, although it is seldom, if ever, demonstrated pathologically. What is peculiar and puzzling is the phenomenon itself—why should infarcts develop in the growing epiphyses of young patients? Why, for example, should a circumscribed area of avascular necrosis appear in the capital femoral epiphysis (as shown in Fig. 14-23, *A*) or in both femoral heads (as illustrated in Fig. 14-23, *B*)? The answer may lie in the realm of pathophysiology of the available vasculature, and Trueta has made many relevant observations. Also, the prevalence of lesions of osteochondritis dissecans (in the hip, knee, and elbow) in certain families is well known,[21] but if the condition results from a gene-transmitted trait, again what is the mechanism for avascular necrosis?

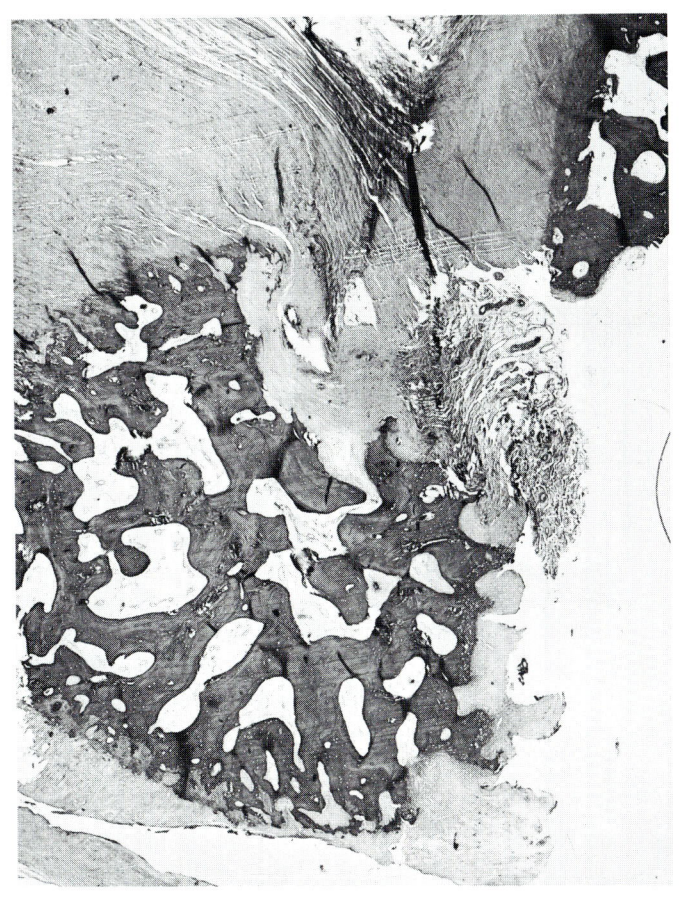

Fig. 14-24. Photomicrograph of a representative section of a specimen removed in a case of Osgood-Schlatter's disease. Note that the tibial apophysis (lower left) does *not* show avascular necrosis. The essential change is rather that of injury and reparative vasculation of the connective tissue between the apophysis and the tibia proper (upper right).

Incidentally, *Osgood-Schlatter's disease* does *not* belong in this category, despite what may be read in the literature. Pathologic examination of intact surgical specimens fails to show avascular necrosis of the tibial apophysis. What one does find is evidence of injury and reparative vascularization, either at the insertion of the patellar tendon or in the connective tissue interface between the apophysis and the tibia proper (Fig. 14-24). Uhry[22] demonstrated this in 1944. His observations were later confirmed and amplified by La Zerte and Rapp.[23] However, it appears that once a mistaken impression gets into the literature, it takes many years to eradicate it.

POSTTRAUMATIC RAREFACTION OF BONE

Following an acute trauma without fracture (and the injury need not be severe), one occasionally sees not only atrophic soft tissue changes including muscle atrophy, but also pronounced local rarefaction of bone. The "acute atrophy of bone" in these circumstances is accompanied by refractory pain and disability, which may persist for many months or even several years. Such changes in the hand and foot bones particularly are commonly designated as *Sudeck's atrophy*.[24] They are reflected roentgenographically in a hazy appearance initially and later by a mottled or spotted rarefaction. The type and extent of the atrophy and the attendant disability go far beyond anything that might be ascribed to the simple atrophy of inactivity or disuse. Occasionally, the rarefaction may be more circumscribed and affect a scaphoid, semilunar, or ulnar styloid.

Comparable changes may appear after an injury in vertebral bodies, which are then prone to collapse insidiously, giving rise to so-called *Kümmell's disease*. Once in a while, posttraumatic rarefaction may develop in a large limb bone, especially the femur, and the roentgenographic changes may be sufficiently pronounced as to suggest infection or a bone tumor. It has been shown pathologically by Jaffe[25] and others that the mottled bone rarefaction seen radiologically reflects thinning and porosity of the compact cortical bone, as well as diminution in the size and number of the spongy trabeculae, and that these changes are associated with striking hypervascularity. The latter is particularly prominent in the cortical bone, where large resorption spaces around eroded haversian systems are filled with loose connective tissue in which numerous dilated and engorged blood vessels are present. As for pathogenesis of the condition, it is generally postulated, in keeping with the view of Leriche, that after a trauma there is initially a vasomotor reflex spasm with injury to one or more bones, followed by a loss of neurovascular tone, persistent vasodilation, and rapid vascular resorption of bone as a consequence.

It is conceivable that so-called *disappearing* or *vanishing bone disease* (phantom bones, massive osteolysis, regional angiomatosis) represents a more severe expression of the same phenomenon, rather than angiomatosis in the sense of a neoplasm, as some have suggested. This peculiar condition has been known clinically for a long time,[26] but it was not until recent years that a spate of articles on the subject appeared, only a few of which are cited here for convenient orientation.[27-30] Disappearing bone disease may affect one or more bones of the shoulder girdle (clavicle, scapula, and upper humerus), the lower extremity, and the pelvis, as well as ribs and vertebrae. Whatever region is involved, there is a tendency to progressive rarefaction and, eventually, lysis of the bone, so that its original contour is no longer discernible. Interestingly enough, the process tends to subside after a time, according to published reports, but not until there has been considerable loss of bone.

In the limited relevant material that I have had occasion to review, the only consistent feature was the presence of congeries of congested capillaries. While one can readily understand how this finding might be construed as indicative of hemangioma or "angiomatosis," I see no compelling reason to do so. There is a vast capillary bed in the marrow, only a small part of which is utilized or even discernible under ordinary circumstances. However, with loss of the normal neurovascular regulatory mechanism, the dilatation and engorgement of the entire potential capillary bed might easily simulate hemangioma.

MYOSITIS OSSIFICANS

Myositis ossificans is actually a misnomer in that (1) inflammatory reaction is the exception rather than the rule, and (2) it is the connective tissue in muscle that ossifies—the muscle tissue itself undergoes atrophy and tends to disappear at the affected site. In pathologic terms, the process is that of metaplastic ossification, and sometimes cartilage formation as well, in the connective tissue of muscle.

The condition is usually localized and is only rarely progressive or generalized. It occurs in children as well as adults. The most common sites of involvement are the thigh (in quadriceps and vastus muscles, particularly) and the arm (especially in the brachialis anticus muscle), although these are by no means the only ones (Fig. 14-25). Very often there is a history of prior injury, but this is not invariably the case. Initially, there is a painful swelling of varying size, which can be puzzling or alarming clinically. Only after some 2 weeks or more does one discern focal radiopacity (reflecting bone formation through calcification of osteoid).

When the lesion is deep seated and in proximity to the periosteum, its early roentgenographic picture may arouse a suspicion of malignant neoplasm, although it tends to become smaller and more clearly localized in the ensuing months. Malignant change in myositis ossificans has been recorded, but it is comparatively rare. As experienced orthopedists are well aware, early surgery before the process has become quiescent and static only tends to stir up renewed activity.

Examination of a surgical specimen of a focus of myositis ossificans still in an active phase reveals impressive proliferation of spindle connective tissue cells and, in places, the formation of osteoid and bone, which tends to become organized into trabeculae (Fig. 14-26). In this milieu, one can readily discern

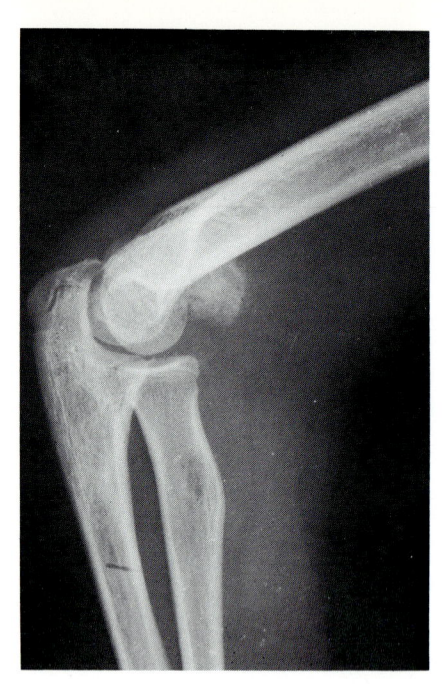

Fig. 14-25. Roentgenogram showing an organized focus of myositis ossificans in the vicinity of an elbow joint, a relatively frequent site of localization.

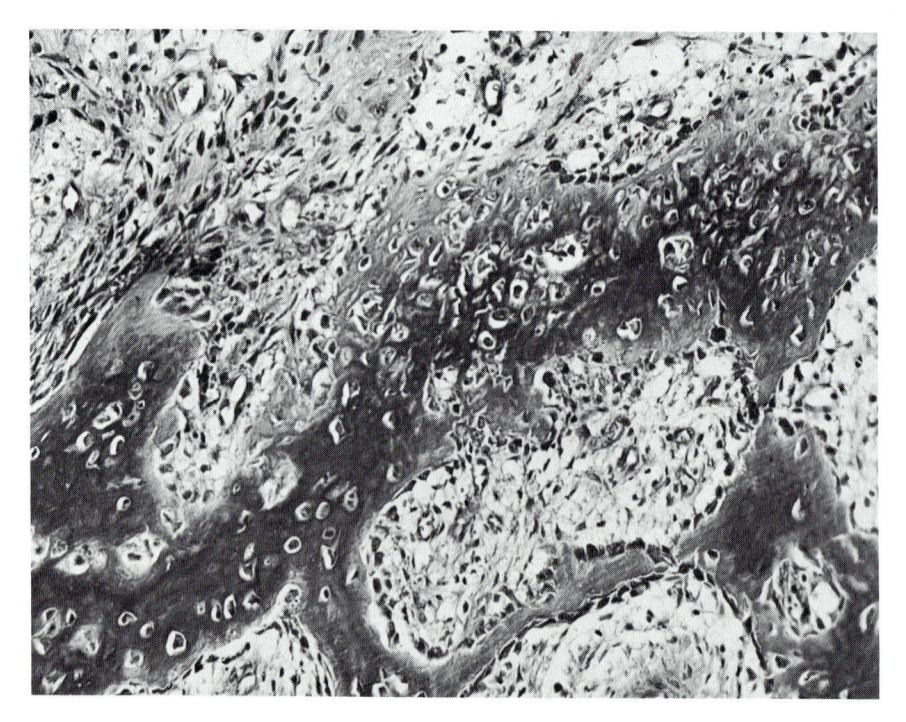

Fig. 14-26. Photomicrograph of a lesion of myositis ossificans still in an active stage. Pictures such as this are sometimes interpreted as osteogenic sarcoma by inexperienced pathologists who fail to take cognizance of the fact that the process has developed *outside* the bone. Note the proliferating connective tissue stroma and the transition to plump osteoblasts, which are actively engaged in laying down new bone.

Pathology of some common and unusual orthopedic conditions

the transition from fibroblasts to osteoblasts. A small amount of cartilage may also be formed; this tends to undergo fairly rapid osseous transformation. In some lesions, giant cells may be prominent in places within the condensed connective tissue areas, as well as in proximity to mineralized matrix. The trabecular organization of bone is most apparent in the older peripheral portion of the lesion. This should be reassuring to a pathologist who is concerned about the possibility of osteogenic sarcoma, apart from the fact that the stroma, while cellular, is not malignant.

In older, mature, or reconstructed lesions of myositis ossificans in which the process has simmered down, active fibroplasia is no longer in evidence, and the bone that has been formed appears to be well organized (Fig. 14-27).

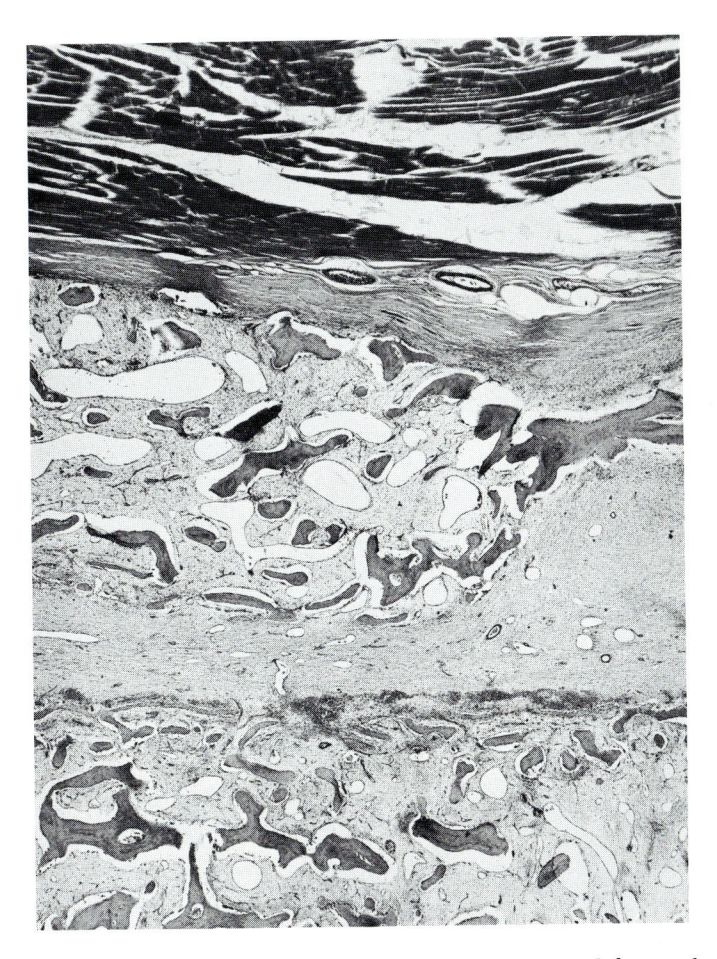

Fig. 14-27. Photomicrograph of an older, mature or reconstructed focus of metaplastic ossification of the connective tissue in muscle (myositis ossificans) (compare with Fig. 14-26).

Diseases of bone and joints

METAPLASTIC OSSIFICATION IN OTHER SITES

Viewed in perspective, myositis ossificans is only one expression of a more general phenomenon in skeletal pathology. Paraskeletal connective tissue, wherever it may be, retains the capacity to form bone and cartilage by metaplasia (perhaps an atavistic throwback to the time when our remote ancestors were armadillos). This trait is apparently more pronounced in some individuals than in others. Thus one observes metaplastic bone, and perhaps cartilage, formation in joint capsules (either spontaneously or, more often, after surgery), in tendons (particularly the Achilles tendon, after injury or previous surgery), in ligaments, fascia, and aponeuroses, and, most importantly, in the cambium layer of the periosteum (after fracture and under other circumstances, to be indicated).

Periosteal ossification may follow an injury without fracture that results in a tear or lifting up of the membrane. It may also be a sequel of subperiosteal hemorrhage, notably in scurvy, hemophilia, or trauma ("ossifying hematomas").

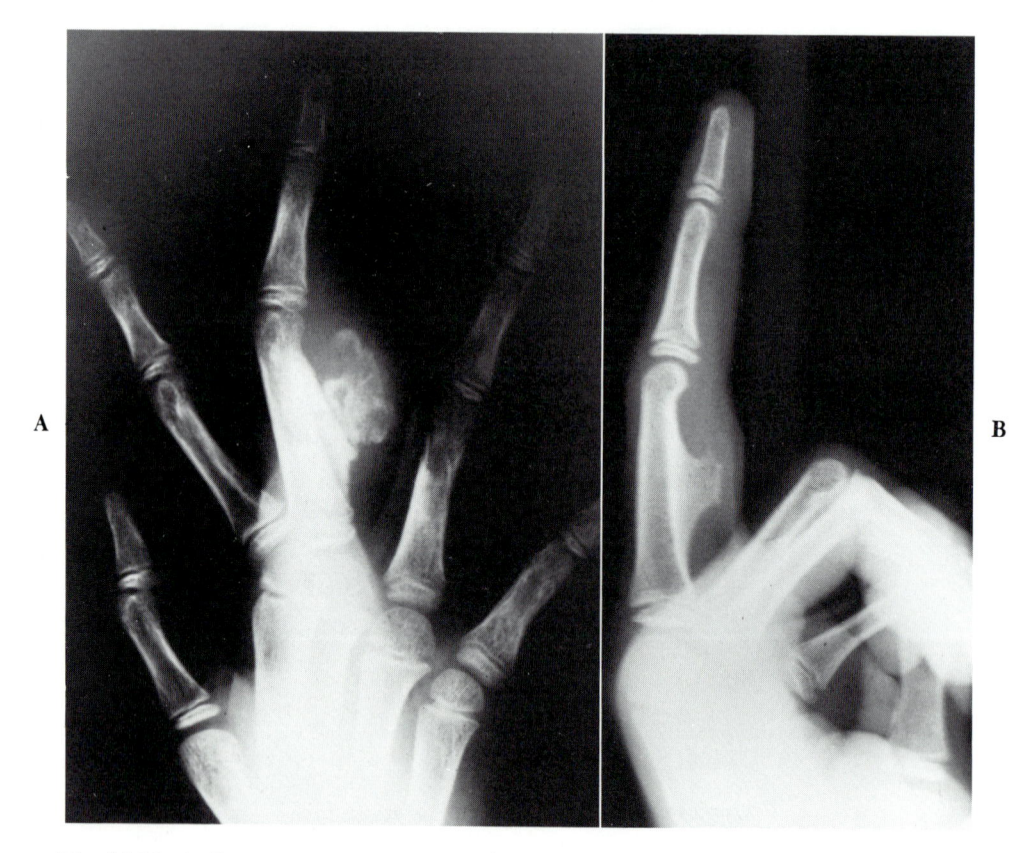

Fig. 14-28. **A,** Roentgenogram of a bone-forming parosteal growth on the proximal phalanx of the long finger of an 11-year-old boy who had injured the finger while playing ball. The x-ray picture aroused some concern over the possibility of osteosarcoma, but biopsy showed only active metaplastic bone formation, and nothing further was done. **B,** Roentgenogram showing bony reconstruction of the lesion illustrated in **A** some 8 months later. (Courtesy Dr. Donald L. Hager, Los Angeles.)

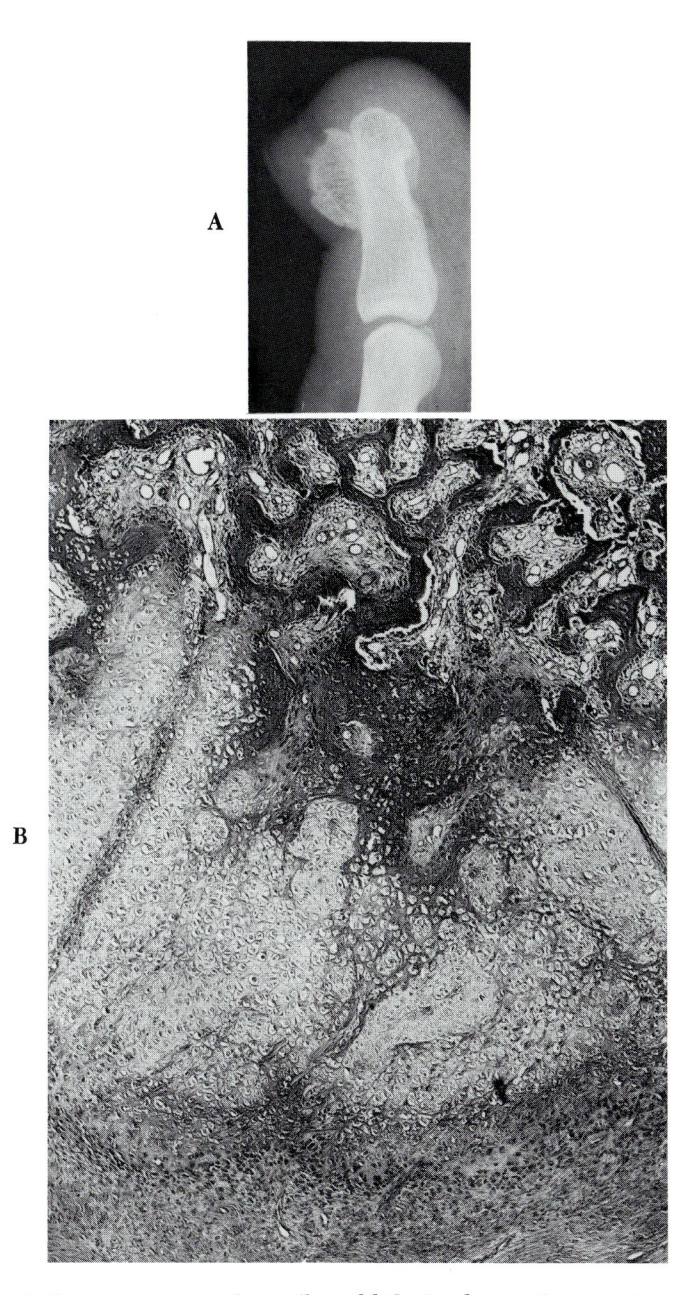

Pathology of some common and unusual orthopedic conditions

Fig. 14-29. **A**, Roentgenogram of a well-established subungual exostosis protruding from the nail bed of the distal phalanx of a toe in a young female patient. **B**, Photomicrograph (low magnification) of a section through a subungual exostosis in a female teen-ager. At the bottom is the active cambium layer of the periosteum (the nail bed of the toe is not included in the picture). Above that is an irregular (pale) zone of newly formed cartilage, which tends to undergo osseous transformation. The bulk of the growth, and the oldest portion of it, was composed of newly formed bone (at the top) undergoing trabecular organization. (×50.)

249

Diseases of bone and joints

Further, any intramedullary lesion of bone that erodes or penetrates the cortex stimulates the periosteum to lay down new bone in an apparent attempt to buttress the weakened cortex. Occasionally, localized periosteal ossification develops without any obvious predisposing cause and may arouse concern over the possibility of osteogenic sarcoma (Fig. 14-28).

Subungual exostosis represents another noteworthy expression of metaplastic bone and cartilage formation by the cambium layer of the periosteum. In this condition, as the name indicates, a hard growth develops in the nail bed (of a toe), which protrudes from the dorsum of the distal phalanx (Fig. 14-29). Over the years I have had occasion to review a substantial number of instances submitted for opinion. In most of them, curiously enough, the patients were young females between the ages of 6 and 20 years—it may be that wearing open-toe shoes predisposes to injury at a time when the periosteum at this site is still potentially active. In any case, sections show the "tumor" to be composed of actively growing, metaplastic bone and cartilage (in varying proportions), which is clearly of periosteal origin. When the process is exuberant, the examining pathologist, if he is not familiar with the condition, may take too serious a view of the findings and interpret them as indicating osteosarcoma or chondrosarcoma (Fig. 14-29, *B*). Actually, I have never seen malignant change in these circumstances.

In *hypertrophic osteoarthropathy*,[31,32] which is associated mainly but not exclusively with pulmonary neoplastic or suppurative disease, the periosteal new bone apposition is more widespread and may be layered on phalanges, metacarpals, and metatarsals and the distal portions of the long bones of the arm or leg (Fig. 14-30). It is usually bilateral and more or less symmetrical. The soft tissues over the joints and the ends of the long bones are warm and tender. The condition is often associated with clubbing of the fingers and toes, and the whole picture may well be a sequel of increased arterial pressure and peripheral blood flow.[33] Pathologic studies have shown[31] that initially there is increased vascularity, edema, and infiltration of the periosteal connective tissue by lymphocytes and plasma cells, and this is soon followed by periosteal new bone formation. The new bone is, at first, cancellous and highly vascular, and later becomes more compact, as it is incorporated in the original cortex.

With successful treatment of the underlying thoracic condition, if that is possible, there is regression of clubbing and a fall in peripheral blood flow. Also noteworthy is the provocative observation[34] that the pain and joint swelling of osteoarthropathy can be dramatically relieved by vagotomy.

UNICAMERAL BONE CYST

Our interest in unicameral bone cyst, a fairly common entity, dates back to 1942, when Jaffe and I[35] described its essential pathology in correlation with the roentgenographic changes, with a view to resolving further the then popular mishmash of "localized fibrocystic disease of bone." It is gratifying that, with the delineation of fibrous dysplasia, bone cyst, and fibrous cortical defect or

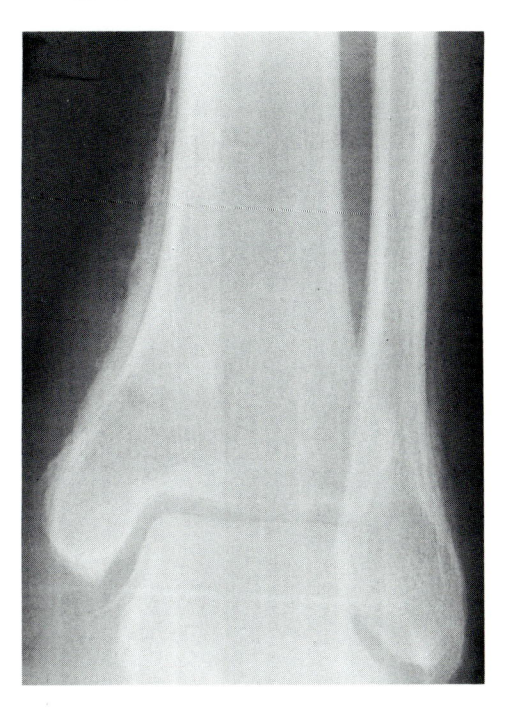

Pathology of some common and unusual orthopedic conditions

Fig. 14-30. An instance of hypertrophic osteoarthropathy showing conspicuous periosteal new bone apposition on the lower tibia and fibula. The patient had chondrosarcoma of bone with a large pulmonary metastasis.

nonossifying fibroma, as well as the osseous manifestations of hyperparathyroidism, this catchall designation has been relegated to the historic shelf of skeletal pathology.

Solitary unicameral bone cyst occurs mainly in children and adolescents, more often in males, and, with few exceptions, develops in the shaft of a long tubular bone. The upper humeral shaft is its most common site (Fig. 14-31) and the upper femur the next most common (Fig. 14-32), although occasional instances are encountered in the lower femur, the upper or lower tibia, and the forearm bones (Fig. 14-33). Only rarely does one see a bone cyst elsewhere, such as in a rib, an iliac bone, or a hand or foot bone. A few have been reported in the talus,[36] and I have seen a large one in a calcaneus (Fig. 14-35, *C*). It appears to be exceptional also for a unicameral bone cyst to involve the epiphyseal end of the bone, although this may happen (Figs. 14-34 and 14-35).

Pathologically, as its designation indicates, the lesion is a fluid-containing unicameral cavity. The fluid may be clear and yellow or serosanguineous, particularly if there has been a recent cortical infarction. The overlying cortex is usually thinned and expanded. The periosteal surface is smooth, and there is no new bone apposition unless there has been a pathologic fracture. Its inner (endosteal) surface may show slight ridging and is ordinarily lined by a thin membrane of connective tissue, yielding no more than one or two curettefuls

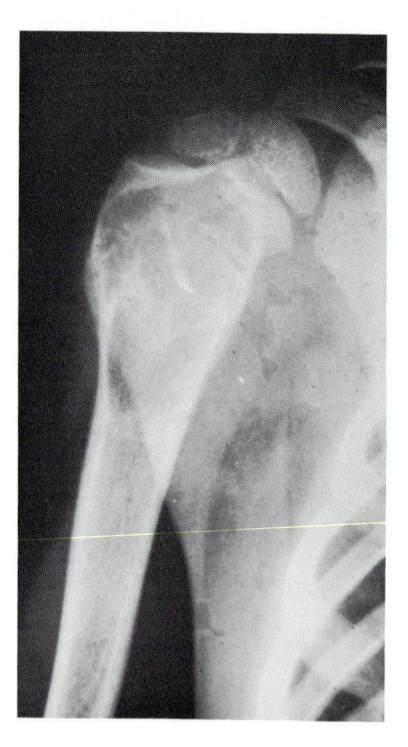

Fig. 14-31. Roentgenogram of a solitary unicameral bone cyst in its most common site, the upper metaphysis of a humerus. It still borders on the growth plate and is therefore in an active stage, capable of further enlargement.

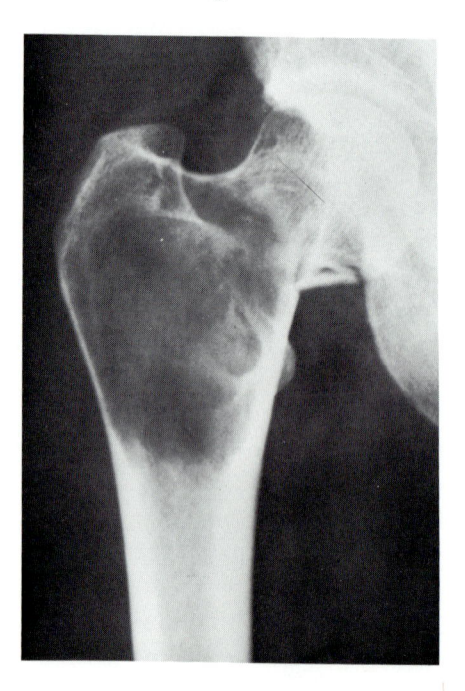

Fig. 14-32. Roentgenogram of a unicameral bone cyst in the upper femur of a young woman of 22, which came to clinical notice because of a pathologic fracture of the femoral neck.

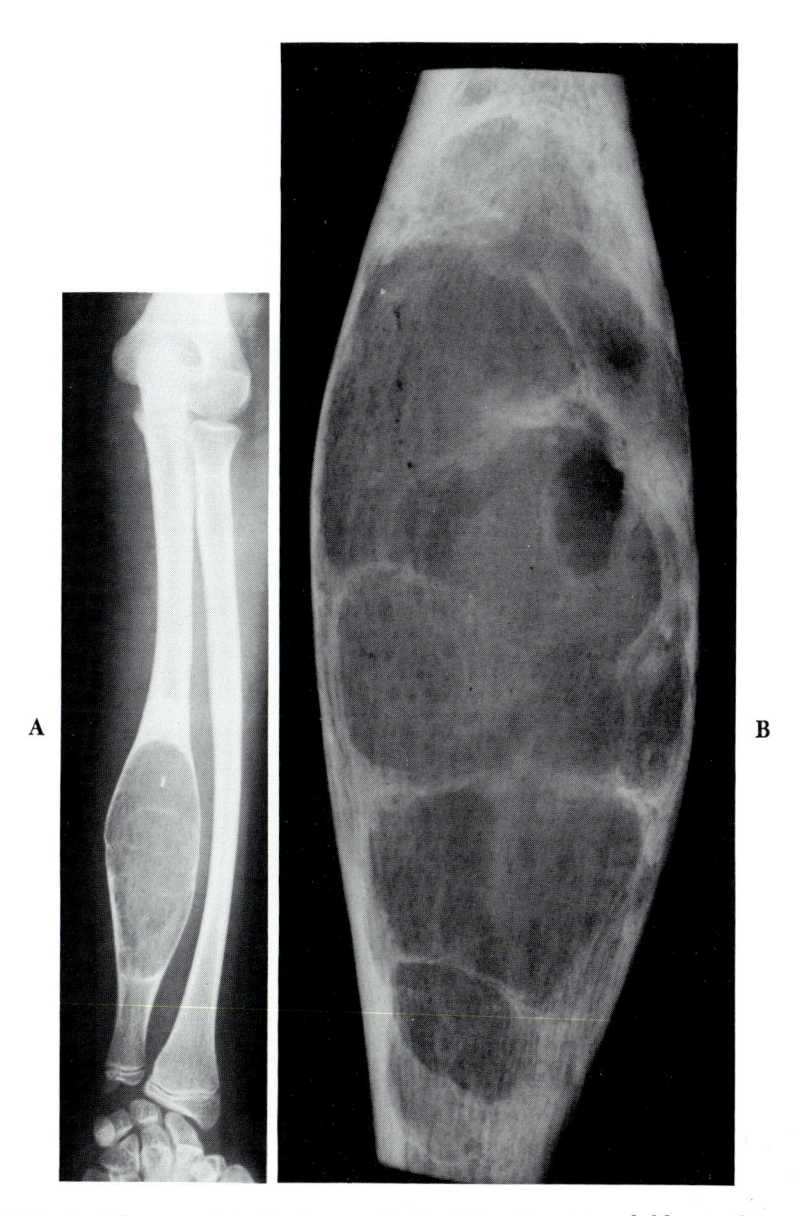

Pathology of some common and unusual orthopedic conditions

Fig. 14-33. **A,** A bone cyst in the lower shaft of the ulna in a child—a rather unusual site for it. This cyst was known to have been present for several years before it was operated on. **B,** Enlargement of the resected bone cyst in the ulna illustrated in **A** to show greater detail.

Diseases of bone and joints

on thorough scraping. Sections of this material may show some new bone formation, blood extravasation, hemosiderin pigment, a scattering of multinuclear macrophages, and often organizing fibrin, which may serve as a substrate for osteoid transformation. Occasionally, especially in older cysts, there may be prominent lipid deposits that take the form of either cholesterol crystals or foam cells containing cholesterol esters (Fig. 14-36).

The evolution of a bone cyst may be seen as developing in two phases: (1) an active phase, in which the lesion in the metaphysis still abuts on the growth plate and is capable of progressive enlargement (Fig. 14-31), and (2) a latent phase, in which the lesion has moved away from the plate down the shaft; the lesion no longer enlarges, but it persists unless it is operated on (Figs. 14-36 and 14-38). The indicated procedure is, of course, thorough curettement and packing with bone chips.[37] Autogenous spongy bone from the iliac crest seems

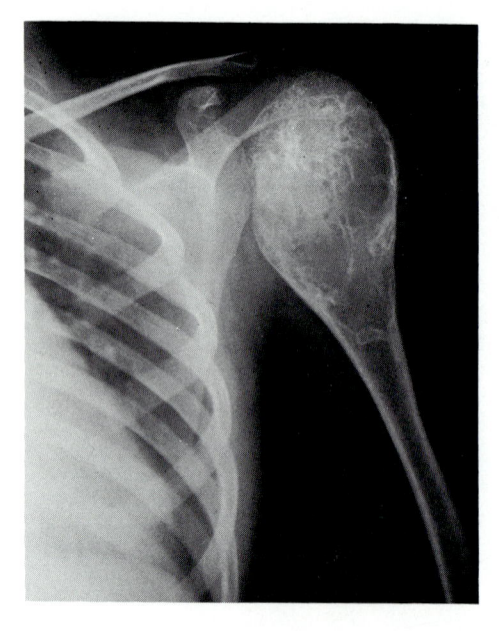

Fig. 14-34. A unicameral bone cyst in a child, which is unusual in that it involved the entire head of the humerus as well as the metaphysis. (The epiphyseal cartilage plate is gone.)

Fig. 14-35. **A**, A remarkable bone cyst in the upper metaphysis of the tibia of a 10-year-old child, which also involved the adjacent epiphysis. There was a 2-cm. defect in the epiphyseal cartilage plate at the site of communication between the two fluid-filled compartments. **B**, Followup roentgenogram taken 3 years after surgery. The reconstructed, previously cystic area has moved away from the plate. **C**, Roentgenogram of an unusual, circumscribed, and rarefied defect in a calcaneus, which proved on tissue examination to be a bone cyst.

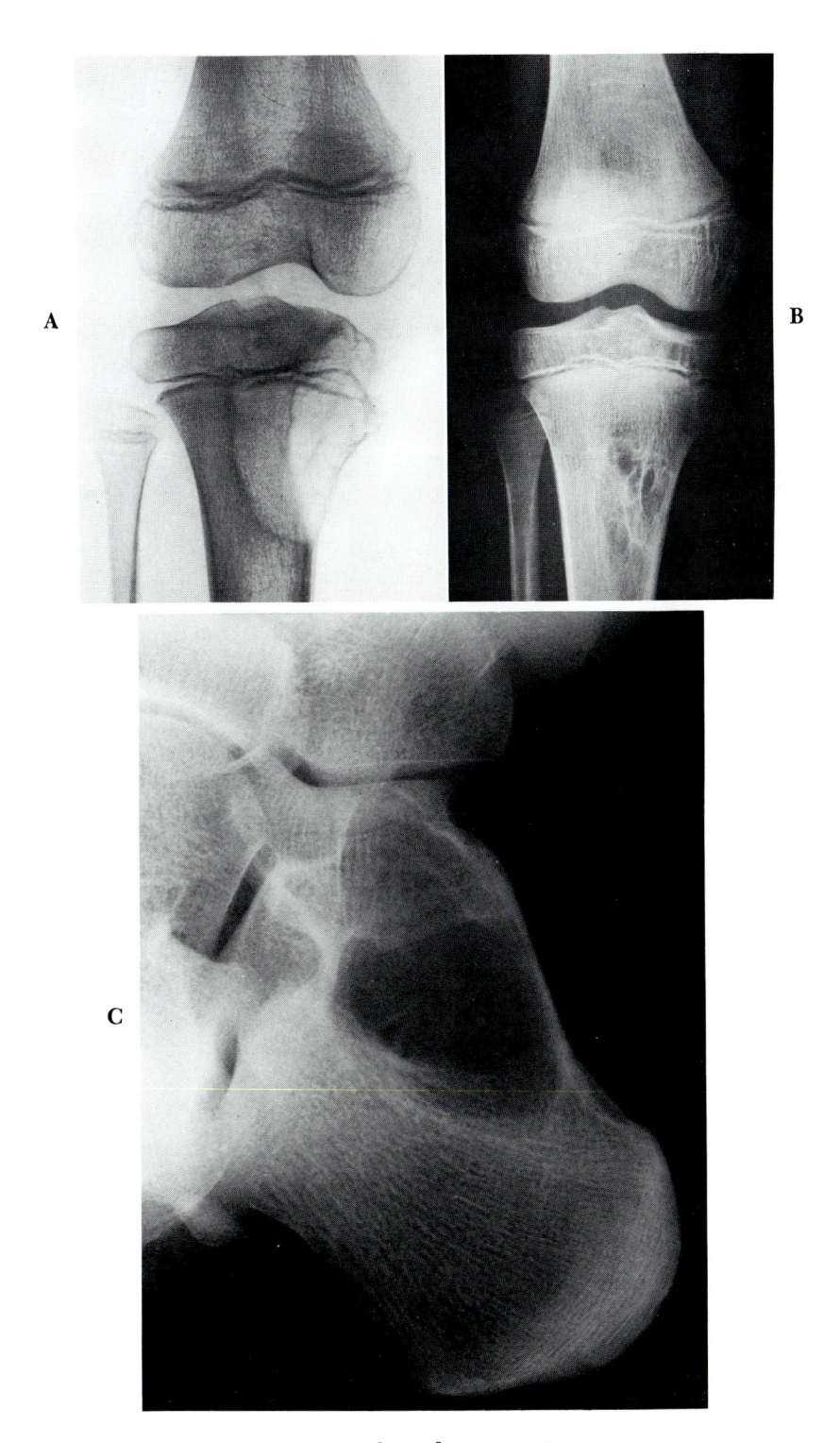

Pathology of some common and unusual orthopedic conditions

Fig. 14-35. For legend see opposite page.

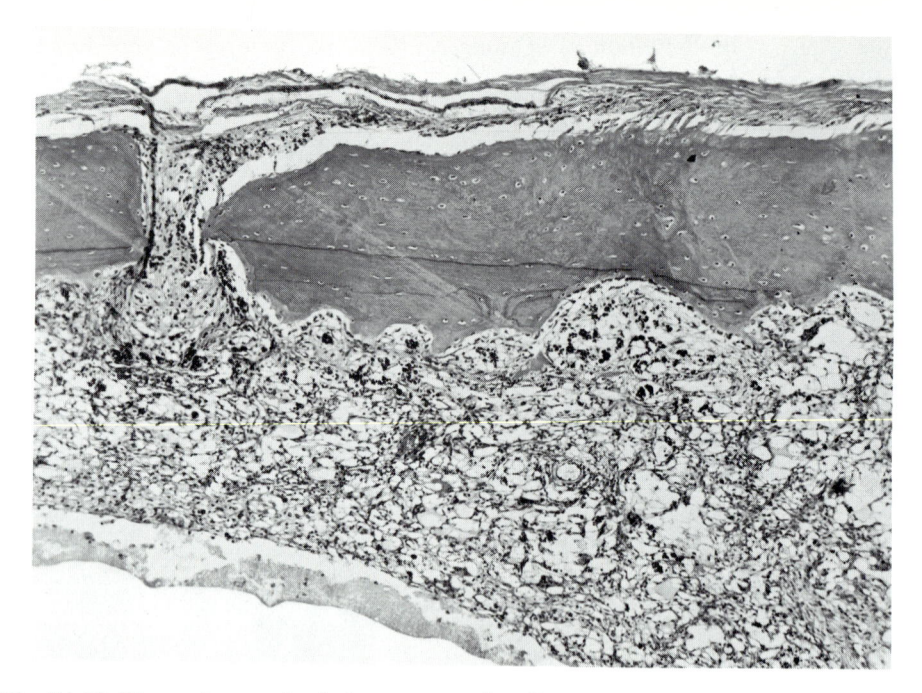

Fig. 14-36. Photomicrograph of the attenuated wall of a bone cyst. The lining tissue in this instance contained abundant lipid in the form of foam cell aggregates.

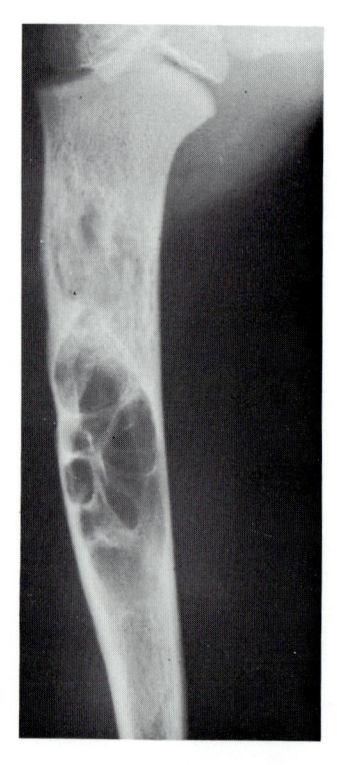

Fig. 14-37. Roentgenogram of a latent bone cyst in the upper shaft of a humerus, persisting after unsuccessful curetment and packing. The cyst moved away from the plate region but did not heal.

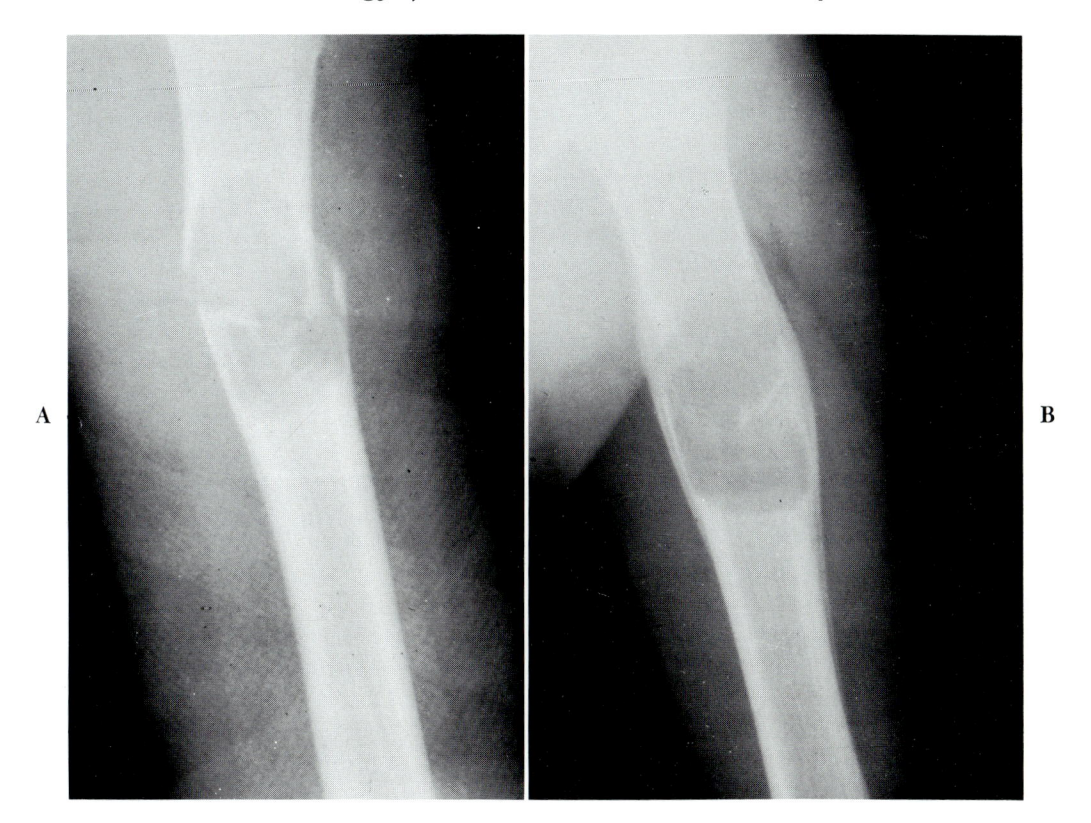

Pathology of some common and unusual orthopedic conditions

Fig. 14-38. **A**, A latent bone cyst in the upper shaft of a humerus with a pathologic fracture through its thin cortical wall. **B**, Healing of the fracture shown in **A**. The cyst itself did not disappear.

clearly to be the material of choice, although, if this is not available, cancellous bank bone can be utilized. Milled bone is not nearly as satisfactory, and the results with Boplant that I have seen have not been encouraging. In any event, it must be recognized that an occasional cyst fails to heal after surgery and may require reoperation or, in a few cases, even a third procedure (Fig. 14-37). Irradiation appears to delay healing and is definitely contraindicated, for this and other reasons.

Pathologic fracture, which often directs attention to the presence of a bone cyst, tends to heal rapidly (Fig. 14-38). While it may be followed by spontaneous healing of the cyst, this happens only occasionally.

The pathogenesis of unicameral bone cyst is not well understood, although it has been the subject of debate and speculation for over 60 years. I can recall wading through a 90-page, old German article by Pommer dealing with this question, only to find toward the end that his theory was based on examination of half of one specimen. Inasmuch as the lesion develops at the epiphyseal plate region, it seems logical to postulate that it has its basis in a local disorder of growth and development. This is begging the question, however—precisely

Diseases of bone and joints

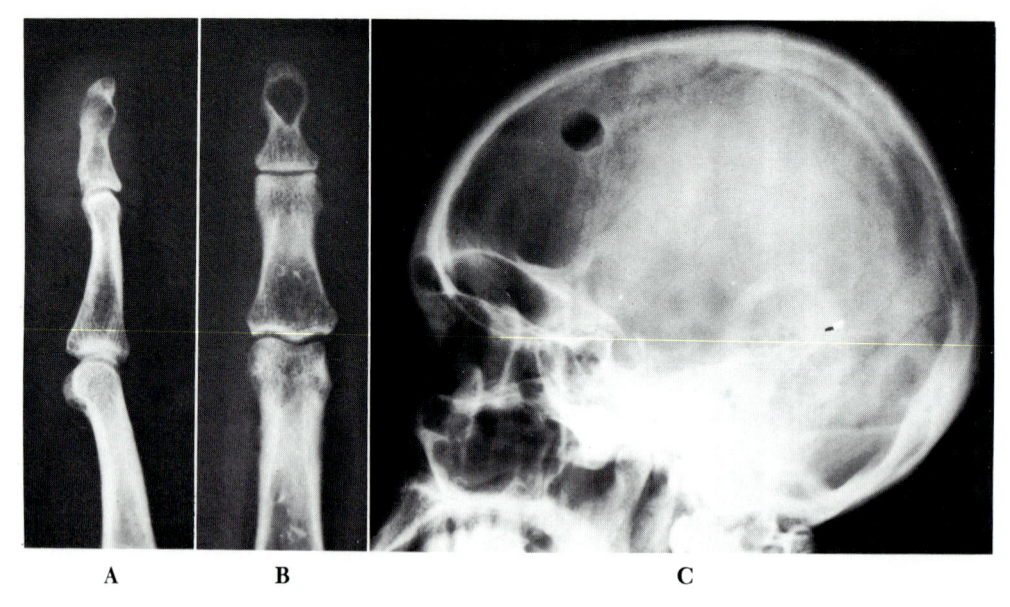

Fig. 14-39. **A** and **B**, Roentgenograms of an epidermoid inclusion cyst in a terminal finger phalanx. There was no history of prior injury. **C**, An epidermoid cyst in the calvarium.

what happens in pathologic terms in the early evolution of a bone cyst is still a matter of conjecture. It has been suggested recently by Cohen[38] that venous obstruction at the metaphysis may be the responsible or initiating factor.

EPIDERMOID CYST IN BONE

Epidermoid inclusion cysts are relatively unusual in bone and are encountered with any appreciable frequency in only two sites: the calvarium[39] and the tufts of terminal finger phalanges. In the latter site particularly, the possible role of antecedent trauma is sometimes raised as a factor in pathogenesis, but it seems clear that the lesion can develop spontaneously, presumably from an embryonal rest or inclusion.

Epidermoid cysts are characterized radiographically by their sharp outline, as though they had been punched out with a drill press (Fig. 14-39). Pathologically, epidermoid cysts in bone are not essentially different than they are anywhere else.

ANEURYSMAL BONE CYST

Aneurysmal bone cyst is a clinical and pathologic entity that we first became aware of in 1942[35] and later described in a series of papers on the basis of further experience with it.[40-43] The condition is probably more common than is generally realized. Its frequency can be judged from the fact that I was able to survey as many as fifty cases in 1957 (most of which were submitted for consultation), and the tally at present exceeds a hundred. Undoubtedly, many instances are not identified prior to surgery and, even after tissue examination,

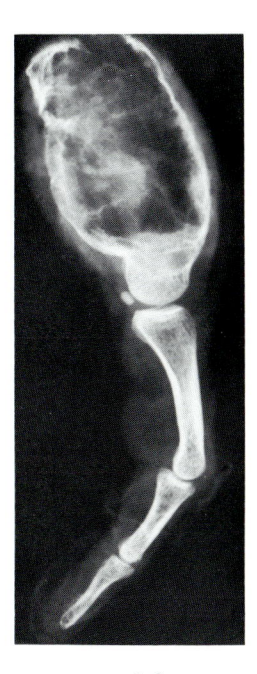

Pathology of some common and unusual orthopedic conditions

Fig. 14-40. Roentgenogram of an amputated finger ray showing an expanded aneurysmal bone cyst in a metacarpal bone. Radical surgery was done on the mistaken premise that the lesion was a malignant tumor. (Courtesy Armed Forces Medical College, Poona, India.)

some are still mistaken for neoplasm, especially giant cell tumor (Figs. 14-40 and 14-42), sometimes with unfortunate results.

While aneurysmal bone cyst has now been observed in virtually every part of the skeleton, the most common sites are the long bones of the upper and lower extremities and the vertebral column. With reference to age incidence, it is noteworthy that approximately two thirds of the patients are children or adolescents.

The affected bone site, whatever its location, is completely transformed and ultimately comes to resemble an expanded, blood-filled sponge, which may in time attain impressive size. The communicating pools of venous blood within this reservoir are bordered by a brownish, fibro-osseous meshwork showing, microscopically, conspicuous giant cell reaction to inordinate vascularity and hemorrhage, as well as fields of osteoid and new bone deposition by way of attempted reconstruction. When such a lesion is explored and the surgeon unroofs its thin expanded dome, he is confronted by blood welling up, though not spurting into the field, which may make thorough curettement difficult (Fig. 14-43).

The roentgenographic picture reflecting these changes is sufficiently distinctive, at least in large limb bones and the vertebral column (the most common sites of localization), to enable one to suspect the condition in the majority of cases, if he is familiar with it.[44] The affected bone area is characteristically

Diseases of bone and joints

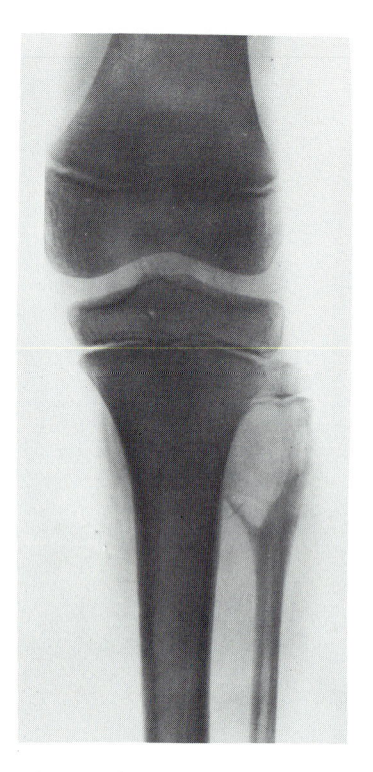

Fig. 14-41. Roentgenogram of an early aneurysmal bone cyst in the upper metaphysis of the fibula of a 9-year-old boy.

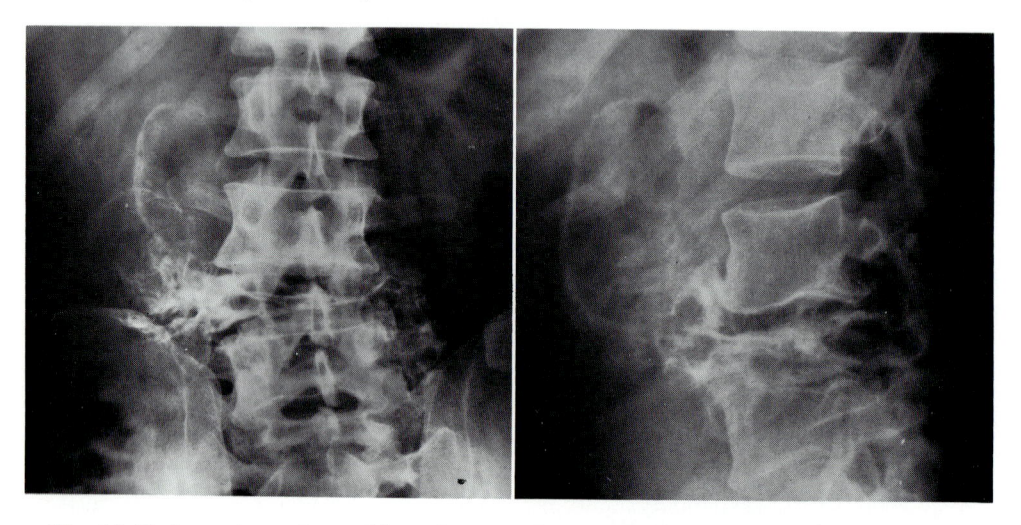

Fig. 14-42. Anteroposterior and lateral views of a remarkable aneursymal bone cyst that originated in a fourth lumbar vertebra (collapsed) and expanded steadily over a period of 5 years, eventually eroding into the duodenum, with fatal exsanguination. At autopsy it was found also to have encroached on the right renal pelvis and encircled the aorta and inferior vena cava. The original biopsy was interpreted as showing a giant cell tumor, and the lesion was said to have been irradiated, but apparently not adequately for effective control. (Courtesy Dr. Tibor Bodi, Jefferson Medical College, Philadelphia.)

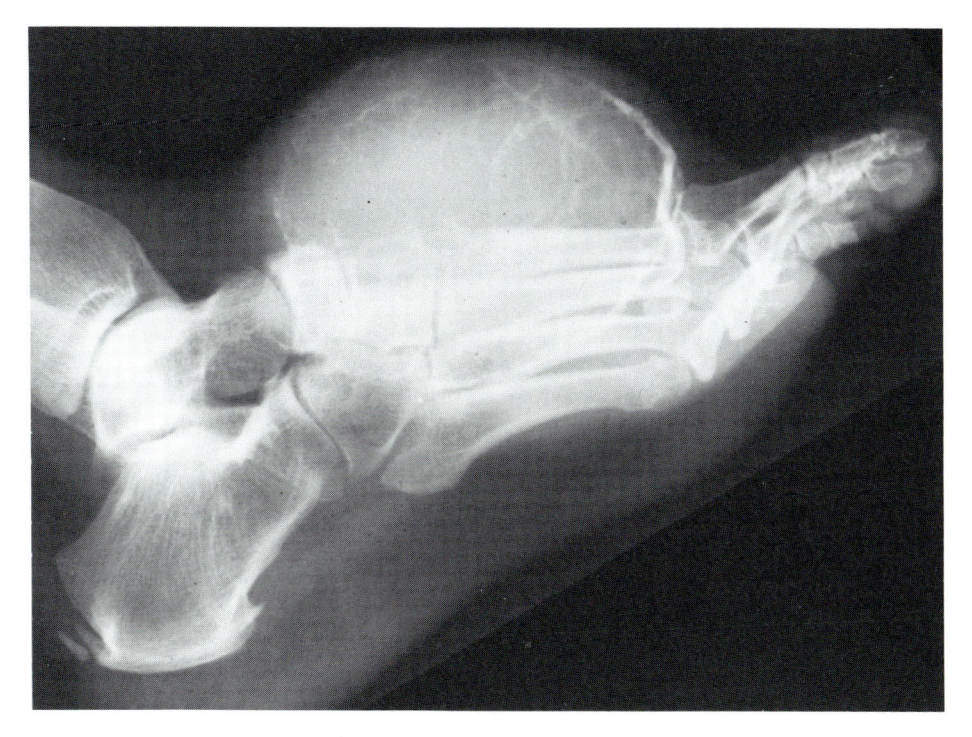

Pathology of some common and unusual orthopedic conditions

Fig. 14-43. Roentgenogram of an expanded aneursymal bone cyst in the foot of a man, aged 55, which had been gradually enlarging over a period of about 4 years. The biopsy sections had been interpreted originally as showing giant cell tumor, although origin of a giant cell tumor in a bone of the foot would be a rarity. (Courtesy Dr. U. Guevara, Nicaragua.)

expanded, appearing cystically transformed and often eccentrically ballooned out to a striking degree (Figs. 14-40, 14-42, and 14-43).

I still adhere to the view that the condition apparently results from some persistent local alteration in hemodynamics leading to increased venous pressure. The anomalous circulation could conceivably result from intraosseous arteriovenous shunts. Radiographic vascular injection studies prior to surgery, with a view to identifying possible abnormal patterns, might well be informative and should be done whenever the condition is suspected.

The progressive enlargement of an aneurysmal bone cyst can be halted and reconstruction initiated by thorough curettement or by roentgen irradiation in moderate dosage. The necessity for *prompt* treatment by whatever means, once the diagnosis is established, must be strongly emphasized. An untreated or poorly treated aneurysmal bone cyst may eventually attain impressive, if not huge, size (Fig. 14-42), sometimes necessitating amputation of a limb,[42] or, in the case of vertebral involvement, resulting in partial destruction of a number of vertebrae[43] and even irreversible paraplegia.

For relatively small or moderately sized lesions in readily accessible sites, curettement and packing with bone chips are calculated to effect a cure and is

Diseases of bone and joints

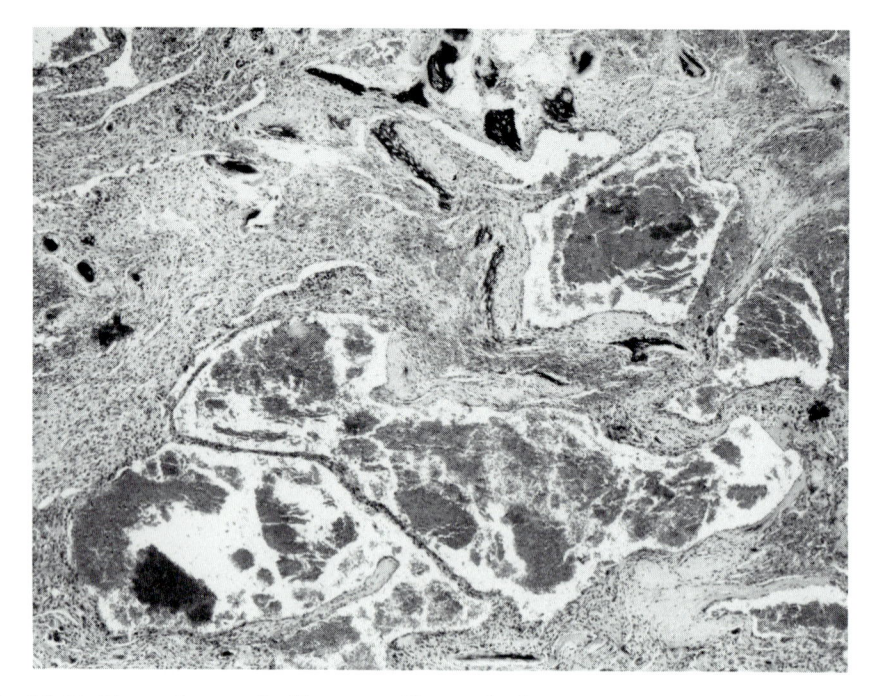

Fig. 14-44. Photomicrograph (low magnification) of a representative section through a huge, expanded aneurysmal bone cyst originating in the proximal ulna. Note the large pools of blood (these do not have an endothelial lining), hemorrhage in the surrounding connective tissue, and the formation of small, irregular trabeculae of new bone. In particular, the strands of calcified, woven bone around some of the blood pools (seen just above center) appear to be characteristic of the lesion. (×50.)

the treatment of choice. Curettement should be as thorough, however, as the situation will permit, since recurrence is possible otherwise. If irradiation is employed, either as the prime modality or to supplement incomplete eradication by surgical means, previous experience has shown that a total of 1,400 rads should suffice for effective control. Substantially larger doses should be avoided because of the potential hazard of postirradiation sarcoma,[43,45] especially in children.

The possibility of spontaneous malignant change without prior irradiation (so-called malignant bone aneurysm) has been postulated by Jacobson,[46] but it is my impression that the lesions he described were actually telangiectatic osteosarcomas to begin with, and not transformed aneurysmal bone cysts.

In dealing with an aneurysmal bone cyst developing in a vertebral body or its neural arch (such as in the cervical spine of young patients), early diagnosis and appropriate prompt treatment are of the utmost importance. As previously indicated,[43] such lesions, although initially small, may enlarge rapidly and extend to contiguous vertebrae within just a few months, so that the problem of treatment becomes much more formidable. If the changes seen in the roentgenograms suggest aneursymal bone cyst, prompt conservative biopsy is indicated to confirm this impression. More extensive surgery with a view to substantially complete extirpation is unnecessarily hazardous and should be avoided. As soon as the diagnosis has been established (by a pathologist familiar with the condition), roentgen irradiation in moderate dosage is indicated before the lesion grows much larger. Undue delay or prolonged neglect may have serious consequences (Fig. 14-42).

REFERENCES

1. Goldman, R. L., and Friedman, N. B.: Ganglia ("synovial" cysts) arising in unusual locations: report of 3 cases, one primary in bone, Clin. Orthop. 63:184, 1969.
2. Hicks, J. D.: Synovial cysts in bone, Aust. N. Z. J. Surg. 26:138, 1956.
3. Crabbe, W. A.: Intra-osseous ganglia of bone, Br. J. Surg. 53:15, 1966.
4. Johnson, W. C., Graham, J. H., and Helwig, E. B.: Cutaneous myxoid cyst—clinicopathological and histochemical study, J.A.M.A. 191:15, 1965.
5. Dandy, W. E.: Serious complication of ruptured intervertebral discs, J.A.M.A. 113:474, 1942.
6. Schmorl, G., and Junghanns, H.: Die gesunde und Kranke Wirbelsäule im Roentgenbild, 1972, Georg Thieme Verlag.
7. Collins, D. H.: The pathology of articular and spinal diseases, London, 1949, Arnold.
8. Gardner, D. L.: Pathology of the connective tissue diseases, Baltimore, 1965, The Williams & Wilkins Co., Chapter 14.
9. DePalma, A. F., and Rothman, R. H.: The intervertebral disc, Philadelphia, 1970, W. B. Saunders Co.
10. Golub, B. S., Rovit, R. L., and Mankin, H. J.: Cervical and lumbar disc disease: a review, Bull. Rheum. Dis. 21:635, 1971.
11. Editorial: The Burnett or milk-alkali syndrome, J.A.M.A. 157:1220, 1955.
12. Stack, H. G.: The palmer fascia, Edinburgh, 1973, Churchill Livingstone.
13. Hueston, J. T., and Tubiana, R.: Dupuytren's disease, Edinburgh, 1974, Churchill Livingstone.
14. Gabbiani, G., and Majno, G.: Dupuytren's contracture: fibroblast contraction? An ultrastructural study, Am. J. Pathol. 66:131, 1972.
15. Pedersen, H. E., and Day, A. J.: Dupuytren's disease of the foot, J.A.M.A. 154:33, 1954.
16. Pickren, J. W., Smith, A. G., Stevenson, T. W., Jr., and Stout, A. P.: Fibromatosis of the plantar fascia, Cancer 4:846, 1951.
17. Sutro, C. J.: Slipping of the capital epiphysis of the femur in adolescence, Arch. Surg. 31:345, 1935.
18. Lacroix, P., and Verbrugge, J.: Slipping of the upper femoral epiphysis: a pathological study, J. Bone Joint Surg. 43-A:371, 1951.
19. Briner, J.: Ultrastructure of congenital pseudoarthrosis of tibia, Arch. Pathol. 95:97, 1973.
20. Jaffe, H. L.: Metabolic degenerative and inflammatory diseases of bones and joints, Philadelphia, 1972, Lea & Febiger, Chapter 19.
21. Stougaard, J.: The hereditary factor in osteochondritis dissecans, J. Bone Joint Surg. 43-B:256, 1961.
22. Uhry, E., Jr.: Osgood-Schlatter's disease, Arch. Surg. 48:406, 1944.
23. LaZerte, G. D., and Rapp, T. H.: Pathogenesis of Osgood-Schlatter's disease, Am. J. Path. 34:803, 1958.
24. Sudeck, P.: Arch: Klin. Chir. 62:147, 1900.
25. Jaffe, H. L.: Bone rarefaction after trauma to large joint regions without fracture, Radiology 33:305, 1939.
26. Jackson, J. B. J.: A singular case of absorption of bone (a boneless arm), Boston Med. Sci. J. 18:368, 1838.
27. Case records of Massachusetts General Hospital: Vanishing or disappearing bone disease, N. Engl. J. Med. 270:731, 1964.
28. Gorham, L. W., and Stout, A. P.: Massive osteolysis (acute spontaneous absorption of bone, phantom bone, disappearing bone), J. Bone Joint Surg. 37-A:985, 1955.
29. Halliday, D. R., Dahlin, D. C., Pugh, D. G., and Young, H. H.: Massive osteolysis and angiomatosis, Radiology 82:637, 1964.
30. Stern, M. B., and Goldman, R. L.: Disappearing bone disease, Clin. Orthop. 53:99, 1967.

31. Gall, E. A., Bennett, C. A., and Bauer, W.: Generalized hypertrophic osteoarthropathy, Am. J. Pathol. **27**:349, 1951.
32. Holling, H. E., and Berman, B.: Pulmonary hypertrophic osteoarthropathy, Arch. Intern. Med. **112**:947, 1963.
33. Mendlowitz, M.: Measurements of blood flow and blood pressure in clubbed fingers, J. Clin. Invest. **20**:113, 1941.
34. Flavell, G.: Reversal of pulmonary hypertrophic osteoarthropathy by vagotomy, Lancet **1**:260, 1956.
35. Jaffe, H. L., and Lichtenstein, L.: Solitary unicameral bone cyst, with emphasis on the roentgen picture, the pathologic appearance and the pathogenesis, Arch. Surg. **44**:1004, 1942.
36. Mohanti, R. C.: Solitary bone cyst: report of an unusual case in talus, Indian J. Surg. **27**:56, 1965.
37. Garceau, G. J., and Gregory, C. F.: Solitary unicameral bone cyst, J. Bone Joint Surg. **36-A**:267, 1954.
38. Cohen, J.: Etiology of simple bone cyst, J. Bone Joint Surg. **52-A**:1493, 1970.
39. Kleinsasser, O., and Albrecht, H.: Die Epidermoide der Schädelknochen, Langenbeck. Arch. Klin. Chir. **285**:498, 1957.
40. Jaffe, H. L.: Aneurysmal bone cyst, Bull. Hosp. Joint Dis. **11**:3, 1950.
41. Lichtenstein, L.: Aneurysmal bone cyst: a pathological entity commonly mistaken for giant-cell tumor and occasionally for hemangioma and osteogenic sarcoma, Cancer **3**:279, 1950.
42. Lichtenstein, L.: Aneurysmal bone cyst: further observations, Cancer **6**:1228, 1953.
43. Lichtenstein, L.: Aneurysmal bone cyst: observations on fifty cases, J. Bone Joint Surg. **39-A**:873, 1957.
44. Sherman, R. S., and Soong, K. Y.: Radiology **68**:54, 1957.
45. Dahlin, D. C., Besse, B. E., Jr., Pugh, D. G., and Ghormley, R. K.: Aneurysmal bone cyst, Radiology **64**:56, 1955.
46. Jacobson, S.: Malignant bone aneurysm, Bull. Pathol. **10**:240, 1969.

chapter 15

Disorders of synovial joints

The linings of synovial joints are very labile and react to a wide variety of changes and noxious influences originating locally or elsewhere in the body. In its response, the multipotent capacity of the synovium becomes evident. Quite apart from the usual manifestations of response to injury, the lining cells can multiply and become several or many layers in thickness; they can phagocytose hemosiderin and lipid, urates and ochronotic pigment, as well as bacteria[1,2] and foreign particles; they can give rise to histiocytes (or macrophages) in response to infection, rheumatoid inflammation, and pigmented villonodular synovitis, among other conditions; they can give rise to fibroblasts, resulting in synovial or subsynovial scarring; and they can elaborate a mucinous fluid rich in hyaluronic acid, excess of which leads to effusion or hydrarthrosis. In addition, the synovium is capable of forming cartilagenous and osseous bodies by metaplasia, as in osteochrondromatosis. On occasion, it may undergo neoplastic change, giving rise to synovial sarcoma and even synovial chondrosarcoma.

The articular cartilages, too, are vulnerable to trauma, degeneration (as in osteoarthritis), prolonged hemarthrosis (as in hemophilia), changes in certain metabolic disorders (gout, hereditary ochronosis), infections, overgrowth by inflammatory pannus (as in rheumatoid arthritis), and injury from whatever cause initiates a sequence of events that will be indicated presently.

The articular bone ends (within the joint capsule) may be involved initially by infection (osteomyelitis or tuberculosis spreading to the capsule), bone infarcts (especially in the hip, leading to subsequent arthritic changes), lipid storage (as in Gaucher's disease), and so on. More often, though, they become implicated secondarily in the familiar changes of osteoarthritis, as a sequel of some process that damages or destroys the articular cartilage.

The discussion that follows will attempt in an orderly sequence to indicate the basic pathologic changes that ensue in the more common disorders of joints and in some that are more unusual. A number of these conditions have already been discussed in other chapters and will be mentioned again only briefly for the sake of completeness. The clinical background of each of these disorders

Diseases of bone and joints

will be considered insofar as it appears essential for clear definition or orientation.

CHRONIC NONSPECIFIC VILLOUS SYNOVITIS

Chronic nonspecific villous synovitis is a descriptive designation commonly used by pathologists for the nonspecific reaction of the synovial lining of a joint, such as a knee, to a wide variety of irritating factors. It may be induced by anything that causes internal derangement of a joint, and it is therefore observed frequently in routine orthopedic surgical specimens. It is sometimes seen in children with capsular thickening and arthralgia, especially after enteric infections. It may also be seen at times in women at menopause, in which case there may be remission after estrogen therapy. In some instances, trauma may be a factor. In still others, no predisposing factor can be implicated.

Whatever the cause of the reaction, one observes a varying degree of villous hypertrophy (this is the only way in which the synovium can expand or enlarge). Usually associated with it is slight thickening of the lining, capillary vascularization, a sprinkling of chronic inflammatory cells, and slight synovial or subsynovial fibrosis (Fig. 15-1). At times, the inflammatory reaction may be more intense, even with the formation of focal nodular aggregates, without this necessarily implying rheumatoid etiology (Fig. 15-2).

JOINT CHANGES FOLLOWING TRAUMA

Intraarticular fractures frequently injure the articular cartilage as well as the joint capsule. When there is comminution of the bone, compression with telescoping, or dislocation with extensive tearing of ligaments so that protracted immobilization is required, fibrous ankylosis with pain and loss of motion and sometimes even bony ankylosis may be the end result.

Trauma to joints without fracture may likewise induce certain deleterious effects in the articular capsule. The articular cartilage may be injured in one or more areas; while the defects are slowly repaired, they are filled with fibrous connective tissue rather than regenerated hyaline cartilage (Fig. 15-3). A number of changes may also be observed in the synovium, namely, some thickening of the lining, villous hypertrophy, fibrosis, slight fibrin exudate at times, possibly occasional nests of foam cells, and discoloration of the lining (to yellow-brown or darker brown) by hemosiderin pigment resulting from hemorrhage. Actually, it takes surprisingly little hemosiderin to impart gross coloration to the lining. When there is abundant hemosiderin deposition, pathologists sometimes consider the possibility of pigmented villonodular synovitis, although the essential component of active histiocytic proliferation is lacking.

Altogether, the synovial changes described are usually not specific enough in themselves to justify a diagnosis of *posttraumatic synovitis* (or arthritis), it seems to me, although one may suspect that they result from an injury, particularly when the latter is well documented.

Injury to joint regions may also cause the formation of *joint bodies,* whose

Disorders of synovial joints

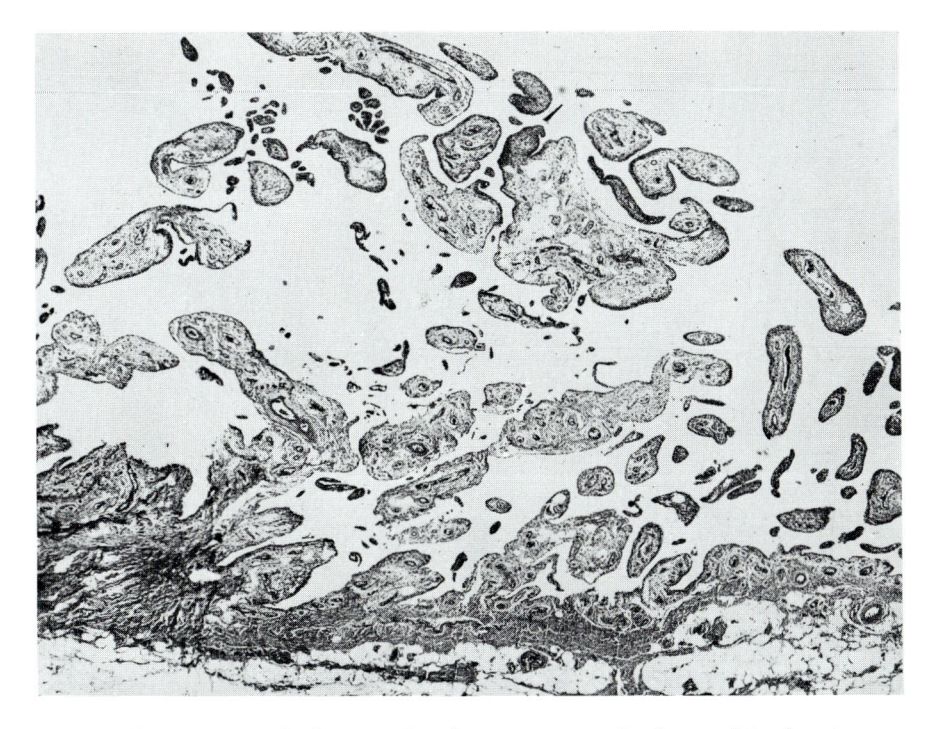

Fig. 15-1. Photomicrograph showing the changes commonly observed in chronic nonspecific villous synovitis.

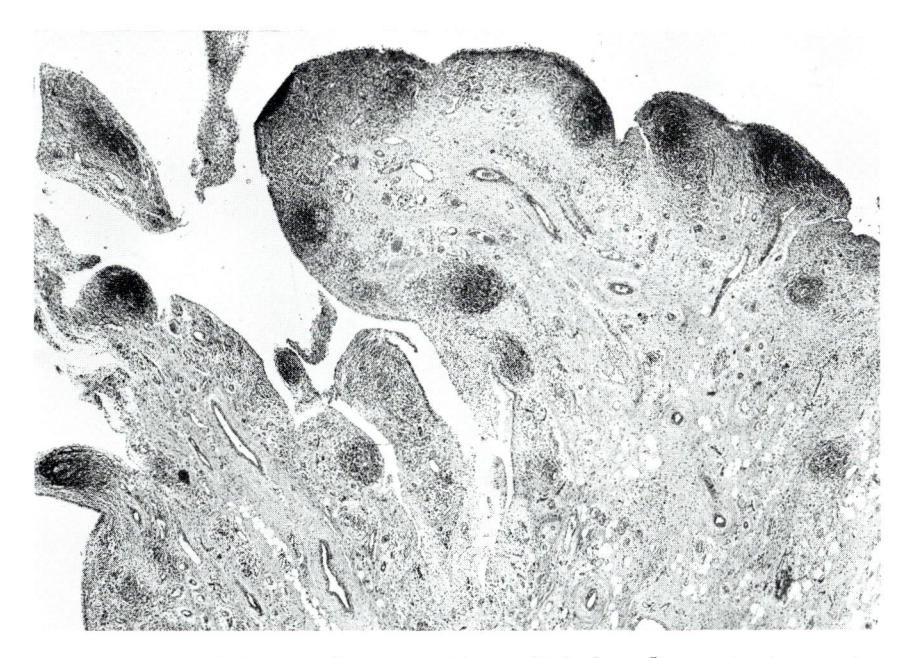

Fig. 15-2. Instance of chronic villous synovitis in which the inflammation is more intense than in Fig. 15-1. In the absence of abundant fibrinoid exudate, this picture should not be interpreted as necessarily suggesting rheumatoid disease.

Diseases of bone and joints

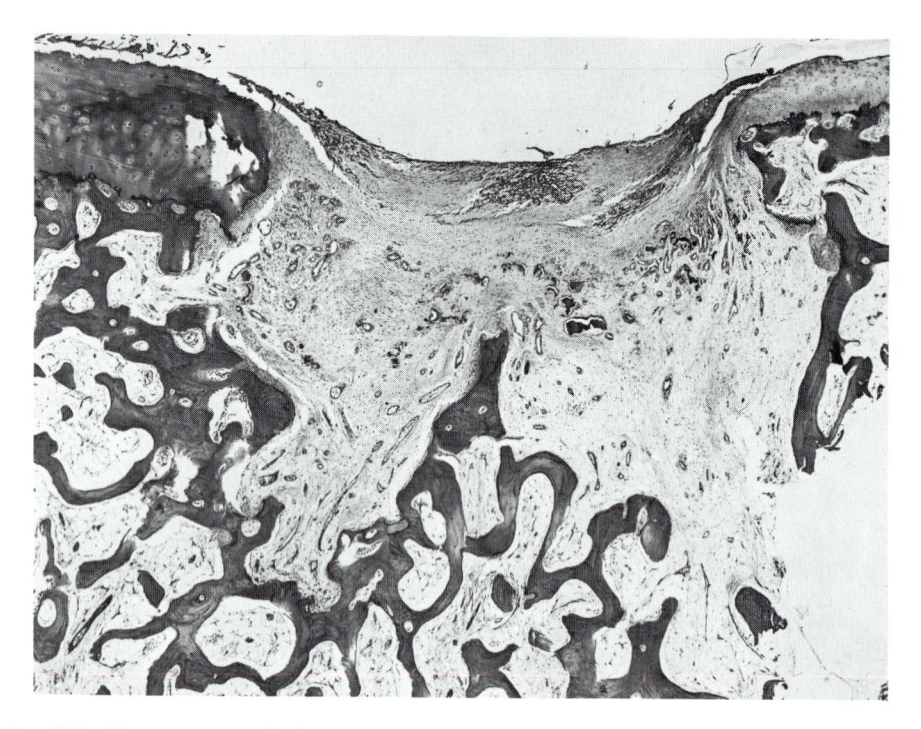

Fig. 15-3. Photomicrograph showing focal injury to an articular cartilage surface and its organization by granulation tissue.

long-term effect is to favor articular damage (like foreign bodies in a closed gearbox). Such joint mice may represent detached bits of articular cartilage, or small osteoarticular fracture fragments, or marginal osteophytes. To be sure, there are other sources of joint bodies—osteochondromatosis of the synovium or a focus of osteochondritis dissecans of the knee that has become free—but we are not concerned with these at the moment.

Whatever the origin of joint bodies, they are nourished by the synovial fluid and grow slowly by the accretion of layers of cartilage on their surface. Eventually, they may become several or many times their original size. The cartilage component can become calcified, but ossification does not occur, since this would require a blood supply (Figs. 15-4 and 15-5).

Fig. 15-5. An osteochondral joint body (from a knee) with a necrotic osseous core and a cartilage periphery, which has increased in thickness from the deposition of successive layers of cartilage. A "joint mouse" such as this could conceivably represent a broken-off marginal osteophyte or an old osteoarticular fracture fragment.

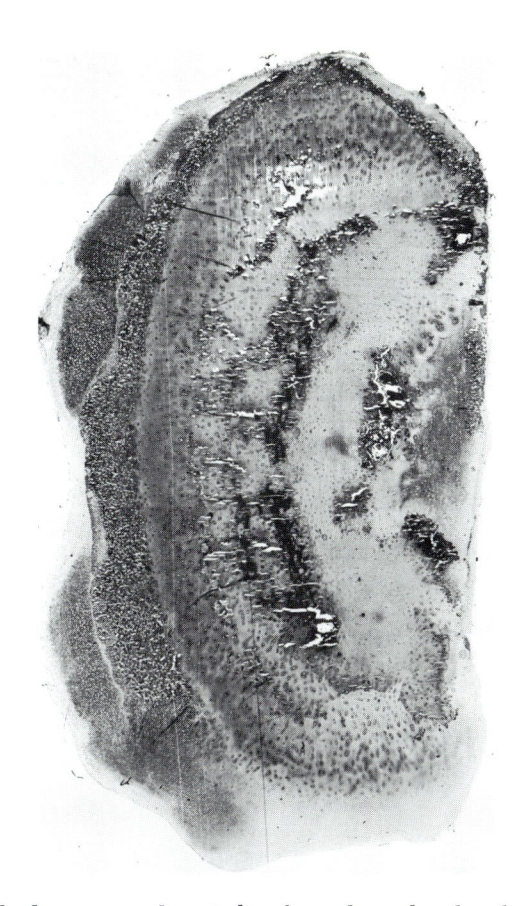

Fig. 15-4. A joint body composed entirely of cartilage that has become calcified. On its surface (particularly at the left), one sees successive layers of cartilage formed by accretion.

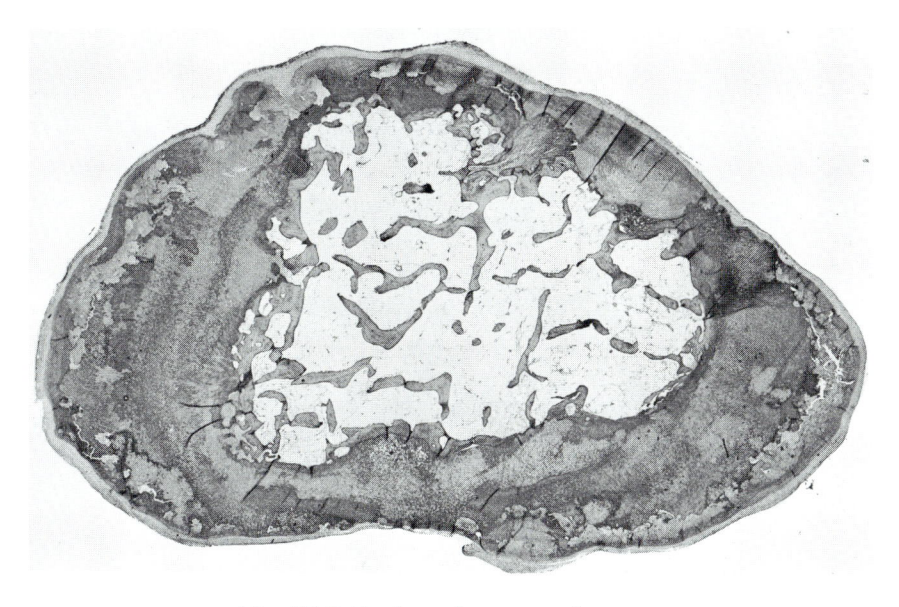

Fig. 15-5. For legend see opposite page.

Diseases of bone and joints

INFECTIONS OF JOINTS

Infections of joints, on the whole, are of distinctly varied nature and may be associated with sepsis, tuberculosis, syphilis, mycoses (especially coccidiomycosis), and even certain viral infections. Many aspects of joint infection have already been considered in Chapter 3 and will not be reiterated here. As previously indicated, it is often difficult, if not impossible, to draw a sharp line of demarcation between infections of bone and those of joints, inasmuch as the two are frequently associated. Also mentioned briefly will be certain conditions of as yet undetermined etiology, such as Reiter's disease, since there is a clinical presumption that they are of infectious nature.

Pyogenic arthritis (septic arthritis; acute infectious arthritis; suppurative arthritis; pyarthrosis). Pyogenic arthritis, which is usually monarticular, is most often associated with bacteremia or with irruption of a focus of infection in bone into a neighboring joint. Occasionally, it may be a complication of penetrating wounds or joint surgery or of intraarticular injections[2] or aspiration. As in osteomyelitis, the major pathogenic microorganisms are *Staphylococcus aureus* and *Streptococcus hemolyticus,* although occasionally *Gonococcus, Meningococcus, Diplococcus pneumoniae, Haemophilus influenzae, Brucella,* and still others may be responsible for joint infection. While the widespread use of antibiotics has sharply reduced the incidence of pyarthrosis, it may still be a problem in vulnerable premature infants, in those on prolonged massive steroid therapy, in cancer patients receiving marrow-depressing chemotherapeutic agents predisposing to unusual infections, and in patients infected with resistant strains of staphylococci.

The affected joint is usually red, hot, swollen, and very tender. Constitutionally, as one might expect, there is associated fever, leukocytosis, and elevated sedimentation rate. The situation calls for prompt blood culture, as well as culture of aspirated synovial fluid or pus, and bacterial sensitivity studies. Penicillin or tetracycline may well be the antibiotic of choice, although others are often required when dealing with resistant strains of staphylococci. In any event, systemic therapy is usually indicated, in addition to local aspiration, irrigation, and instillation of antibiotic agents. These measures apparently have largely obviated the necessity for incision and drainage, which were once common practice.

The synovial lining of the infected joint capsule is edematous, hyperemic, and acutely inflamed (Fig. 15-6). Study of the synovial membrane in experimental pyogenic arthritis by electron microscopy[1] shows a marked increase in lysosomes within the synovial cells, and their enzymes are thought to be an important factor in bacteriolysis and in necrosis of synovial tissues. Apart from this, the tendency to rapid lysis of the articular cartilage by the proteolytic enzymes of pus cells is of paramount importance and underscores the necessity for early diagnosis and treatment if one is to avoid serious damage to the articular bone ends and bony ankylosis. With staphylococcal infection particularly, destruction of cartilage may ensue rapidly. Some of the most solidly fused joints I have ever seen have been the result of healed staphylcoccal pyarthrosis in the preantibiotic era. Other

Disorders of synovial joints

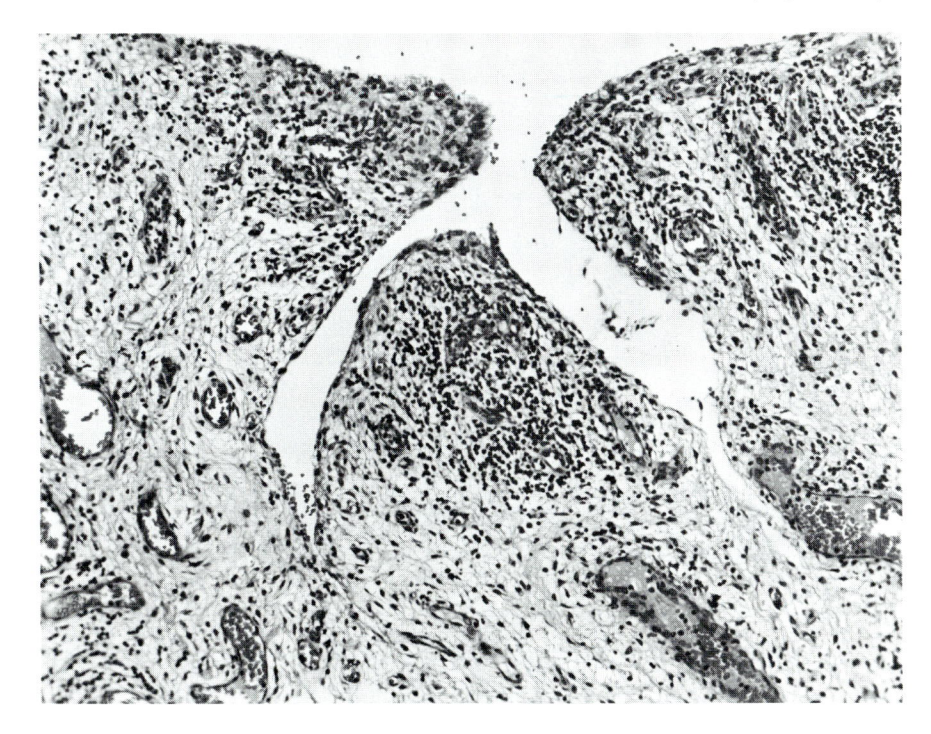

Fig. 15-6. Photomicrograph of the synovial lining of a knee joint infected by *Streptococcus hemolyticus*, showing marked edema, engorgement of blood vessels, and intense inflammatory exudate. Most of the inflammatory cells are polymorphonuclear leukocytes.

possible complications of untreated or poorly treated severe pyogenic arthritis, now fortunately uncommon, are rupture of abscess into extracapsular soft parts, extension of infection into the articular bone ends, infarction of bone from interference with blood supply (in a femoral head, for example), and, in children, dislocation and epiphyseal separation.

Gonococcal arthritis deserves special mention here, although the effectiveness of penicillin in treating the primary infection of the urethra or cervix has sharply reduced its incidence. In untreated or resistant cases, after a latent period of some 2 to 4 weeks, severe manifestations of arthritis may suddenly appear. Initial polyarthralgia is soon followed by localizing signs in one joint, usually the knee, hip, ankle, or wrist. Occasionally, tendon sheaths may be involved without associated arthritis.[3] If there is a cervical or urethral discharge, Gram stain of a smear affords a valuable clue to the specific diagnosis, which may otherwise be overlooked. Gonococci can sometimes be cultured from the joint fluid or exudate, but even if they are not, penicillin in large doses should be administered systemically in addition to appropriate local therapy. Here again, one must stress the importance of effective early treatment in view of the hazards of serious damage to articular cartilage surfaces and of extensive bone atrophy.

Tuberculosis of joints. Apart from spondylitis, with its sequelae of caseation, gibbus, paravertebral cold abscess, and possibly spinal cord compression, one of

Diseases of bone and joints

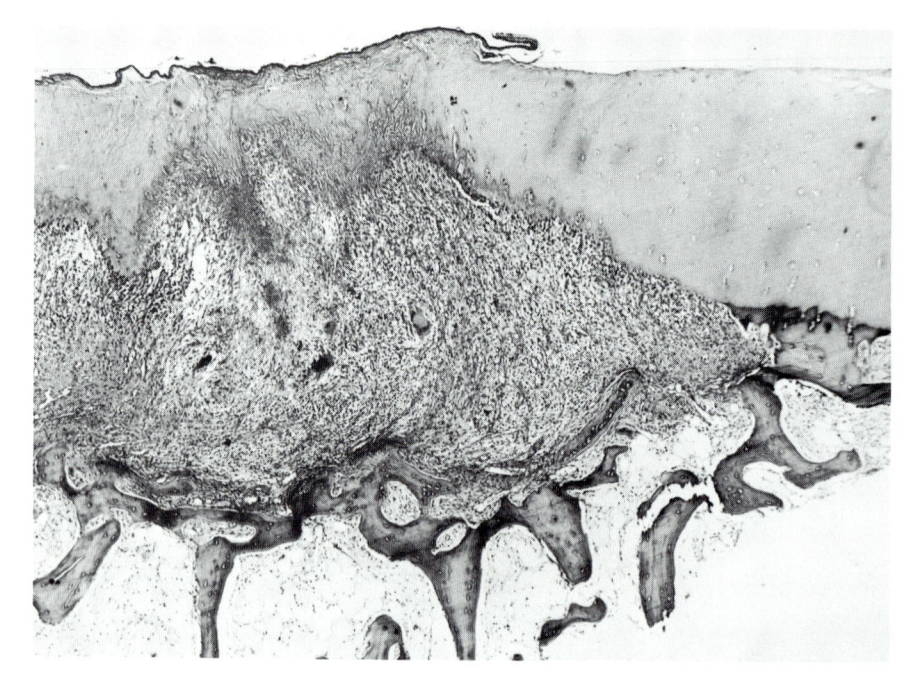

Fig. 15-7. Photomicrograph showing spread of tuberculous granulation tissue beneath articular cartilage, which is substantially necrotic and in the process of being sequestrated.

the more common expressions of skeletal involvement by tuberculosis is arthritis. The knee joint is most often involved in adults and the hip in children, although occasionally the shoulder, elbow, wrist, or some other joint may be affected (Fig. 3-7). The onset of infection is usually insidious, and the course generally indolent and protracted, leading to progressive destruction of the capsule and articular bone ends, unless the disease is controlled by specific chemotherapy, immobilization, and surgery, when indicated.

Arthritis of long standing affecting a single joint must be presumed to be tuberculous until proved otherwise. A positive tuberculin skin test indicates exposure and hypersensitivity essentially and in itself is not conclusive. The roentgenographic changes, while helpful, may be varied and unusual and, by the same token, are not infallible. For that matter, frozen section of a synovial biopsy is not always dependable either, because of the random distribution of tubercle. However, a firm diagnosis may often be established preoperatively by culture or guinea pig inoculation of aspirated synovial fluid. The latter is likely to show a low total white cell count, few pus cells, a low sugar concentration, and high protein content.

While tuberculous lesions in joints may start in the synovium, they usually begin in one or both osteoarticular bone ends. In the latter event, there is a tendency for tuberculous granulation tissue sooner or later to dissect beneath the

Disorders of synovial joints

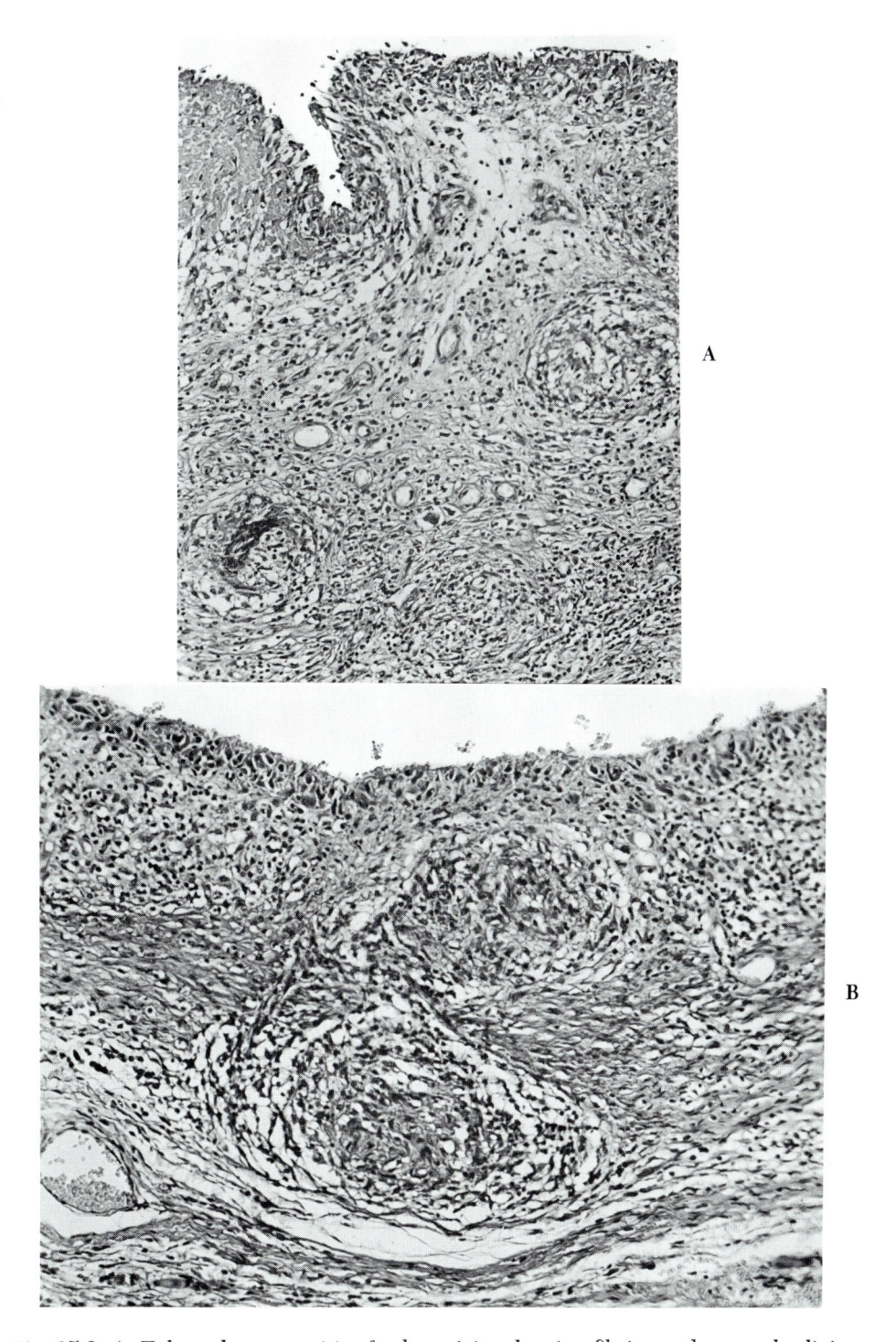

Fig. 15-8. **A,** Tuberculous synovitis of a knee joint showing fibrin exudate on the lining surface and chronically inflamed granulation tissue containing a number of tubercles. **B,** Photomicrograph showing tuberculous reaction in the wall of a subdeltoid bursa.

Diseases of bone and joints

articular cartilage, which becomes necrotic, softened, and uplifted (Fig. 15-7). Spread of infection over the synovial lining leads to effusion, relatively abundant fibrin exudate, and the development of tuberculous granulation tissue (Fig. 15-8, A). Eventually, if the process is not checked, one may see thickening and induration of the capsule and periarticular soft tissues (Fig. 15-8, B), burrowing fistulae, and extensive secondary destruction of bone, with irreparable damage to the function of the joint as a whole. As previously indicated, arthrodesis may well be the surgical treatment of choice for badly damaged weight-bearing joints.

Coccidiomycosis of joints. The subject of skeletal coccidiomycosis in general has been previously discussed (Chapter 3). As for joint involvement specifically, two relevant observations may be cited here. The manifestation of "desert rheumatism"—the development of transient painful, tender, and slightly swollen joints in the course of primary pulmonary disease, often associated with erythema nodosum—is well known in endemic areas. This would seem to be a manifestation of hypersensitivity.

What is perhaps not common knowledge is that there may be chronic indolent involvement in a single joint lasting for years, without clinically demonstrable disease elsewhere.[4] The affected joint is likely to be swollen and painful, with

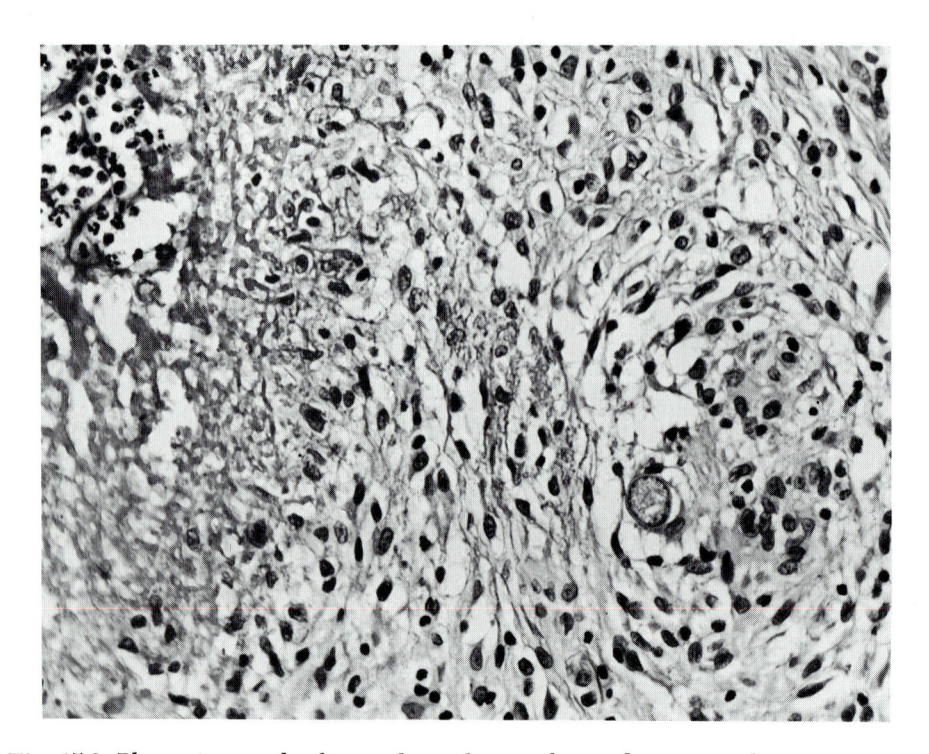

Fig. 15-9. Photomicrograph of an arthritic lesion of coccidiomycosis showing acute inflammation and necrosis (on the left) as well as histiocytic response and the formation of a tuberclelike nodule containing a doubly refractile spherule of *Coccidioides immitis* (see also Fig. 3-12, B).

some limitation of motion. Prior to tissue examination the condition may simulate tuberculous arthritis. I have seen material from at least four cases in point; in three a knee joint was affected and in another an ankle (Fig. 15-9). In one such instance, in which the tissue reaction closely resembled that of tuberculosis, it was only after a persistent search that a single spherule of *Coccidioides immitis* was found within a giant cell in a granulomatous tuberclelike nodule. In the matter of treatment, amphotericin B is the antibiotic currently used, but it is not always as effective as it might be.

Joint manifestations in syphilis. In congenital lues, osteochondritis appearing at or soon after birth may be responsible for joint disability. Involvement of the upper humeral epiphysis, for example, can result in flaccidity of the arm (Parrot's pseudoparalysis). In older children (between the ages of 8 and 16 years), a painless bilateral synovitis of the knee may sometimes develop (Clutton's joints) in association with keratitis, periostitis, and other manifestations.

During the secondary stage of acquired syphilis, painful swollen joints (suggesting rheumatoid arthritis) may occasionally appear, but this too is an infrequent manifestation. By all odds the most common joint disorder is that encountered in tertiary syphilis, namely, the Charcot joint, the neurotrophic changes of which result from dorsal column sclerosis in the spinal cord, as seen in tabes. The pathogenesis and evolution of these changes have already been described in Chapter 9.

Joint manifestations in viral diseases. In this area, there is more clinical inference available than hard pathologic fact. While arthralgias are common in influenza and epidemic viral arthritis[5] and are an occasional feature of other viral infections, little is known apparently about their synovial reflection. Perhaps this is because the pathologist does not ordinarily examine the joints at autopsy when the opportunity arises, even though the sternoclavicular joint and the knee at least are readily accessible.

The development of migratory polyarthralgias and arthritis some 2 weeks after mumps parotitis (and orchitis) has been well documented clinically.[6,7] In rubella, a synovial mononuclear reaction has been noted on biopsy,[8] but there is apparently no record of examination of an entire involved joint.

It is interesting to note also, that some children inoculated with rubella vaccine for immunization develop swelling and tenderness of small joints.[9] Joint infection has also been observed as an unusual complication of chickenpox, but this is apparently of secondary pyogenic nature. Transitory painful swelling of joints in children with varicella, possibly due to viral infection, has also been observed.[10] Continuing, polyarthritis may occur during the course of infectious mononucleosis—in biopsy specimens examined thus far, only nonspecific synovitis has been recognized.[11] Transient polyarthritis sometimes occurs in cases of infectious hepatitis associated with circulating Australian antigen. Joint involvement, sometimes leading to ankylosis and deformity, may be a sequel of smallpox.[12] This comprehensive list is not intended to be complete, but it suffices to indicate that joint involvement of one type or another is by no means an unusual manifestation of viral disease.

Diseases of bone and joints

Reiter's syndrome. Arthritis is a feature of Reiter's syndrome, along with urethritis, conjunctivitis, and, often, a peculiar dermatitis as well. While its etiology is not clear, a strong suspicion of some infectious agent prevails (pleuropneumonia-like organisms or mycoplasma, and *Bedsonia* have been implicated). It is for that reason that the disease is tentatively considered here under the head of joint infections.

Usually a number of joints are affected, particularly the knees and ankles, although occasionally only a single joint may be involved. Inflammatory changes in the heel cord are also common. The pathologic changes in the synovium have been described[13] as those of chronic nonspecific inflammation with a lymphocytic and plasma cell infiltrate. While the arthritic condition is usually self-limited, it may recur and sometimes becomes chronic. In the latter event, the late roentgenographic changes are indicative of cartilage damage and the development of secondary osteoarthritis. Occasional cases are said to progress to true rheumatoid arthritis or ankylosing spondylitis.[13] This observation, along with reports of cardiac complications and the favorable response to steroid therapy, would suggest that the syndrome may conceivably be a peculiar expression of rheumatic disease.

Joint involvement in sarcoidosis (Besnier-Boeck-Schaumann's disease). While the etiology of sarcoidosis is still uncertain, it is mentioned here for want of a better place to categorize it. Sokoloff and Bunim,[14] in reporting on five cases proved by synovial biopsy in which polyarthritis was a conspicuous specific feature, point out that joint involvement in sarcoid disease may be more common than is generally realized. Some instances in point may be mistaken for rheumatoid arthritis or rheumatic fever. Their article is valuable also for its bibliography.

As previously mentioned (Chapter 14), extensive regional involvement of tendon sheaths may also occur as an unusual major manifestation of sarcoidosis.

JOINT DAMAGE RESULTING FROM CHRONIC HEMARTHROSIS

While a single hemorrhage into a joint can be resorbed readily, leaving only light hemosiderin staining of the synovial lining as a residuum, repeated, long-term hemarthrosis (or hemosiderosis) from whatever cause can have deleterious effects. That it may lead to serious permanent damage to small and large joints in untreated hemophilia and hemophilialike conditions has already been indicated (Chapter 10). It may also be a factor in diffuse pigmented villonodular synovitis of the knee joint, and occasionally other joints, if the condition is allowed to continue long enough without effective therapy, be it synovectomy or irradiation. In advanced or terminal hemochromatosis, one may find joint effusion in the knee, for example, as well as obvious brown hemosiderin staining of the articular cartilage and synovium.[15,16] In scurvy, as previously noted (Chapter 4), painful hemorrhages occur within and about the joints, among many other sites, although these are usually overshadowed by the lesions in the epiphyses of limb bones. Finally, one may occasionally see comparable hemorrhages about a joint or even into the joint itself (such as a knee or an elbow) in severe purpura (hemorrhagic arthritis or arthritic purpura).

It would appear that injury to the articular cartilage in these circumstances results from a number of contributing factors. Impregnation of the cartilage by blood pigment is apparently harmful in itself. In experimental hemarthrosis of comparatively long standing, it has been shown by electron microscopy that iron-containing bodies are deposited in chondrocytes and that this may be associated with intracellular degeneration.[17] It seems reasonable to postulate also that the addition of substantial amounts of blood or its derivatives to the synovial fluid may well interfere with adequate nutrition of the articular cartilage. Still another factor to be considered is overgrowth of the articular cartilage by the folds of the brownishly discolored synovial membrane, which, in time, undergoes matting from extensive villous hypertrophy.

ARTHRITIC MANIFESTATIONS OF CERTAIN METABOLIC DISORDERS

We are concerned here specifically with gout, hereditary ochronosis, and (indirectly) Gaucher's disease. The skeletal alterations in general of these inborn errors of metabolism have already been discussed (Chapter 6), and the observations made will not be reiterated here. A number of illustrative photomicrographs have been introduced, however, to highlight the joint changes, particularly in chronic tophaceous gout and in ochronosis (Figs. 15-10 and 15-11, respectively).

NEUROTROPHIC JOINT DISORDERS

The skeletal changes that may occur in neurotrophic disorders, of which tabes dorsalis and syringomyelia are the most common, have already been considered in Chapter 9.

OSTEOARTHRITIS

Osteoarthritis (degenerative arthritis, degenerative joint disease, senescent arthritis, hypertrophic arthritis, arthritis deformans, osteoarthrosis) is by all odds the most common expression of arthritic change. It is characterized pathologically by degenerative alterations in the articular cartilage. This is eventually combined with hypertrophic changes in the bone ends, leading to deformation of the articular surfaces. Inflammatory reaction in the synovial membrane, so conspicuous in rheumatoid arthritis, is usually insignificant.

Articular cartilage, despite its old reputation of being inert, is a complex and metabolically active tissue. There has been a good deal of experimental work in recent years, designed to study the structure, synthesis, and metabolism of the essential biochemical constituents of articular cartilage, especially the sulfated acid polysaccharides bound to protein (protein-polysaccharide) and collagen, as well as water, minerals, and enzymes, and to determine, with particular reference to osteoarthritis and rheumatoid disease, how these constituents are affected by aging, heredity, stress, injury, hormonal factors (particularly steroids),

Diseases of bone and joints

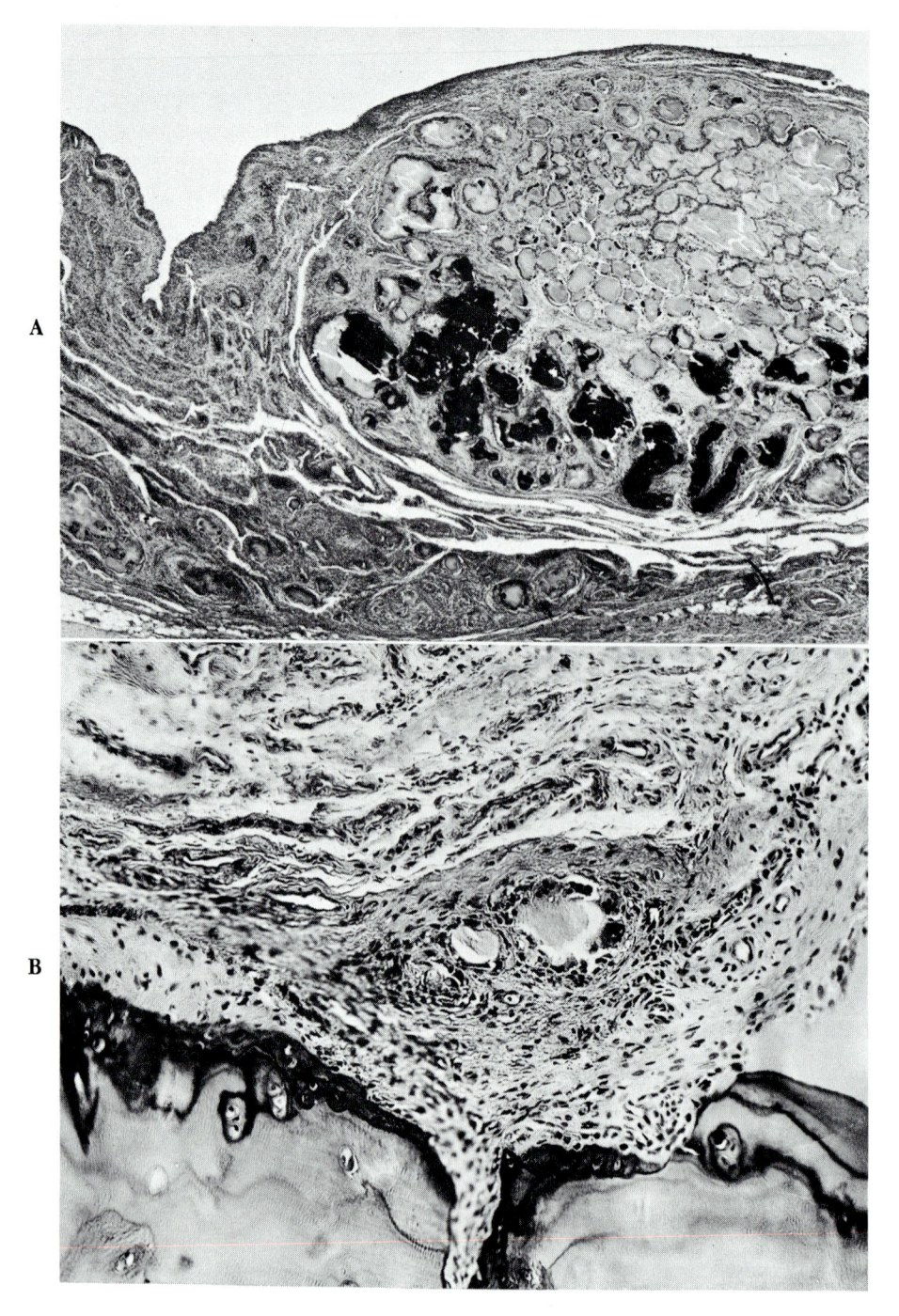

Fig. 15-10. **A,** Photomicrograph showing partially calcified urate deposits within the synovial lining of the knee joint of a patient with moderately severe gout. **B,** From the surface of a patella in a case of gout showing a urate-containing connective tissue pannus over the modified articular cartilage.

Disorders of synovial joints

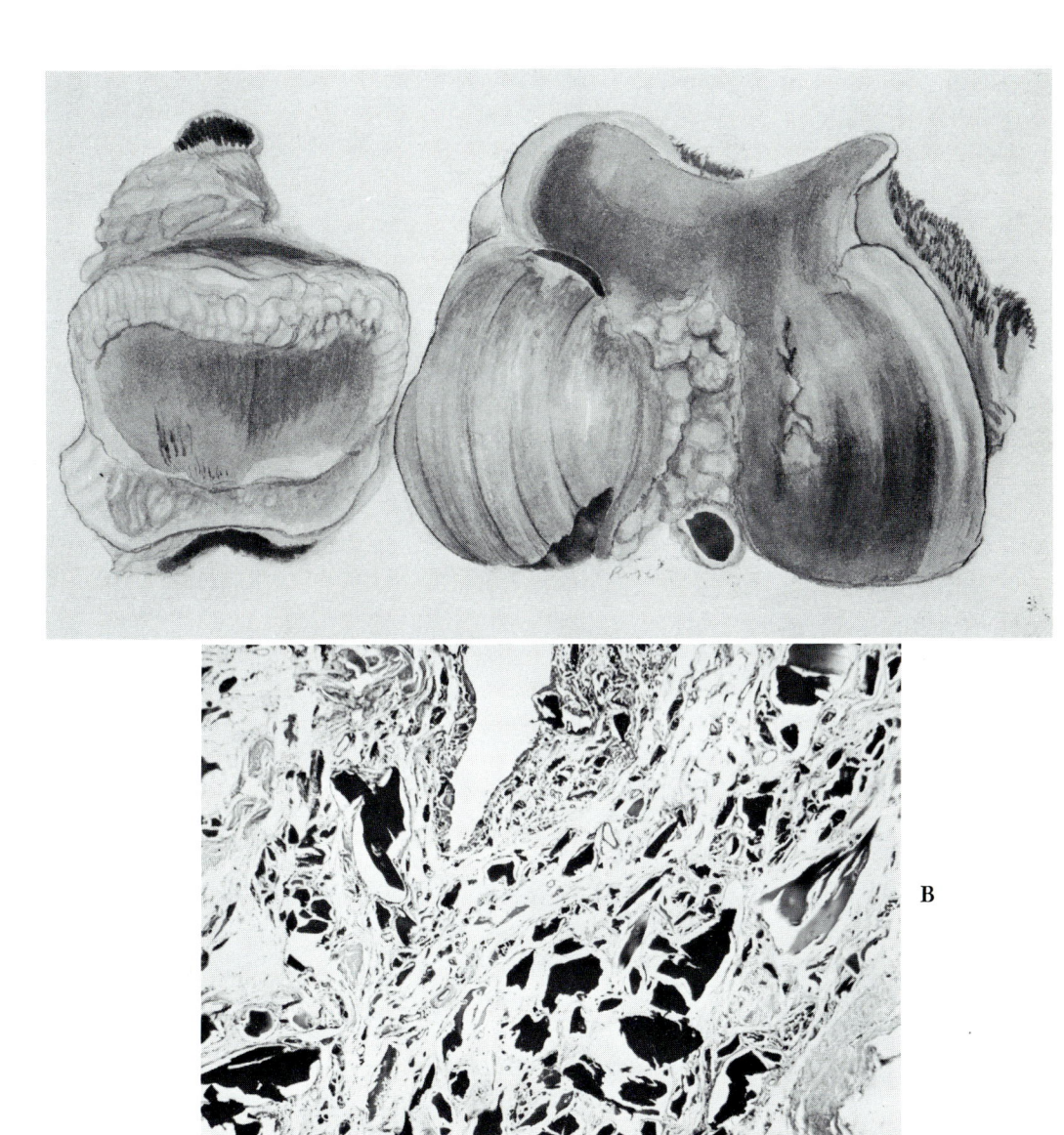

Fig. 15-11. **A,** Drawing showing the striking changes of ochronotic arthritis in a knee joint. The darker areas were discolored blue or blue-black. There is also extensive erosion, or loss of articular cartilage. (Courtesy Dr. E. Mathias.) **B,** Photomicrograph of a section of synovium of a knee joint in a case of hereditary ochronosis showing numerous fragments of broken-off, heavily pigmented articular cartilage ground into the synovial lining and the sublining tissues.

Diseases of bone and joints

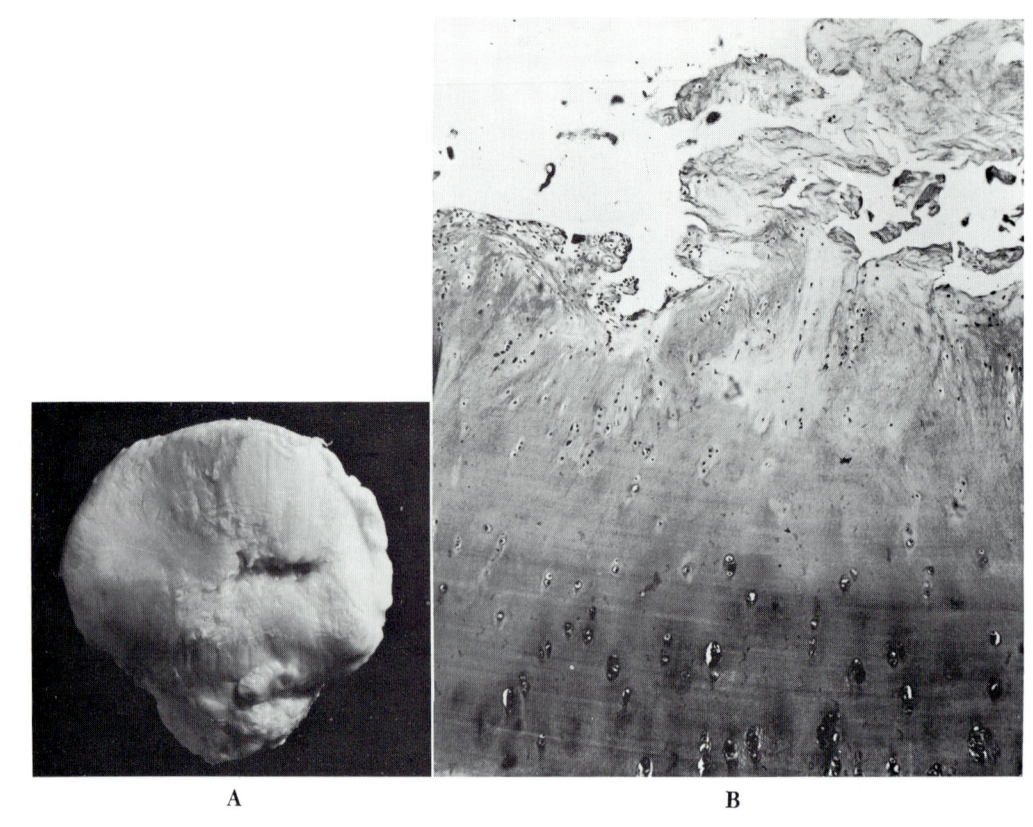

Fig. 15-12. A, Photograph of articular surface of a patella showing flaking and fibrillization of the cartilage, as seen in so-called chondromalacia of the patella. The linear horizontal depression apparently resulted from an injury. (The patient also had a bucket-handle tear of a meniscus.) **B,** Low-power photomicrograph of a specimen of chondromalacia of the patella showing fraying and degeneration of its articular surface (reflected in a yellowish nap in the gross).

and such substances as papain. Although much has been accomplished in a relatively short time, there are still wide uncharted areas, and any attempt to formulate hypotheses at this early stage appears to be premature and subject to early revision. For helpful reviews of our current knowledge, the reader may have recourse to the discussion by Mankin[18] and Moskowitz and associates[19] in *Bulletin on the Rheumatic Diseases*. The concise account that follows will deal with the familiar pathologic changes, as seen in surgical specimens and in autopsy material.

The alterations in the articular cartilage may reflect primary degenerative or senescent change, or they may follow in the wake of damage to the articular cartilages from other causes (secondary hypertrophic arthritis), such as previous infection or trauma with intraarticular fracture (Figs. 15-12 to 15-16). In the hip joint, for example, slipped epiphysis, Perthes' disease, Gaucher's disease, or caisson disease may be significant initiating factors; in the knee, joint mice,

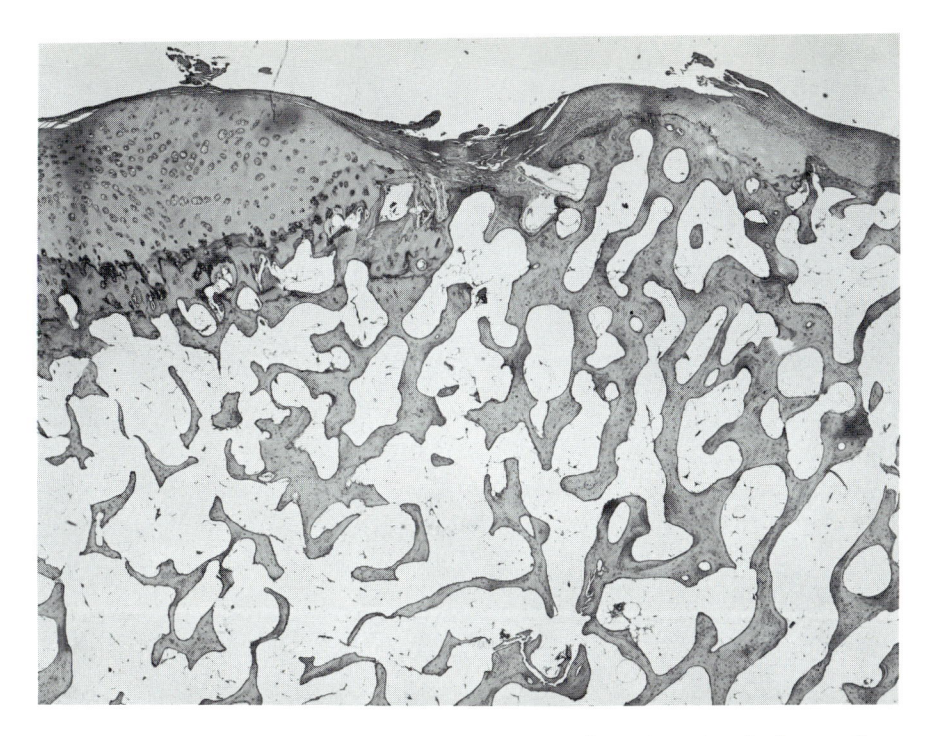

Fig. 15-13. Photomicrograph showing degeneration and erosion of articular cartilage, as seen in osteoarthritis.

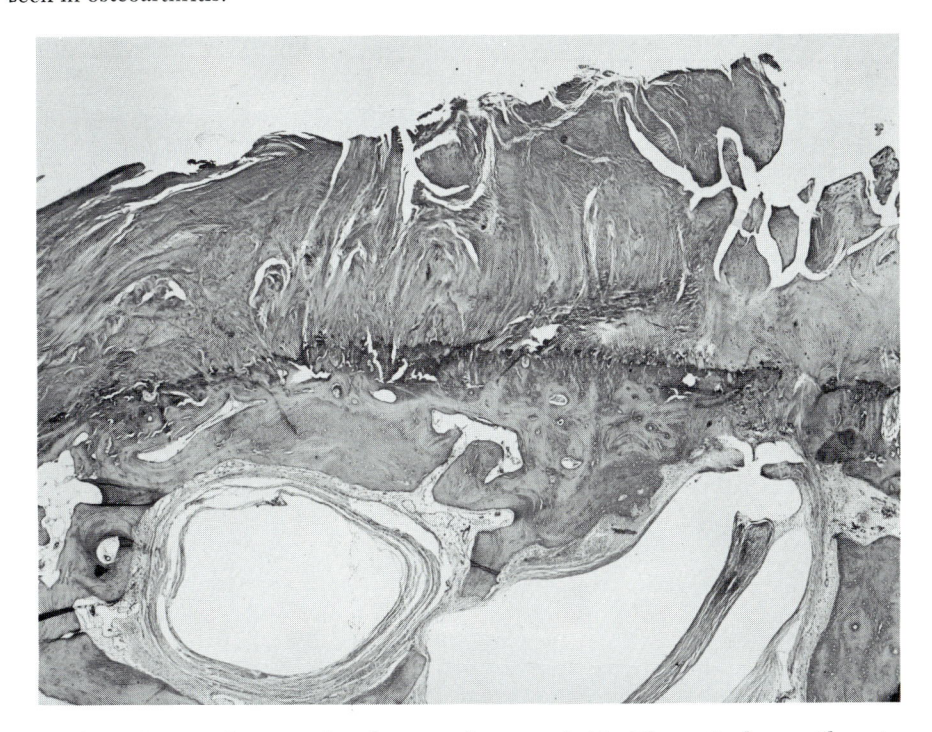

Fig. 15-14. Section showing the changes of osteoarthritis. The articular cartilage is extensively degenerated and frayed (in other areas it was eroded down to the bone). Within the thickened subchondral bone, one sees fibrous connective tissue that has undergone cystic softening.

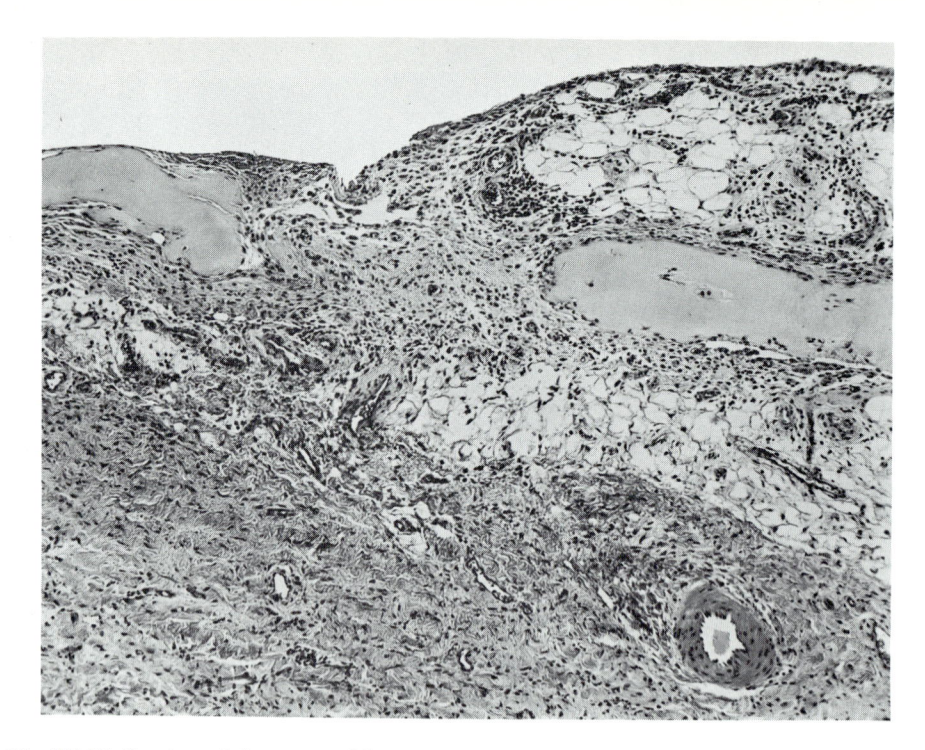

Fig. 15-15. Section of the synovial lining of a knee joint in a case of osteoarthritis. There are two bits of articular cartilage embedded in it, and around them there is some fibrosis and chronic irritative reaction. Note, however, that the lining is not hyperplastic and that there is no fibrinoid exudate such as one might expect in rheumatoid synovitis.

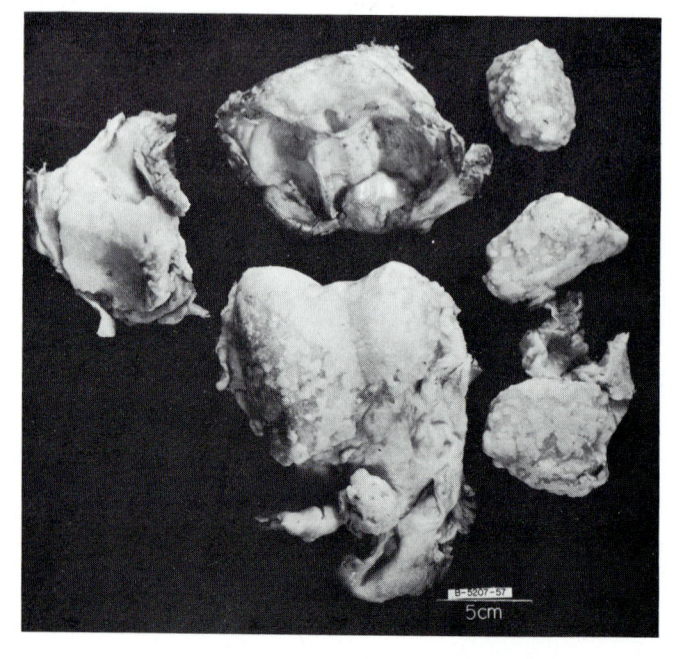

Fig. 15-16. Photograph (reduced) showing changes of severe osteoarthritis in a knee of a patient who 50 years previously had fallen down an elevator shaft. The smaller bodies on the right represent old modified osteoarticular fracture fragments.

osteochondritis dissecans, osteochondromatosis, or torn menisci of long standing may be responsible.

Whatever its basis, the primary change in osteoarthritis is in the articular cartilage, which becomes yellowish, fibrillized, nappy, rubbed down, or denuded (Fig. 15-12). The nature of the yellow (or yellow-brown) senescent pigmentation in biochemical terms has been investigated, but it is not yet fully understood.[20] As for changes in the ground substance of the articular cartilage in general, that of osteoarthritic hips has been found to contain significantly increased amounts of chondroitin 4-sulfate and decreased amounts of keratin sulfate, with little alteration in the total mucopolysaccharide (glycosaminoglycan) content. Increased wear and tear through weight bearing and excessive or abnormal use of a joint is known to accelerate the tendency to degenerative changes, but the latter may be observed at times in comparatively young adults, in so-called chondromalacia of the patella, for example (Fig. 15-12).

Where the cartilage is denuded and blood vessels reach the surface, there is a localized advance in the line of ossification. Marginal exostoses (osteophytes) develop, usually around the periphery. When the latter are well established, they may cause extensive deformity of the articular bone ends, pain, and limitation of motion. The central contact surfaces tend to become eburnated and often highly polished, like the surface of a billiard ball. The synovium, quite understandably, becomes thickened and modified as a result of chronic irritation; but, as noted, there is no real inflammation, as there is in rheumatoid arthritis (Fig. 15-15), nor do the muscles undergo atrophy. What happens to the subchondral bone depends on whether there is motion in the affected joint: if there has been some motion, the subchondral bone tends to become sclerotic; if there is no appreciable motion, the bone undergoes atrophy. Foci of fibrous tissue may develop in the subchondral bone, and these can undergo degeneration and cystic softening (Fig. 15-14), appearing as cystlike rarefactions in roentgenograms (if they become large enough to be visualized).

This sequence of events may be observed in the large mushroomed femoral head of osteoarthritis of the hip (malum coxae senilis); in spondylosis deformans, when the vertebral bodies are fused by exostoses extending across the altered intervertebral discs; in Heberden's nodes, reflecting marginal exostoses about the terminal interphalangeal joints; and in other comparable situations. With reference to Heberden's nodes, however, it should be added that not all the osteophytes are associated with osteoarthritis of the distal interphalangeal joints; some are tendon osteophytes.[21]

RHEUMATOID ARTHRITIS

Rheumatoid arthritis (atrophic arthritis, ankylosing arthritis, proliferative arthritis) is a major member of a group of inflammatory systemic connective tissue diseases ("collagen" diseases), which also includes rheumatic fever, disseminated lupus erythematosus, periarteritis (polyarteritis) nodosa, dermatomyositis, systemic sclerosis (scleroderma), and possibly other conditions.

Diseases of bone and joints

While the target sites vary in these disorders, in their pathologic reaction they exhibit certain features in common: namely, swelling and modification of the ground substance, fibrinoid degeneration or necrosis, fibroblastic proliferation, and a predominantly mononuclear inflammatory response. It has been suggested that this response may reflect altered immune reactions, and this area is a subject of active investigation.[22-24] In some of the disorders at least, a tissue hypersensitivity reaction to specific agents can be logically postulated, as in the case of rheumatic fever and certain forms of periarteritis nodosa, as indeed Klinge indicated back in the early 1930's. Furthermore, the observation of occasional cases with overlapping clinical and pathologic manifestations referable to two or more of the systemic connective tissue diseases would suggest that the latter have certain pathogenetic factors in common.

In rheumatoid arthritis, the linings of the synovial joints are the principal target site, although tendon sheaths and bursal sacs may also be affected, as well as the eye, lungs, pleura, heart, and occasionally other visceral sites. Also, subcutaneous rheumatoid nodules develop at one time or another in some 20% of all cases. We are concerned here primarily with the inflammatory joint lesions and especially with the pathologic changes. The clinical picture is well known from countless articles and monographs and hardly needs exposition.

Commonly, there is multiple joint involvement, but there are undoubtedly some cases in which apparently one a single joint is affected, clinically at least. Joints of the hands and feet are involved most often, but many others in both upper and lower extremities and in the vertebral column are commonly implicated. Whatever the site, the process starts as a synovitis (in contrast to osteoarthritis, in which the initial lesion is damage to the articular cartilage). Later, there is extension of inflammatory pannus over the articular cartilages (Fig. 15-17), and eventually loss of function and often severe and disabling deformity.

The roentgenographic alterations parallel and reflect the pathologic changes. The early manifestations are those of soft tissue swelling, thickening of the affected joint capsule, and significant osteoporosis unrelated to steroid therapy and presumably resulting from disuse and perhaps inflammatory hyperemia. Later, destruction of articular cartilage is reflected in narrowing of the joint space and, with the advent of secondary osteoarthritis following in the wake of denudation of cartilage, in such changes as marginal osteophytes and small subchondral rarefactions. In the late stage of severe disease, one may eventually see subluxation, flexion contracture, ankylosis, and other deformities (Fig. 15-18). In a terminal, burned-out stage (as seen in joint specimens obtained at autopsy) it may be difficult to distinguish clearly the sequelae of earlier rheumatoid arthritis from the heavy overlay of secondary osteoarthritis after the inflammatory reaction has subsided. In these circumstances, one must have recourse to a good clinical history to determine the probable sequence of events.

The pathologic picture of the synovitis varies somewhat, depending on the stage of the disease at the time of examination. The inflammation may be subacute or more chronic. In general, the synovium is thickened and congested and

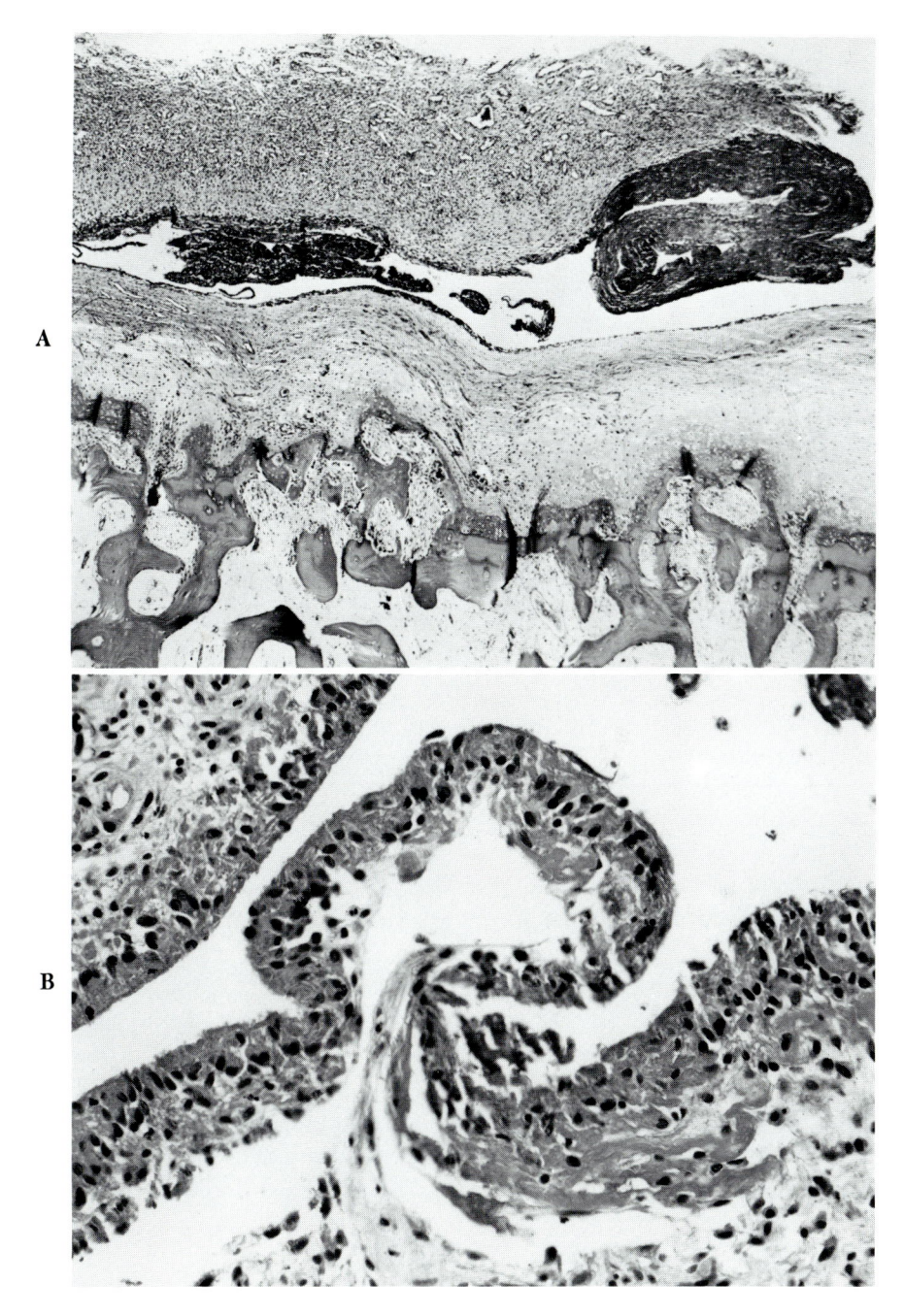

Fig. 15-17. **A,** Photomicrograph of an articular bone end in rheumatoid arthritis showing extension of vascularized, inflammatory pannus containing abundant fibrinoid exudate (dark staining) over the damaged and disappearing articular cartilage. **B,** Photomicrograph of a field of a lesion of rheumatoid synovitis of a knee joint, selected to show conspicuous fibrinous exudate or deposits within and just beneath the folded synovial lining. In other fields of this villous lesion there were numerous histiocytes (some of them multinuclear), fibroblasts, and collections of plasma cells filled with immune globulins. (×250.)

Diseases of bone and joints

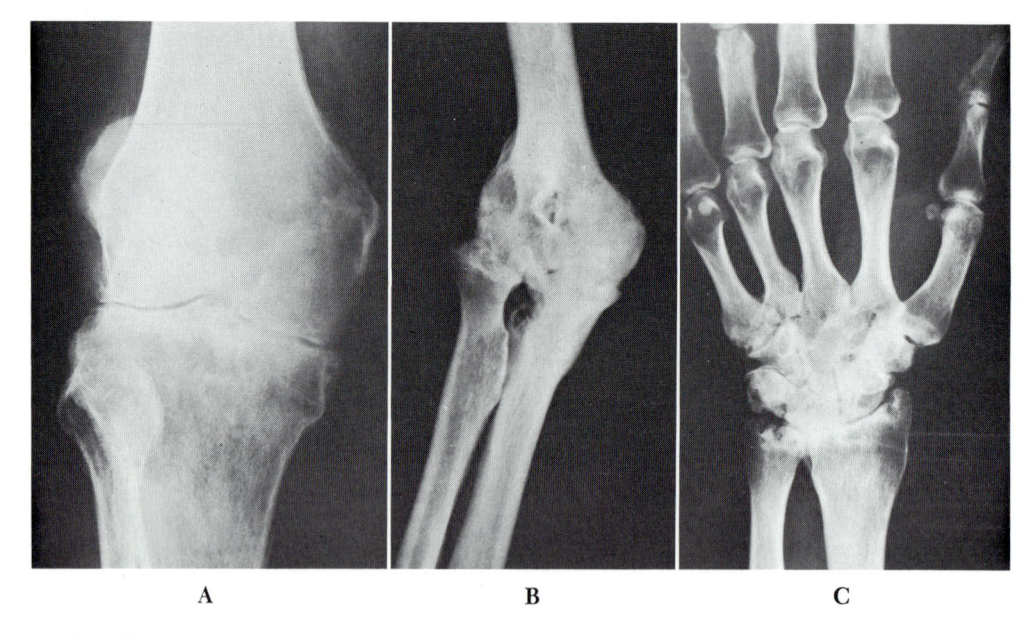

A B C

Fig. 15-18. Roentgenograms from well-established cases of rheumatoid arthritis affecting the knee, elbow, and wrist joints respectively and showing distinct narrowing of the joint space (reflecting loss of articular cartilage), osteoporosis, and evidence of secondary osteoarthritis.

shows villous hypertrophy, extensive fibrinoid deposits on the lining (Fig. 15-17, B), and infiltration of the synovium and sublining connective tissue by large numbers of inflammatory cells, sometimes clumped in aggregates. These inflammatory cells are mainly lymphocytes, macrophages (of synovial origin), and plasma cells. If the joint is "hot" at the time of synovectomy or biopsy, there may also be a sprinkling of polymorphonuclear leukocytes. The plasma cells contain abundant cytoplasmic ribonucleic acid, which reacts with methyl green–pyronin to produce a deep, red-purple color.[25] These are also the cells that are rich in immune globulins; this can be demonstrated by appropriate immunofluorescent techniques.

It should be emphasized that none of the features of the inflammatory reaction are specific in themselves, since one may find them in other conditions. As for fibrinoid deposits (and rice bodies) in particular, they are by no means peculiar to rheumatoid lesions. They are seen with regularity not only in tuberculous synovitis but also in ordinary, chronically irritated bursae. What is helpful is the composite picture, particularly the intensity of the reaction. In most situations, the pathologist is well advised to state simply that the reaction observed microscopically is consistent with rheumatoid arthritis, if such is the case, implying that the diagnosis must be based upon clinical evidence as well (Fig. 15-19). For that matter, the demonstration of "rheumatoid factor" (gamma globulin) by a variety of laboratory techniques, while helpful, is not specific. This is true also of examination of aspirated synovial fluid.

Disorders of synovial joints

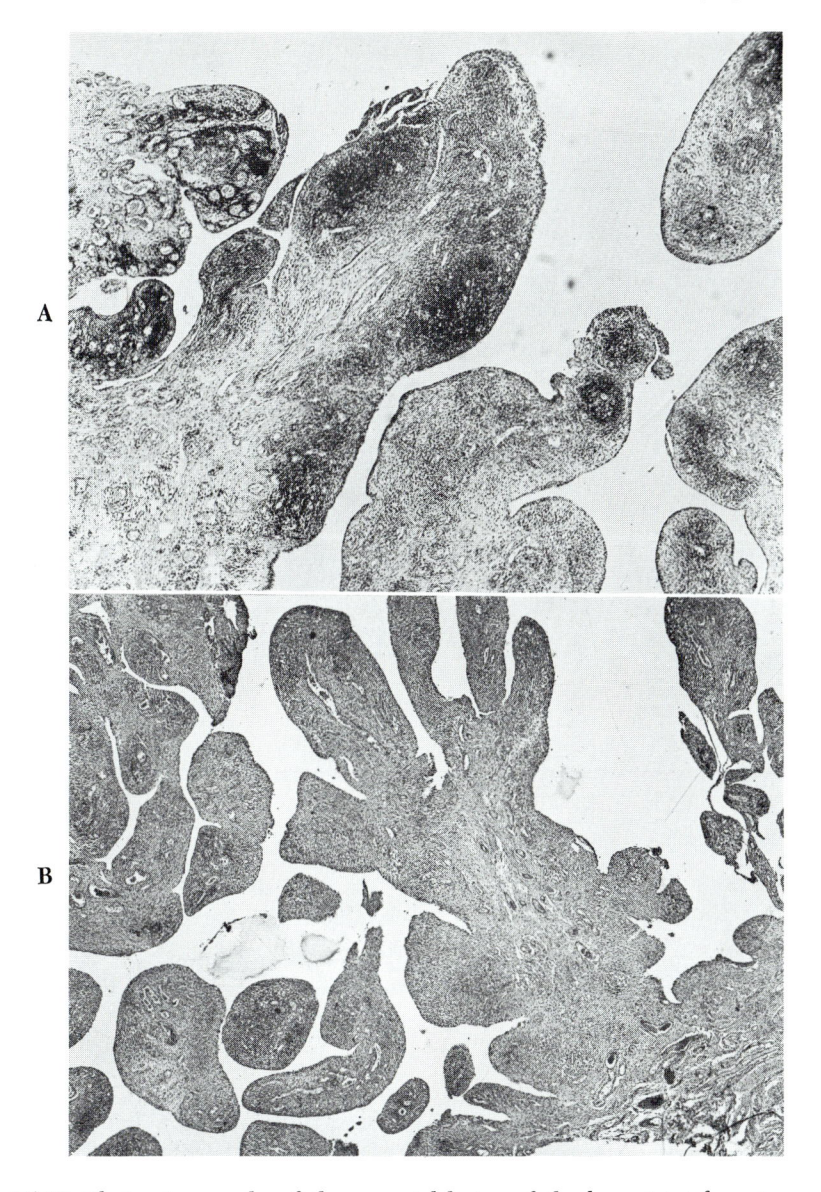

Fig. 15-19. Photomicrographs of the synovial lining of the knee joint from two cases of clinical rheumatoid arthritis showing intense villous synovitis.

The subcutaneous nodule is said to be pathognomonic for rheumatoid arthritis, although a comparable lesion may also occur in rheumatic fever and in systemic lupus erythematosus. They develop most often in the elbow region, the olecranon bursa, the knee region, and the tendon sheaths of fingers and toes but may also be encountered elsewhere. In the early stage of its development, as Sokoloff and his associates[26] indicated, the appearance of vascular granulation tissue is a prominent feature, and the blood vessels may show inflammatory changes and occasionally even necrosis. In routine surgical specimens, however,

Diseases of bone and joints

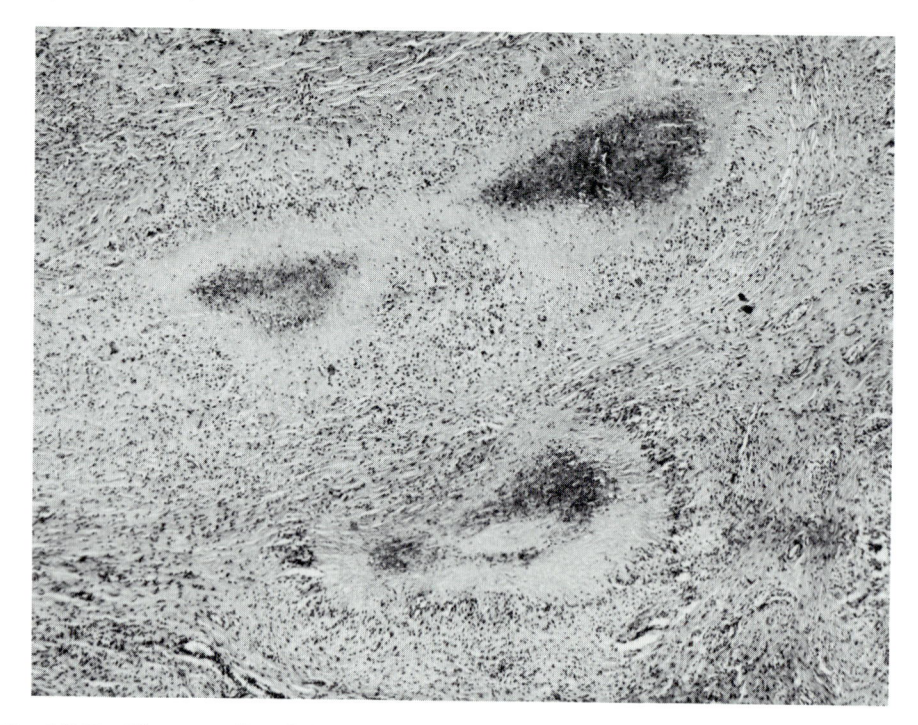

Fig. 15-20. Rheumatoid nodule within vascularized, collagenous connective tissue (elbow region). Note the areas of collagen necrosis, bordered by histiocytes.

these changes are not usually observed. The familiar conventional picture is that of a serpiginous focus of collagen necrosis, bordered by palisaded histiocytes and macrophages (Fig. 15-20). It should be noted also that in autopsied subjects with long-standing but still active rheumatoid arthritis, one may occasionally observe similar granulomas in visceral sites, such as the pleura, lungs, heart, or dura.

The skeletal muscles in the vicinity of affected joints tend to undergo atrophy and wasting. Focal lymphocytic infiltrates have been found in them (as well as in the sheaths of large peripheral nerves), but one must be wary of ascribing any specificity to them, inasmuch as collections of mononuclear cells may be found in muscle tissue in a wide variety of orthopedic conditions unrelated to rheumatoid arthritis.

Attention may also be directed here to two other relevant pathologic observations of significance. First, in Great Britain at least, rheumatoid arthritis is the most common cause of amyloidosis at the present time.[25] This ties in well with the concept of an altered immune reaction featuring the formation of abnormal globulins. Second, the repeated intraarticular therapeutic injection of cortisone or hydrocortisone entails a distinct hazard, since it may be followed by accelerated joint destruction, sometimes so extensive as to suggest Charcot arthropathy[27] (although no neurologic disease is present). The pathogenesis of this curious phenomenon is not well understood.

"Rheumatoid" spondylitis (ankylosing spondylitis, Marie-Strümpell arthritis, von Bechterew's arthritis, spondylitis rhizomelica, pelvospondylitis ossificans[28]) is often classified as a special manifestation of rheumatoid arthritis, although there is still apparently some uncertainty about the correctness of this view. It is true that some 20% of these patients present changes in peripheral joints resembling those seen in rheumatoid arthritis. On the other hand, there are dissimilar features: the predilection for males, its familial incidence at times, the rarity of subcutaneous nodules, the beneficial response to roentgen therapy, and the negative agglutination tests. In any case, the intervertebral articulations show fibrous or bony ankylosis with osseous bridges between the bodies. These changes, together with demineralization of the vertebral bodies and calcification of the lateral spinal ligaments, are eventually reflected in the picture of the "bamboo spine" or the "poker back," which may require corrective osteotomy for improved function.

Still's disease (juvenile rheumatoid arthritis) is a chronic progressive polyarthritis in children, usually below the age of 10 years, associated with generalized lymphadenopathy (inguinal, axillary, cervical, epitrochlear), and often fever, secondary anemia, and splenomegaly. Cutaneous symptoms are prominent in some patients who may manifest frequent attacks of urticaria or erythema and sometimes erythema multiforme. The arthritic changes resemble those in rheumatoid arthritis of adults. The joints are usually symmetrically involved and many joints may be affected, particularly shoulders, elbows, wrists, fingers, knees, and feet, and occasionally the vertebral column (cervical), the jaw (temporomandibular joint), and the sternoclavicular articulation. Some of the earliest and most severely affected joints may be the proximal interphalangeal joints of the fingers. The clinical course is usually progressive for months and sometimes years. While crippling may ensue, spontaneous remission and substantial recovery are not unusual.

Felty's syndrome (rheumatoid arthritis with hypersplenism) is an old designation for rheumatoid arthritis in adults, associated with splenomegaly and leukopenia. These patients usually have severe arthritic manifestations.

Association of rheumatoid arthritis with psoriasis. While it may be coincidental, in certain patients (approximately 3%) with severe rheumatoid arthritis there appears to be a peculiar, more intimate relationship designated as *"psoriatic arthritis."*[29,30] In such patients the exacerbations and remissions of the two diseases are likely to coincide, the distal interphalangeal joints are involved, and there is roentgenographic evidence of resorption of bone at the articular margins.

Xanthogranulomatous osteoarthropathy. Cognizance should be taken here of occasional cases of chronic polyarthritis having many clinical and pathologic features in common with rheumatoid arthritis, but with the addition of xanthomatous infiltration of the synovial tissue and of the bones.[31,32] The latter show focal rarefaction and even extensive destruction of their articular ends, leading to a mutilating form of arthritis. The lipid deposits are presumably secondary, but their significance is not clear.

Diseases of bone and joints

JOINT MANIFESTATIONS IN OTHER SYSTEMIC CONNECTIVE TISSUE DISEASES

More clinical observations than informative pathologic data are available in the area of systemic connective tissue diseases. There is definitely a need for more synovial biopsies in relevant cases and for the pathologist who has an unusual opportunity to perform an autopsy in any of these diseases to examine as many joints as possible and to obtain specimens of synovium for microscopic examination.

Rheumatic fever. Rheumatic fever, an acute or chronic inflammatory disease, is initiated by a preceding group A hemolytic streptococcal infection. It has also been induced by streptococcal vaccination (type 3 streptococcal M protein) in healthy siblings of patients with rheumatic fever.[33] In this connection also, one may recall the old animal experiments of Rich and Gregory[34] indicating that lesions having the basic characteristics of rheumatic carditis can result from anaphylactic hypersensitivity. Clinical rheumatic fever affects not only synovial joints but also the heart (pancarditis), the meninges (chorea), and possibly other connective tissue structures. As noted, subcutaneous nodules are also observed, as is erythema marginatum. There is apparently an important familial factor. While its peak incidence is in children above the age of 5 years, there is said to be an appreciable incidence in adults.

The joint manifestations, while acute in onset, are usually not severe, and the number of joints involved is generally small. Those most frequently affected are the ankles, knees, small joints of the foot, wrists, or elbows, and they are usually attacked in succession rather than simultaneously. Sometimes the symptoms are limited to a single joint, such as a hip, knee, or ankle. At times, they are less in the joints themselves than in the periarticular tissues and muscles, so that they are dismissed as "growing pains."

The affected joints show transient acute inflammatory reaction. Microscopically, the synovium is infiltrated by neutrophilic leukocytes and histiocytes, although at a later stage lymphocytes and plasma cells may predominate.[35]

Disseminated lupus erythematosus. Among the many protean manifestations of systemic lupus erythematosus, joint involvement is noted in more than 75% of patients. The arthralgias, however, are likely to be migratory, so that permanent clinical or roentgenographic evidence of arthritis is said to be found in only 35% of patients. The arthritis of systemic lupus erythematosus is held by some to be different from that of rheumatoid arthritis, although this is disputed.[36] According to Gardner,[25] the cellular synovial reaction is less intense, but more fibrinoid exudate is likely to be present.

Recent investigation of the connective tissue in systemic lupus erythematosus, using electron and fluorescent microscopy, has demonstrated widespread deposition of abnormal protein material resembling that in the "wire loops" in the kidneys, within the walls of many small blood vessels, and also between the collagen fibers, where it is associated with inflammation, necrosis, and fibrinous exudate. This material is presumed to represent abnormal proteins, possibly immunoglobulins or antigen-antibody complexes, and was found within affected joints, as well as many other structures.[37]

It is noteworthy also that rheumatoid nodules or granulomas, indistinguishable pathologically from those in rheumatoid arthritis, have been encountered in some patients with systemic lupus erythematosus.[38] They are found mainly in excised subcutaneous nodules in the elbow region and, occasionally, in synovial or tenosynovial tissues.

Dermatomyositis. Among the varied manifestations of dermatomyositis, those referable to the joints and muscles are noteworthy here. Arthralgias are mild, and the pathologic changes that they reflect are apparently not well understood, although Aegerter and Kirkpatrick[39] state (without offering supporting evidence) that they resemble those of mild rheumatoid arthritis. Involved muscles may undergo marked degeneration and atrophy, and joint deformities from flexion contractures develop late in the disease.

Scleroderma. Among the skeletal changes in scleroderma that may be cited are sclerodactyly and Raynaud's phenomenon, sometimes associated with calcinosis of the skin (see Fig. 14-8). Arthralgias are less frequent, but the tightening of the skin that ensues may eventually result in diminished joint motion. Certain dental changes have been described, particularly widening of the periodontal space, disappearance of the lamina dura, and, occasionally, loosening of teeth.

Periarteritis (polyarteritis) nodosa. As noted, some cases of polyarteritis may be triggered by hypersensitivity reaction to numerous drugs (for example, sulfanilamides) and other substances. The essential pathologic lesion is that of focal inflammation and necrosis of small and medium-sized arteries throughout the body. Skeletal muscle lesions are quite common, and biopsy of an affected muscle may serve to establish a diagnosis, although random sampling may not be rewarding. Arthritis is a very unusual manifestation, although arthralgias associated with polyneuritis and myositis are not infrequently observed.

SOME REMARKS ON THE CLASSIFICATION AND PATHOLOGY OF NONARTICULAR "RHEUMATISM"

It has been stated[40] that some 25% of patients seeking help ostensibly for arthritis do not have intrinsic joint disease at all, but rather some form of "nonarticular rheumatism." This designation proves on close scrutiny to be little more than a catchall category for the assorted aches, pains, and miseries (stiff neck, lumbago, painful shoulder, myalgia, bursitis, and the like) that for generations have provided a bonanza for patent medicine vendors.

Clinicians specializing in arthritis and rheumatology have over the years devised many names to designate certain symptom complexes, with a view to more effective treatment utilizing available potent drugs and numerous physiotherapeutic modalities. This is all right insofar as it goes, provided we do not deceive ourselves for we know next to nothing about the pathology of so-called fibrositis, myalgia, neuralgia, fasciitis, periarthritis, and so forth. Nor has any clarification

Diseases of bone and joints

or definition of these names in pathologic terms been forthcoming in recent years, that I am aware of.

It is my impression also that, in attempting broad coverage of problems in differential diagnosis, rheumatologists have apparently overextended themselves. Conditions such as calcification of tendons (especially the supraspinatus), "frozen" shoulder, Sudeck's atrophy, and infarcts of bone hardly fall within the purview of "rheumatism," while still others, such as fibroplasia of palmar fascia (leading to Dupuytren's contracture), stenosing tenovaginitis, chronic bursitis, joint bodies, neoplasms, pigmented villonodular synovitis, and tenosynovitis, which are also discussed in primers on rheumatic diseases, are perhaps best left to the orthopedist, particularly since the treatment of choice may well be surgery.

JOINT MANIFESTATIONS IN SOME HYPERSENSITIVITY REACTIONS

One can produce a simple hypersensitivity reaction in the rabbit's knee joint as an experimental model by sensitizing the animal to scarlatinal toxin and then, after 10 days, injecting a drop or two of the toxin into the joint. Within a few days the synovial lining shows edema and an eosinophil infiltrate. This reaction disappears within a week if the challenge is not repeated, leaving only slight subsynovial fibrosis as a residuum.

In man, hypersensitivity reactions in joints may occur in susceptible individuals following the administration of *drugs,* such as the sulfonamides and penicillin, as well as in *serum sickness*. Such affected joints may be paniful and tender, but the reaction is apparently self-limited. The opportunity to examine tissue specimens in these circumstances seldom presents itself, and the precise nature of the pathologic response appears to be conjectural.

The phenomenon of *intermittent hydrarthrosis* can, in some cases at least, reflect hypersensitivity or allergy to certain foods—shellfish and English walnuts specifically have been implicated as offending allergens. There are well documented cases in which their ingestion precipitated ephemeral knee joint effusion and in which this could be reproduced at will by dietary indiscretion.

As previously noted, rheumatic fever is commonly initiated by an antecedent group A hemolytic streptococcal infection. In some of the other systemic connective tissue diseases with joint manifestations, it would appear that a hypersensitivity factor is operative, although the problem of pathogenesis as a whole is variable and complex.

CHONDROCALCINOSIS *(pseudogout)*

In chondrocalcinosis, a peculiar apparently familial disease described in recent years,[41] there is a tendency for roentgenographically discernible calcium salts to be deposited intermittently in articular cartilage of the knee and other joints, and occasionally elsewhere. In the acute phase, there may be painful swelling of one or more affected joints. As in gout, the attacks may be triggered by a variety of predisposing circumstances, including surgery.[42] Crystals of cal-

Disorders of synovial joints

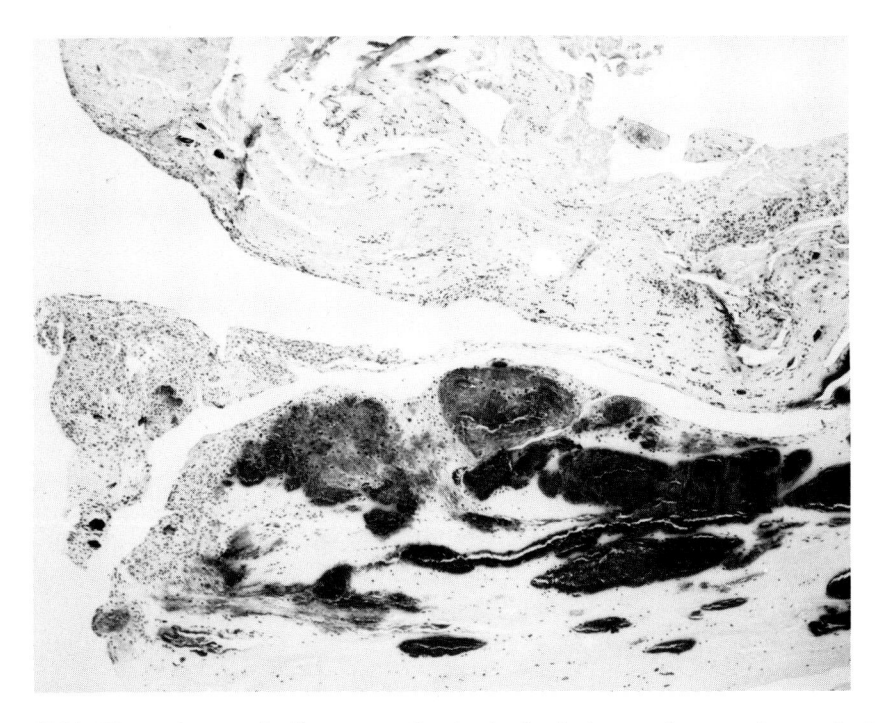

Fig. 15-21. Photomicrograph (low magnification) of a lesion in the carpal tunnel of an adult woman showing the deposition of a granular or crystalline (dark-staining) substance within and around tendon sheaths. These deposits proved to be calcium pyrophosphate, as seen in pseudogout. (×45.)

cium combined with phosphate as calcium pyrophosphate dihydrate are found also in the synovial fluid within leukocytes; this apparently is of diagnostic value. The crystals exhibit a positive birefringence with polarized light.[43] They have been shown to activate Hageman factor, which apparently triggers the acute arthritic reaction.[44] The disorder pursues a prolonged course generally through adult life, and its pathogenesis in precise genetic and biochemical terms is still speculative. For the quick relief of acute attacks, joint aspiration and intra-articular corticosteroid injection have been recommended.[42]

I have seen material from an unusual instance of pseudogout in a woman aged 64 who developed an acute carpal tunnel syndrome 2 days after a minor operation. In the surgical specimen, chalky white flecks were apparent in the gross and sections showed doubly refractile, crystalline deposits within the inflamed tenosynovium (Fig. 15-21).

RELAPSING POLYCHONDRITIS

In relapsing polychondritis, an unusual recurrent disorder, reports of which are to be found in German and English literature dating back to 1923, there is a remarkable tendency for cartilage structures in many sites to undergo inflammation, dissolution, and, eventually, connective tissue replacement. In articular car-

Diseases of bone and joints

tilage, this may lead to clinical arthritis, sometimes deforming and severe. Other untoward sequelae are collapse or distortion of the external ears, the cartilaginous portion of the nose, the laryngeal cartilages, the cartilage rings of the trachea and bronchi (complicated by suffocation and infection), and sometimes the cartilage of the ribs and spinal articulations. That this is more than a papainlike effect is evidenced by the fact that certain noncartilaginous structures, such as the middle ear, the sclera, and the anterior uveal tract, are often involved.

The etiology of this disease remains obscure, although it is noteworthy that corticosteroids are effective in controlling the disease. For a more detailed, informative account, the reader may have recourse to the paper by Pearson and his associates.[45]

CHONDROMATOSIS OF JOINTS

On occasion, innumerable small foci of hyaline cartilage (and sometimes of bone as well) may be formed by nodular condensation and metaplasia of the synovial and subsynovial connective tissue of joints. The most frequent site for this is the knee joint, although occasionally a hip, elbow, or some other joint may be affected. Essentially the same process may develop in the linings of bursal sacs or tendon sheaths, but this is comparatively uncommon.

When a knee joint is involved, for example, one may observe on surgical exploration that the synovium of the joint proper—and perhaps of the suprapatellar pouch and posterior compartment as well—is studded by small, firm, flat or slightly raised, gray-yellow nodules. These have a tendency to be extruded so that the joint may contain numerous, sometimes hundreds of, free chondral bodies. Whether or not they are visualized roentgenographically depends upon whether they show sufficient calcification or osseous transformation to be radiopaque (Fig. 15-22).

On microscopic examination of the lining of an affected joint, one observes numerous foci of cartilaginous or osseous metaplasia in varying stages of devel-

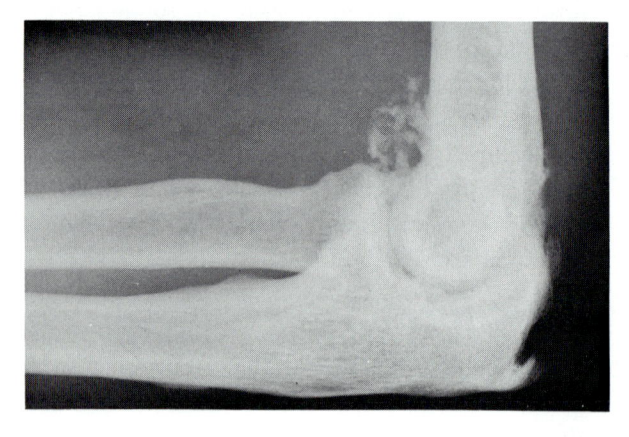

Fig. 15-22. Roentgenogram showing synovial chondromatosis (or osteochondromatosis) in an elbow.

Disorders of synovial joints

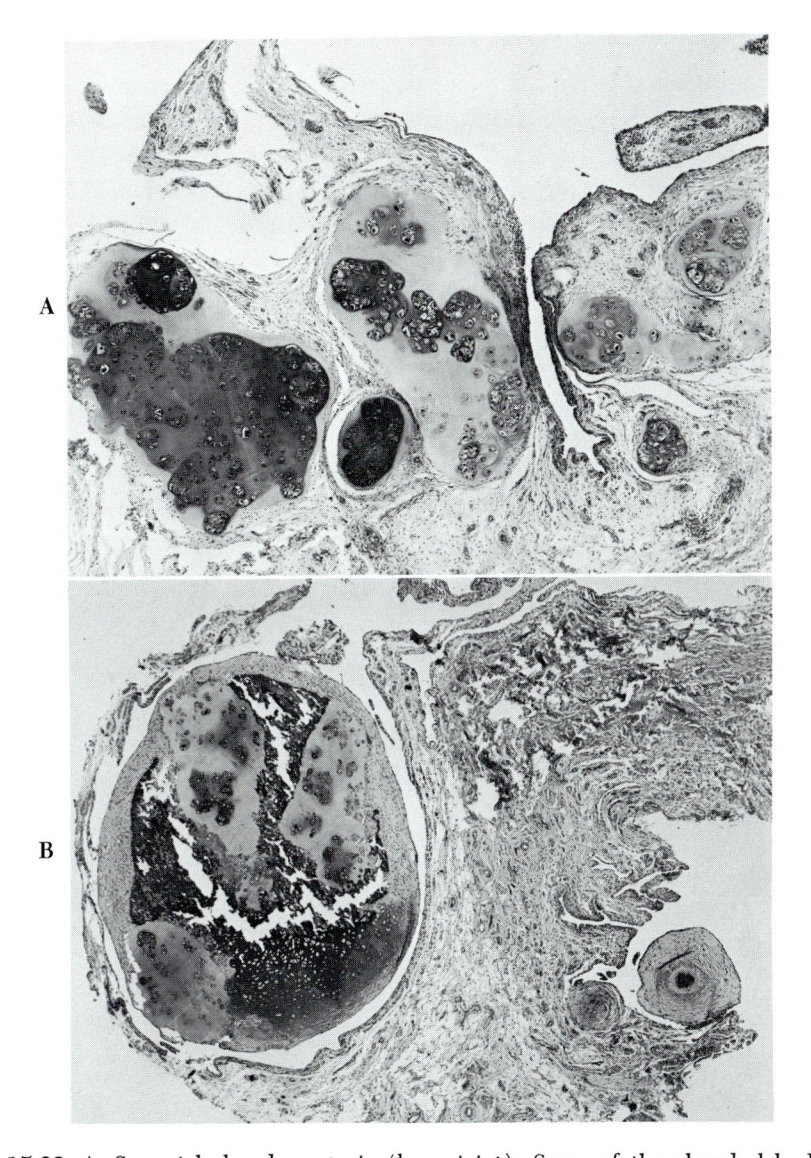

Fig. 15-23. **A,** Synovial chondromatosis (knee joint). Some of the chondral bodies are partially calcified, but there was no osseous metaplasia in this particular instance. **B,** Another example of synovial chondromatosis. The large, calcified chondral body (on the left) is ready to be extruded. The two small bodies (on the right) have been formed through focal nodular condensation of the synovial connective tissue, and the larger of the two shows incipient bone formation in its center.

opment. The cartilage foci, as noted, may become calcified or converted to bone (Fig. 15-23).

The treatment of choice is synovectomy, as complete as possible, and of course flushing out of all free joint bodies. Malignant change (to chondrosarcoma) has been reported,[46] but it is very unusual.[47]

Diseases of bone and joints

PIGMENTED VILLONODULAR SYNOVITIS

Pigmented villonodular synovitis, which Jaffe, Sutro, and I described and christened in 1941[48] represents essentially a peculiar, self-limited histiocytosis of as yet undetermined etiology, affecting the linings of joints (as well as tendon sheaths and occasionally bursae) in either localized or more diffuse forms. The proliferating stromal cells, which are of dual synovial and adventitial reticular origin, may flourish in tumorlike aggregates early in the cycle of evolution. However, even at this stage, they manifest their phagocytic nature by taking up hemosiderin pigment granules and sometimes lipid. While a variable number of multinuclear (giant) cells may be present, these constitute a minor, secondary feature. Eventually, many lesions tend spontaneously to involute, in part or throughout, and undergo extensive fibrosis and collagenization. This cycle may go on to substantial completion (as it commonly does in tendon sheath nodes of long standing), or it may renew itself, as it does in the more exuberant diffuse

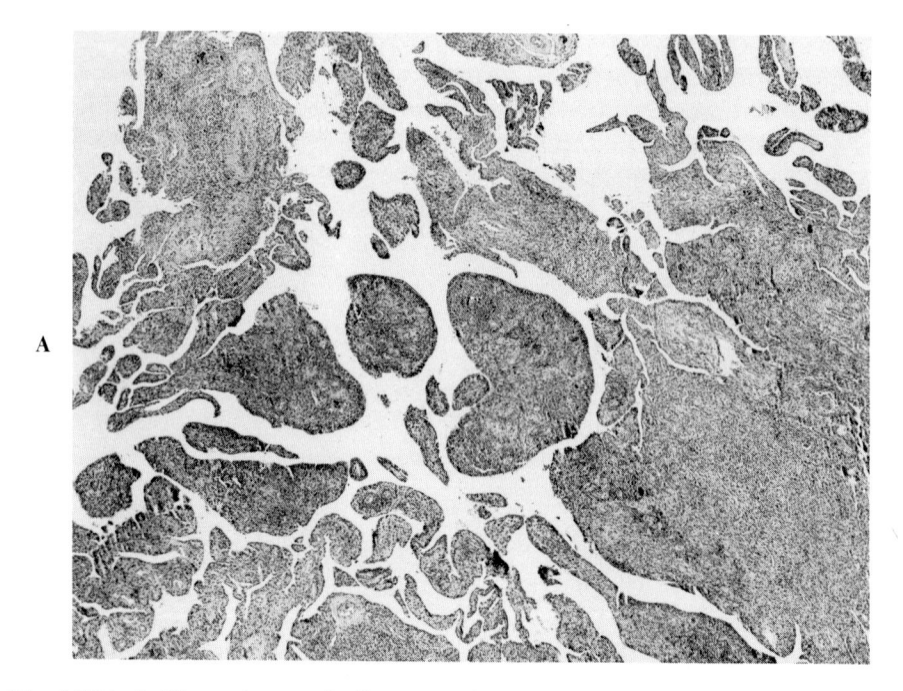

Fig. 15-24. **A,** Photomicrograph (low magnification) of a representative field of a lesion of pigmented villonodular synovitis of a knee joint, illustrating the general pattern and showing both villous and more compact, nodular areas (toward the right). Elsewhere there was intense focal hemosiderin pigmentation. (×25.) **B,** Higher magnification of the lesion illustrated in **A,** showing a field of proliferating histiocytes (beneath the hypertrophied synovial lining) that characterize the lesion. These cells may phagocytize hemosiderin and lipid and have a tendency also to form occasional syncytial aggregates or giant cells (seen on the left). (×350.) **C,** Photomicrograph of a field from a lesion of pigmented villonodular synovitis of a knee joint illustrating prominent synovial-lined spaces within the thickened synovial membrane. (Other fields showed appreciable collagenization, scattered multinuclear giant cells, and abundant hemosiderin deposition.)

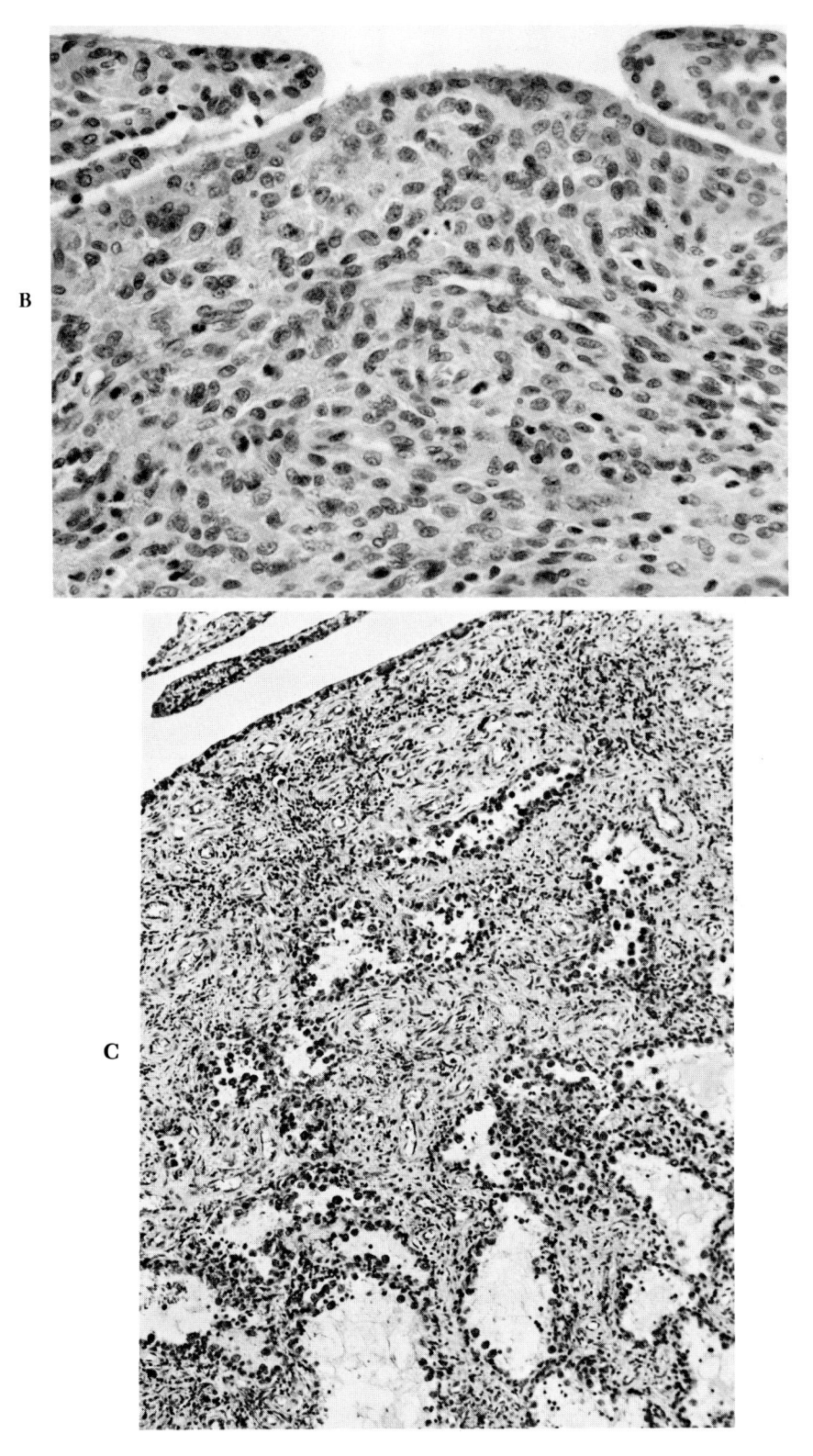

Fig. 15-24, cont'd. For legend see opposite page.

Diseases of bone and joints

lesions in the knee joint. In the process, the synovium and the sublining tissues are more or less deeply pigmented, often becoming deep red-brown or a chocolate-brown. Collaterally, in the diffuse lesions at least, the affected area is transformed into a tangled, spongy mat or web, often intricately associated with protruding sessile or pedicled nodules (Figs. 15-24 and 15-25). These nodules protruding from the synovium are indistinguishable histologically from tendon sheath nodes (pigmented nodular tenosynovitis or so-called giant-cell tumor in the old terminology). Incidentally, some tendon sheath nodes may reappear after excision and require further surgery, and a few recur a second or even a third time. This should not be construed, necessarily, as indicating aggressiveness or malignant change.

The condition is not nearly so common in synovial joints as it is in tendon sheaths. The knee joint is most often involved, although occasionally a hip, ankle, or some other joint may be affected. The symptoms are pain, swelling, and sometimes locking of the joint; they may persist for months or even several years before the condition is recognized. Clinically and radiographically there is evidence of a thickened, swollen joint capsule with effusion. The latter tends to recur after tapping and to be serosanguineous; this fact often affords a valuable diagnostic lead. In recent years, it has become increasingly evident that the lesion may extend into the contiguous articular bone ends,[49] apparently through eroded apertures in the cortex, in much the same way that tendon sheath nodes of long standing may erode adjacent bones (Figs. 15-25, B, and 15-26).

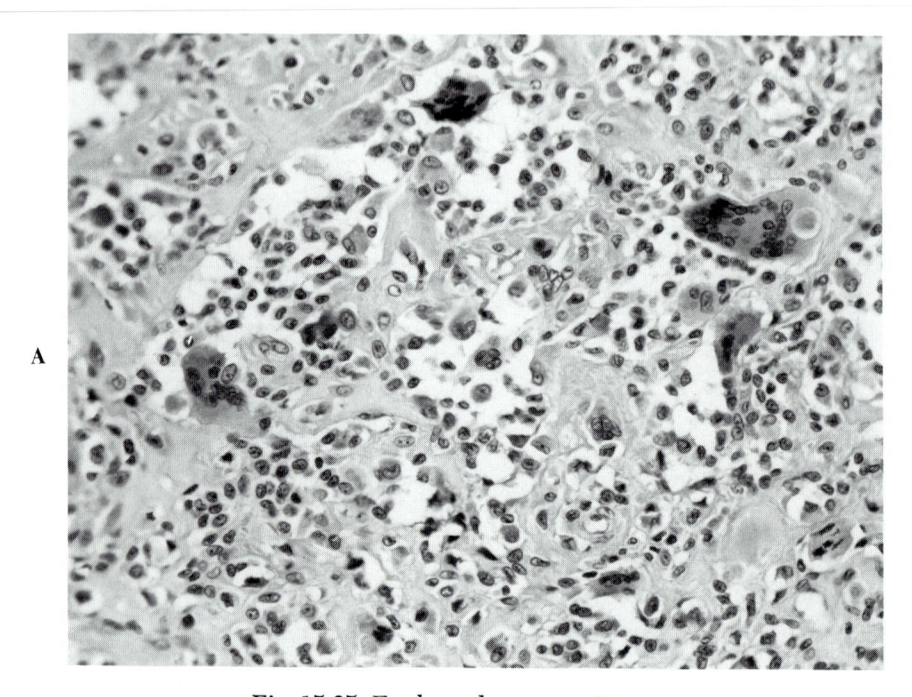

Fig. 15-25. For legend see opposite page.

Disorders of synovial joints

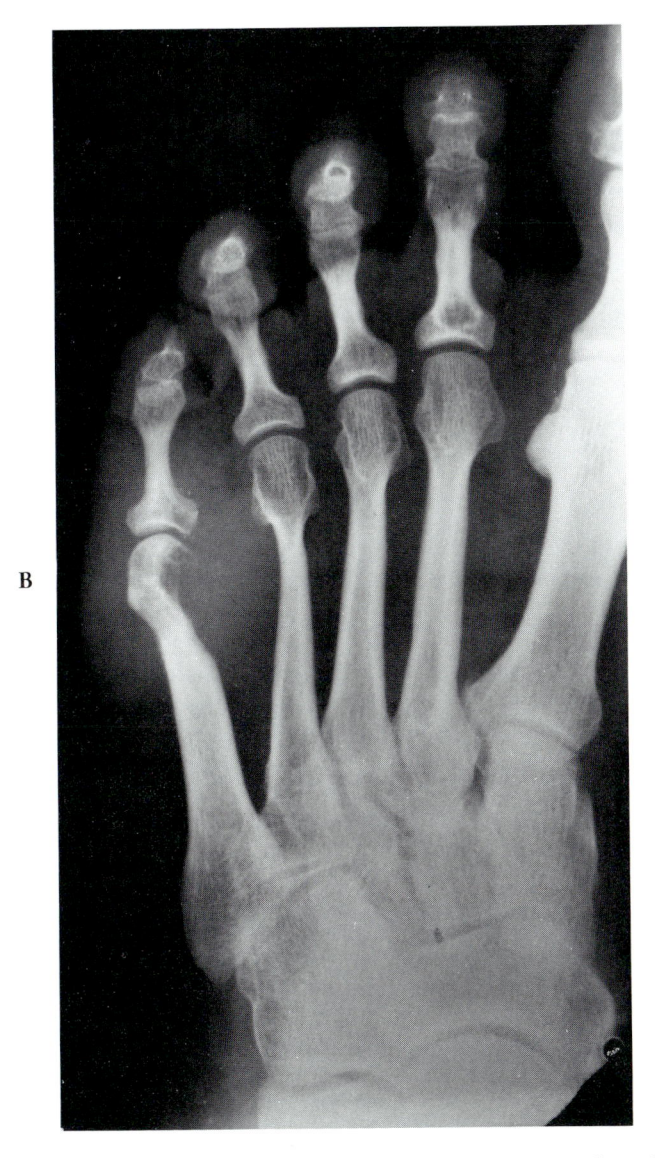

Fig. 15-25. A, Photomicrograph of a representative field of a tendon sheath node of the nature of pigmented nodular tenosynovitis (giant cell tumor in old terminology). Here again one finds histiocytes, often bordering open spaces, and occasional syncytial aggregates within a stroma that is becoming collagenized. Elsewhere there was focal hemosiderin pigmentation. (×250.) B, Roentgenogram showing erosion of the proximal end of a fifth metatarsal bone by a tendon sheath node of long standing (pigmented nodular tenosynovitis).

Diseases of bone and joints

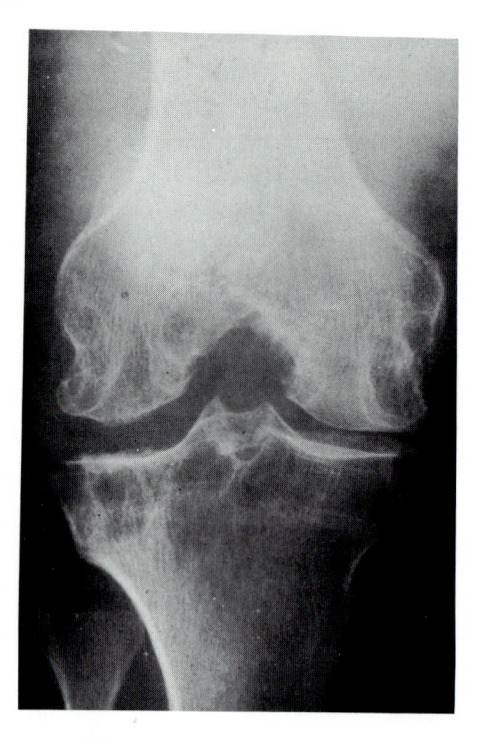

Fig. 15-26. Roentgenogram of knee joint region in a case of long-standing pigmented villonodular synovitis. From this picture, one may anticipate finding extension of the lesion into the articular bone ends.

In referring to the condition, some commentators drop the qualifying adjective "pigmented," but I find this objectionable since "villonodular synovitis" is too nondescript in itself to constitute a meaningful designation. Also, with reference to dissent, we reject the suggestions that the lesion represents a sclerosing hemangioma, that it represents a benign (giant cell) synovioma in the sense of a genuine neoplasm, or that it results from chronic hemarthrosis. The weight of pathologic evidence is against these views, as has been previously indicated.[48] With reference to the last notion particularly, it may be emphasized that while repeated hemorrhage into a joint does, to be sure, induce villous hypertrophy and hemosiderin deposition in the lining, it does *not* provoke diffuse histiocytic proliferation. This is as true in experimental models as it is in hemophilia.

Localized lesions of pigmented villonodular synovitis can be readily excised. For diffuse lesions, total synovectomy is the treatment of choice, although the condition may recur. For these exuberant, recurrent lesions, and for lesions that cannot be totally extirpated surgically for whatever reason, roentgen therapy affords effective control. As small a tissue dose as 1,500 rads may suffice, but at times a total of 2,000 to 2,500 rads may be necessary. As for malignant change, it is conceivable that this may happen (as it does on rare occasions in old, neglected tendon sheath nodes),[50] but it would be remarkable. I have not observed it to date in my own experience.

REFERENCES

1. Bhawan, J., Tandon, H. D., and Roy, S.: Ultrastructure of synovial membrane in pyogenic arthritis, Arch. Pathol. 96:155, 1973.
2. Johnson, A. H., Campbell, W. G., Jr., and Callahan, B. C.: Infection of rabbit knee joints after intra-articular injection of *Staphylococcus aureus*, Am. J. Pathol. 60:165, 1970.
3. Medical Staff Conference: Gonococcal sepsis and arthritis, Calif. Med. 114:18, 1971.
4. Sotelo-Ortiz, F.: Chronic coccidioidal synovitis of knee joint, J. Bone Joint Surg. 37-A:48, 1955.
5. Anderson, S. G., Doherty, R. L., and Carley, J. G.: Med. J. Aust. 1:173, 1961.
6. Caranasos, G. J., and Felker, J. R.: Mumps arthritis, Arch. Intern. Med. 119:394, 1967.
7. Filpi, R. G., and Houts, R. L.: Mumps arthritis, J.A.M.A. 205:216, 1968.
8. Chambers, R. J., and Bywaters, E. G. L.: Rubella synovitis, Ann. Rheum. Dis. 22:263, 1963.
9. Chin, J., Werner, S. B., Kusumoto, H. H., and Lennette, E. H.: Complications of rubella immunization in children, Calif. Med. 114:7, 1971.
10. Ward, J. R., and Bishop, B.: Varicella arthritis, J.A.M.A. 212:1954, 1970.
11. Gardner, D. L.: Pathology of the connective tissue diseases, Baltimore, 1965, The Williams & Wilkins Co.
12. Cockshott, P., and MacGregor, M.: Osteomyelitis variolosa, Q. J. Med. 27:369, 1958.
13. Committee of the American Rheumatism Association: Primer on the rheumatic diseases: part III, J.A.M.A. 171:1680, 1959.
14. Sokoloff, L., and Bunim, J. J.: Clinical and pathological studies of joint involvement in sarcoidosis, N. Engl. J. Med. 260:841, 1959.
15. Case records of the Massachusetts General Hospital, N. Engl. J. Med. 263:93, 1960.
16. Collins, D. H.: Haemosiderosis and haemochromatosis of synovial tissues, J. Bone Joint Surg. 33:436, 1951.
17. Roy, S.: Ultrastructure of articular cartilage in experimental hemarthrosis, Arch. Pathol. 86:69, 1968.
18. Mankin, H. J.: The structure, chemistry and metabolism of articular cartilage, Bull. Rheum. Dis. 17:447, 1967.
19. Moskowitz, R. W., Klein, L., and Mast, W. A.: Current concepts of degenerative joint disease (osteoarthritis), Bull. Rheum. Dis. 17:459, 1967.
20. Van der Korst, J. K., Sokoloff, L., and Miller, E. J.: Senescent pigmentation of cartilage and degenerative joint disease, Arch. Pathol. 86:39, 1968.
21. Stecher, R. M.: Heberden's nodes, the clinical characteristics of osteo-arthritis of the fingers, Ann. Rheum. Dis. 7:1, 1948.
22. Hollander, J. L., McCarty, D. J., Astorga, G., and Castro-Marillo, E.: Studies on the pathogenesis of rheumatoid joint inflammation: the "R.A. cell" and a working hypothesis, Ann. Intern. Med. 62:271, 1965.
23. Rawson, A. J., Quismoria, F. P., and Abelson, N. M.: The induction of synovitis in the normal rabbit with Fab: a possible experimental model of rheumatoid arthritis, Am. J. Pathol. 54:95, 1969.
24. Graham, R. C., Jr., and Shannon, S. L.: Peroxidase arthritis: an immunologically mediated inflammatory response with ultrastructural cytochemical localization of antigen and specific antibody, Am. J. Pathol. 67:69, 1972.
25. Gardner, D. L.: The pathology of polyarthritis. In Symposium; polyarthritis, The Royal College of Physicians of Edinburgh, 1964.
26. Sokoloff, L., McCluskey, R. T., and Bunim, J. J.: Vascularity of the early subcutaneous nodule of rheumatoid arthritis, Arch. Pathol. 55:475, 1953.
27. Chandler, G. N., Jones, D. T., Wright, V., and Hartfall, S. J.: Charcot's arthropathy following intra-articular hydrocortisone, Br. Med. J., p. 952, 1959.
28. Romanus, R.: Pelvo-spondylitis ossificans, Chicago, 1968, Year Book Medical Publishers.
29. Bauer, W., Bennett, G. A., and Zeller, J. W.: The pathology of joint lesions in patients with psoriasis and arthritis, Trans. Assoc. Am. Physicians 56:349, 1941.
30. Sherman, M. S.: Psoriatic arthritis: observations on the clinical, roentgenographic and pathological changes, J. Bone Joint Surg. 34-A:831, 1952.
31. Graham, G., and Stanfield, A. G.: A case of hitherto undescribed lipoidosis simulating rheumatoid arthritis, J. Pathol. 58:545, 1946.

32. Golden, G. N., and Richards, H. G. H.: Xanthogranulomatous disease of bone with polyarthritis, J. Bone Joint Surg. 35-B:275, 1953.
33. Massell, B. F., Honikman, L. H., and Amezcua, J.: Rheumatic fever following streptococcal vaccination, J.A.M.A. 207: 1115, 1969.
34. Rich, A. R., and Gregory, J. E.: Experimental evidence that lesions with basic characteristics of rheumatic carditis can result from anaphylactic hypersensitivity, Bull. Johns Hopkins Hosp. 73:239-264, 1943.
35. Bennett, G. A.: Comparison of the pathology of rheumatic fever and rheumatoid arthritis, Am. Int. Med. 19:111, 1943.
36. Cruickshank, B.: Lesions of joints and tendon sheaths in systemic lupus erythematosus, Ann. Rheum. Dis. 18:111, 1959.
37. Grishman, E., and Churg, J.: Connective tissue in systemic lupus erythematosus: demonstration of disseminated vascular and extravascular "wire loop" deposits, Arch. Pathol. 91:156, 1971.
38. Dubois, E. L., Friou, G. S., and Chandor, S.: Rheumatoid nodules and rheumatoid granulomas in systemic lupus erythematosus, J.A.M.A. 220:515, 1972.
39. Aegerter, E., and Kirkpatrick, J. A., Orthopedic diseases, Philadelphia, 1963, W. B. Saunders Co., p. 753.
40. Freyberg, R. H.: Nonarticular rheumatism: the musculoskeletal system: a symposium, New York, 1952, The Macmillan Co., p. 271.
41. McCarty, D. J., Jr., Kohn, N., and Faires, J.: The significance of calcium phosphate crystals in the synovial fluid of arthritic patients: the "pseudogout syndrome," Ann. Intern. Med. 56:711, 1962.
42. O'Duffy, J. D.: Pseudogout syndrome in hospital patients, J.A.M.A. 226:41, 1973.
43. Bluhm, G. B.: Laboratory diagnosis of crystalline arthritis, Bull. Path. Amer. Soc. Clin. Pathol. 10:91, 1969.
44. McKay, D. G.: Participation of components of the blood coagulation system in the inflammatory response, Am. J. Pathol. 67:181, 1972.
45. Pearson, C. M., Kline, H. M., and Newcomer, V. D.: Relapsing polychondritis, N. Engl. J. Med. 263:51, 1960.
46. Mullins, F., Berard, C. W., and Eisenberg, J. H.: Chondrosarcoma following synovial chondromatosis, Cancer 18: 1180, 1965.
47. Goldman, R. L., and Lichtenstein, L.: Synovial chondrosarcoma, Cancer 17: 1223, 1964.
48. Jaffe, H. L., Lichtenstein, L., and Sutro, C. J.: Pigmented villonodular synovitis, bursitis and tenosynovitis, Arch. Pathol. 91:731, 1941.
49. Breimer, C. W., and Freiberger, R. H.: Bone lesions associated with villonodular synovitis, Am. J. Roentgen. 79:618, 1958.
50. Lichtenstein, L.: Bone tumors, ed. 4, St. Louis, 1972, The C. V. Mosby Co., p. 416.

GENERAL REFERENCE

Collins, D. H.: The pathology of articular and spinal diseases, Arnold, London, 1949.

Index*

A

Abscess
  bone, chronic, 52, *54-56*, 58, *60*
  Brodie's, 58
Achondroplasia, **35-37**, *36*
Acidosis
  chronic, in chronic renal insufficiency, 138-139
  renal tubular, 142
Aclasis, diaphyseal; *see* Hereditary multiple exostosis
Acquired syphilis, 70-72, *71*
Acromegalic arthritis, 102
Acromegaly 101, 102, *102*
  joint changes in, 102
  osteoporosis in, 150
Actinomycosis, 75
Adenomas, parathyroid, 107
Adolescent coxa vara, 233; *see also* Slipped capital femoral epiphysis
Adrenal glands, skeletal changes caused by, **104**
Agenesis, ovarian, 106
Albers-Schönberg disease; *see* Osteopetrosis
Albright's syndrome, 19; *see also* Fibrous dysplasia of bone
Allopurinol for gout, 125
Amaurotic idiocy, 119
Aminoaciduria with renal tubular reabsorption defects, 142
Amphotericin B for coccidiomycosis of joints, 275
Amputation neuroma, **230**, *230*
Amyloid deposition, 133
Amyloidosis, 133
  rheumatoid arthritis as cause of, 288
  as sequel of chronic osteomyelitis, 61
Anemia
  Cooley's erythroblastic, 169, *170*
  hemolytic
    chronic, **167**
    familial; *see* Spherocytic anemia
  Mediterranean, 169

Anemia—cont'd
  sickle cell, 167-168, *169*
    Salmonella osteomyelitis in, 168-169, *169*
  spherocytic, 170-171
Aneurysmal bone cyst, **258-263**, *259-262*
Angiomatosis, regional, 244-245
Ankylosing arthritis; *see* Rheumatoid arthritis
Ankylosing spondylitis; *see* Rheumatoid spondylitis
Anomalies, systemic, of skeletal development, **16-49**
Antibiotics
  for brucellosis, 61
  for pyogenic osteomyelitis, 52
Arthralgias caused by viral diseases, 275
Arthritis
  acromegalic, 102
  atrophic; *see* Rheumatoid arthritis
  degenerative; *see* Osteoarthritis
  gonococcal, 271
  manifestations of, in metabolic disorders, **277**, *278-279*
  Marie-Strümpell; *see* Rheumatoid spondylitis
  psoriatic, 289
  pyogenic, 270, 271, *271*
  in Reiter's syndrome, 276
  rheumatoid; *see* Rheumatoid arthritis
  in tuberculosis, 272-274, *272-273*
  von Bechterew's; *see* Rheumatoid spondylitis
Arthritis deformans; *see* Osteoarthritis
Arthropathy, acromegalic, 102
Articular bone ends, disorders of, 265
Articular cartilage, 277, 280
  alterations in, **280-283**, *280, 281-282*
  degeneration of, *281*
  disorders of, 265
  injury to, 266, *268*
Atrophic arthritis; *see* Rheumatoid arthritis
Atrophy, Sudeck's, 244
Avascular necrosis, *10*, **234-239**, *235, 238*
  in juvenile osteochondritis, **239-244**, *240-243*
Avitaminosis C; *see* Scurvy
Azotemic osteodystrophy; *see* Renal insufficiency, chronic

B

Baker's cyst, **232-233**

---

*Page references to illustrations appear in italics. The more important references are in boldface.

303

Index

Bamboo spine, 289
Basedow's disease, 104
Basophilism, pituitary, 100
Bedsonia causing Reiter's syndrome, 276
Beryllium, effect of, on bone, 213
Besnier-Boeck-Schaumann's disease; *see* Sarcoidosis
Biliary cirrhosis, osteoporosis in, 150
Bismuth, effect of, on bone, 210-211
Blastomyces dermatitidis, 75
Blastomycosis, 75
Blood diseases, skeletal changes in, **164-171**
Bodies
  joint, formation of, 266, 268, *269*
  Reilly, 39
  rice, 286
Bone(s)
  abscess of, chronic, 52, *54-55*, 58, *60*
  brittle; *see* Osteogenesis imperfecta
  changes in; *see* Skeletal changes
  chemical effects on, **210-214,** *211, 213*
  cyst of
    aneurysmal, **258-263,** *259-262*
    epidermoid, **258,** *258*
    unicameral, **250-258,** *252-255*
      solitary, 251-252
  disease of
    associated with chronic renal insufficiency, **138-142,** *139-141*
    associated with renal tubular reabsorption defects, **142-143**
    disappearing or vanishing, 244-245
    Paget's, **173-194;** *see also* Paget's disease of bone
  effect on
    of beryllium, 213
    of bismuth, 210-211
    of cadmium, 213
    of fluoride, 211-213, *213*
    of lead, 210, *211*
    of mercury, 213
    of phosphorus, 211
  fibrous dysplasia of; *see* Fibrous dysplasia of bone
  histiocytosis X
    chronic disseminated, **206-209,** *204, 206-208*
    disseminated in, **203-206,** *203, 205*
    localized in, **198-203,** *199-202*
  infarcts of, **234-239,** *235-238*
  in Gaucher's disease, 119-122, *121-122*
  infections of, **52-80**
  lesions of, caused by parasitic disease, **76**
  posttraumatic rarefaction of, **244-245**
  radiation effects on, **214-217,** *215*
    external, 214-216
    internal, 216
  resorption of, 107
  spotty; *see* Osteopoikilosis
Bone ends, articular, disorders of, 265
Brittle bones; *see* Osteogenesis imperfecta
Brodie's abscess, 58
Brown tumor, 108, *110, 111, 113*

Brucella
  osteomyelitis caused by, 58, 61
  causing pyogenic arthritis, 270
Brucellosis, 58, 61
Bucket-handle tear of meniscus, 218, 219, *219*
Bursitis, chronic, **219-221**

C

Cadmium, effect of, on bone, 213
Caffey's disease; *see* Infantile cortical hyperostosis
Calcification
  of fingers, *227-228*
  from irradiation, 214, *215*
  of patellar tendon, 226, *226*
  of soft tissues, 227, *228-229*
  of tendons, 226-229, *228-229*
Calcitonin, 105
  for Paget's disease, 177, 178
Callus
  fibrocartilaginous, 2
  formation of, 2, 3, *3*
  osseous, 2
  primary, *4, 5*
Calvarium, cotton-wool, *187*
Capital femoral epiphysis, slipped, 233, *233*
Cartilage
  articular, 277, *278-279*, 280
    alterations in, 280-283, *280-282*
    degeneration of, *281*
    disorders of, 265
    injury to, 266, 268, *268*
  formation of, at fracture site, *4-5, 5, 6*
Cartilaginous exostoses, multiple; *see* Hereditory multiple exostosis
Cat-scratch fever, skeletal changes in, 77
Charcot elbow, *160*
Charcot hip, *159*
Charcot knee, *159, 161*
Charcot neuroarthropathy, 156
Charcot spine, *159*
Chemicals, effects of, on bones, **210-214,** *211, 213*
Chemotherapy for skeletal tuberculosis, 64
Cherubism causing hyperostosis, *191*, 192
Chickenpox
  joint changes after, 275
  skeletal changes in, 78
Chief cell hyperplasia, parathyroid adenoma, *114*
Children, effects of radiation on, 215-216
Chloramphenicol for granuloma inguinale, 68
Cholesterol deposition in xanthoma tuberosum multiplex, 123, *123*
Chondrocalcinosis, **292-293,** *293*
Chondrodystrophia fetalis; *see* Achondroplasia
Chondrodystrophic dwarfism; *see* Achondroplasia
Chondromalacia of patella, *280*
Chondromatosis of joints, **294-295,** *294-295*
Chondroosteodystrophy, Morquio-Brailsford type; *see* Morquio's disease
Chondrosarcoma in osteocartilaginous exostosis, **24-28,** *26-27*

Index

Cirrhosis, biliary, osteoporosis in, 150
Classification of histiocytosis X, 196
Cleidocranial dysostosis, 40, *42*
Coccidioides immitis, 72-75, *73-74*, 274-275
Coccidiomycosis, 72-76
    of joints, 274-275, *274*
Colchicine for gout, 125
Collagen diseases, 283-284
Congenital porphyria erythropoietica, 132
Congenital pseudoarthrosis of tibia, **233-234**, *234*
Congenital syphilis, 68-70, *69-70*
    causing hyperostosis, 192
    manifestations of, 70
Congenital torticollis, 232
Connective tissue diseases, systemic, joint manifestations in, **290-291**
Contracture
    Dupuytren's, **230-232**, *232*
    Volkmann's, **230**, *231*
Cooley's erythroblastic anemia, 169, *170*
Copper deficiency, 134
Cortical hyperostosis, infantile, **77-80**, *78-79*
    skeletal changes in, 77-78
Corticotropin for gout, 125
Cortisone for rheumatoid arthritis, 288
Cotton-wool calvarium, *187*
Coxa anteverta, 233, *233*
Coxa vara, adolescent, 233
Cretinism, 105, *105*
Cryptococcosis, 75-76
Cushing's syndrome, 100, 104
Cutaneous myxoid cysts, 223
Cystine storage disease, 131, 142
Cystinosis; *see* Cystine storage disease
Cysts
    Baker's, **232-233**
    bone
        aneurysmal, **258-263**, *259-262*
        epidermoid, **258**, *258*
        unicameral, **250-258**, *252-255*
            solitary, 251-252
    cutaneous myxoid, 223
    meniscal and parameniscal, 219, *220*, 222
    synovial, 223

D

Dactylitis
    sickle cell, 168
    tuberculous, 63, *64*
Damage, joint, from chronic hemarthrosis, **276-277**
de Toni-Debré-Fanconi syndrome; *see* Vitamin D–resistant rickets
Defects
    genetic, of skeletal development, 16-17
    renal tubular reabsorption, bone disease associated with, **142-143**
Deficiency
    copper, 134
    manganese, 134
    vitamin A, skeletal changes in, **83-84**

Deficiency—cont'd
    vitamin C, skeletal changes in, **85-88**, *86-87*
    vitamin D
        in renal disease, 137-138
        skeletal changes in **88-96**, *89*
    zinc, 134
Degeneration
    of articular cartilage, *281*
    of tendons, 228, *229*
Degenerative arthritis; *see* Osteoarthritis
Degenerative joint disease; *see* Osteoarthritis
Dental fluorosis, 212
Deposition
    amyloid, 133
    cholesterol, in xanthoma tuberosum multiplex, 123, *123*
Deposits
    fibrinoid, in rheumatoid arthritis, 286, *287*
    urate, in gout, 125, *125-126*, 127, *278*
Dermatomyositis, 291
Desert rheumatism, 274
Development, skeletal, systemic anomalies of, **16-49**
Diabetes, renal, 142
Diabetes mellitus, 106
    neurotrophic foot in, 156, *157*
Diamidines for blastomycosis, 75
Diaphyseal aclasis; *see* Hereditary multiple exostosis
Diaphyseal dysplasia, progressive, **47**
    skeletal changes in, *46*
Diaphyseal sclerosis, hereditary multiple; *see* Progressive diaphyseal dysplasia
Diphosphonates for Paget's disease, 177, 178
Diplococcus pneumoniae causing pyogenic arthritis, 270
Disappearing bone disease, 244-245
Discoid meniscus, 219, *220*
Discs, intervertebral
    in hereditary ochronosis, 128, *128-131*
    tissue of, herniated, **223-225**, *224*
Disease
    Albers-Schönberg; *see* Osteopetrosis
    Basedow's, 104
    Besnier-Boeck-Schaumann's; *see* Sarcoidosis
    blood, skeletal changes in, **164-171**
    bone
        associated with chronic renal insufficiency, **138-142**, *139-141*
        associated with renal tubular resorption defects, **142-143**
        disappearing or vanishing, 244-245
        Paget's, **173-194**; *see also* Paget's disease of bone
    Caffey's; *see* Infantile cortical hyperostosis
    collagen, 283-284
    connective tissue, systemic, joint manifestations in, **290-291**
    cystine storage, 131, 142
    Engelmann's; *see* Progressive diaphyseal dysplasia
    Gaucher's, 119-122, *121-122*
        bone infarct in, *122*
        skeletal changes in, *120-121*

Index

Disease—cont'd
  Graves', 104
  Hurler-Pfaundler; see Gargoylism
  joint, degenerative; see Osteoarthritis
  Kienböck's; see Juvenile osteochondritis
  Köhler's; see Juvenile osteochondritis
  Kümmell's, 244
  Legg-Perthes'; see Juvenile osteochondritis
  Lignac-Fanconi; see Cystine storage disease
  marble bone; see Osteopetrosis
  Möller-Barlow's; see Scurvy
  Morquio's, **37-39**, *38*
  Niemann-Pick, 118, 119
  Ollier's; see Skeletal enchondromatosis
  Osgood-Schlatter's, *243*, 244
  parasitic, bone lesions caused by, **76**
  Pott's; see Tuberculous spondylitis
  renal, skeletal changes in, **137-143**; see also Renal disease
  Schüller-Christian; see Histiocytosis X, chronic disseminated
  sickle cell, 167-168, *169*
  Simmond's, 104
  Still's, 289
  Tay-Sachs, 119
  viral, joint manifestations in, 275
  Voorhoeve's, 39, *41*
Disorders
  of articular bone ends, 265
  of articular cartilages, 265
  endocrine, skeletal changes in, **100-115**
  of lipid metabolism, primary, **118-123**
  metabolic
    arthritic manifestations of, 277, *278-279*
    skeletal changes in, **118-134**
  neurotrophic, skeletal changes in, 156-162
  of synovial joints, 265-300
  systemic, of mucopolysaccharide metabolism, 132-133
Disseminated lupus erythematosus, 290-291
Dupuytren's contracture, **230-232**, *232*
Dwarfism
  chondrodystrophic; see Achondroplasia
  from hypothyroidism, 105
  Lorain type of, 102, *103*
  from primary hypogonadism, 106
  renal, 141
Dysostosis
  cleidocranial, 40, *42*
  metaphyseal, 48
Dysostosis multiplex; see Gargoylism
Dysplasia
  familial metaphyseal, 48
  fibrous; see Fibrous dysplasia of bone
  progressive diaphyseal, *46*, **47**
Dysplasia epiphysealis multiplex, 48
Dysplasia epiphysealis punctata, 48
Dystrophia adiposogenitalis, 104

E

Eccentroosteochondrodysplasia; see Morquio's disease
Echinococcosis, 76

Elements, trace, influence of, on skeleton, 134
Enchondromatosis, skeletal, **28-30**, *28-30*
Endocrine disorders, skeletal changes in, **100-115**
Engelmann's disease; see Progressive diaphyseal dysplasia
Eosinophilic granuloma, **198-203**, *199-205*, 206; see also Histiocytosis X
Epidermoid cyst in bone, **258**, *258*
Erythroblastic anemia, Cooley's, 169, *170*
Essential hypercholesterolemia; see Xanthoma tuberosum multiplex
Eunuchism, 106
Excess
  vitamin A, skeletal changes in, **84-85**, *84*
  vitamin D, skeletal changes in, **96-97**
Excretion, renal, failure of; see Renal insufficiency, chronic
Exophthalmic goiter, 104
Exostosis
  hereditary multiple, **24-28**, *25*
  multiple cartilaginous; see Hereditary multiple exostosis
  osteocartilaginous, 24, *26*, *27*
    chondrosarcoma in, *26*, *27*
  subungual, *249*, 250
External radiation, effect of, on bone, 214-216
Extraskeletal abnormalities with fibrous dysplasia of bone, 19

F

False joint; see Pseudoarthrosis
Familial hemolytic anemia; see Spherocytic anemia
Familial hyperostosis, 193-194, *193*
Familial metaphyseal dysplasia, 48
Familial osteodysplasia, 194
Fanconi syndrome, *94*
Felty's syndrome, 289
Femoral epiphysis, capital, slipped, **233**, *233*
Fever
  cat-scratch, skeletal changes in, 77
  rheumatic, 290
Fibrinoid deposits in rheumatoid arthritis, 286, *287*
Fibromatosis colli, 232
Fibrous dysplasia of bone, **17-24**
  extraskeletal abnormalities of, 19
  causing hyperostosis, 190, *192*
  monostotic lesions of, *18*
  polyostotic, 17, *20*
  solitary lesions of, 17, 19, *22*
Fibrous union, photomicrograph of, *9*
Fingers
  calcification of, 227-228
  trigger, *228*, 229
Fluoride
  effect of, on bone, 211-213, *213*
  intoxication by, 212
Fluorosis, dental, 212
Foot
  Madura, 64-67, *66*
  neurotrophic, in diabetes mellitus, 156, *157*

Index

Formation
   ganglion, **222-223,** *222*
   of joint bodies, 266, 268, *269*
Fracture(s)
   avulsion, *12*
   closed, 1
   compound, 1
   definition of, 1
   healing of
      requirements of, 6-7
      stages of, 1-2
   incomplete, fibrous repair of, *2*
   intraarticular, 266
   open, 1
   pathologic, *11, 12, 13*
      causes of, 11, 14-15
      definition of, 1
   and sequelae, **1-15**
   simple, 1
   stress, 3
Fragilitas ossium; *see* Osteogenesis imperfecta
Freiberg-Köhler's disease; *see* Juvenile osteochondritis
Fungal infections, skeletal involvement in, **72-76**

G

Ganglion
   formation of, **222-223,** *222*
   intraosseous, 223
Gardner's syndrome, 193
Gargoylism, **40-44,** 133
   skeletal changes in, *45*
   skull changes in, *43*
Garré type of osteomyelitis, 55
Gastrectomy causing osteoporosis, 149, *149*
Gaucher's disease, 119-122, *121-122*
   bone infarct in, 122
   skeletal changes in, 120-121
Generalized osteitis fibrosa cystica, 108
Genetic defects of skeletal development, 16-17
German measles, skeletal changes in, 77
Gigantism
   localized, causing hyperostoses, 192
   pituitary, 101, *101*
Glands
   adrenal, skeletal changes caused by, **104**
   parathyroid
      in chronic renal insufficiency, **138-142,** *139-141*
      skeletal changes caused by, **107-115**
   pineal, skeletal changes caused by, **106**
   pituitary, skeletal changes caused by, **100-104**
   thyroid, skeletal changes caused by, **104-106**
Glycosuria with renal tubular reabsorption defects, 142
Goiter, exophthalmic, 104
Gonads, skeletal changes caused by, **106**
Gonococcal arthritis, 271
Gonococcus causing pyogenic arthritis, 270
Goundou, 192

Gout, **124-127**
   chronic tophaceous, 125-127, *125-126*
   lipid; *see* Xanthoma tuberosum multiplex
   urate deposits in, 125, *125-126,* 127, *278*
Granuloma, eosinophilic, **198-203,** *199-205,* 206; *see also* Histiocytosis X
Granuloma inguinale, skeletal involvement in, 68
Granulomatosis, lipoids; *see* Histiocytosis X
Graves' disease, 104
Growth hormone, human, 100

H

Haemophilus influenzae causing pyogenic arthritis, 270
Hands, trident, 35, *36*
Healing of fractures
   requirements for, 6-7
   stages of, 1-2
Hemarthrosis, chronic, joint damage from, **276-277**
Hemolytic anemia
   chronic, 167
   familial; *see* Spherocytic anemia
Hemolytic jaundice, chronic; *see* Spherocytic anemia
Hemophilia, **164-167**
Hepatitis infections, joint changes in, 275
Hereditary multiple diaphyseal sclerosis; *see* Progressive diaphyseal dysplasia
Hereditary multiple exostosis, **24-28,** *25*
Hereditary ochronosis, **127-132**
   skeletal changes in, *128-131*
Hereditary spherocytosis; *see* Spherocytic anemia
Herniated intervertebral disc tissue, **223-225,** *224*
Hip, Charcot, *159*
Histiocytosis X, **196-209**
   acute (or subacute) disseminated, **203-206**
   chronic disseminated, **206-209**
   classification of, 196
   etiology of, 198
   localized in bone, **198-203,** *199-202*
Histoplasma duboisii, 76
Histoplasmosis, 75-76
Human growth hormone, 100
Hunter's syndrome, 43
Hurler-Pfaundler disease; *see* Gargoylism
Hurler's syndrome; *see* Gargoylism
Hydrarthrosis, intermittent, 292
Hydrocortisone for rheumatoid arthritis, 288
Hypercholesterolemia, essential; *see* Xanthoma tuberosum multiplex
Hypercorticism, adrenal, 104
Hyperostoses
   cortical, infantile, 77-80, *78-79*
      skeletal changes in, 77-78
   familial, 193-194, *193*
   affecting skull, **190-194**
Hyperostosis corticalis generalisata, 194
Hyperostosis frontalis interna, 190, 192
Hyperoxaluria, primary, 131-132

307

Index

Hyperparathyroidism
  primary, 107-111, *109-113*
  secondary, in chronic renal insufficiency, 139, 140
Hypersensitivity reactions, joint manifestations in, **292**
Hypersplenism, rheumatoid arthritis with; *see* Felty's syndrome
Hyperthyroidism, 104
Hypertrophic arthritis; *see* Osteoarthritis
Hypertrophic osteoarthropathy, 250, *251*
Hypervitaminosis A, **84-85**, *84*
Hypervitaminosis D, **96-97**
Hypogonadism, primary, 106
Hypoparathyroidism, 114-115
  with renal disease, 137
Hypophosphatasia, 92-93
Hypophosphatemic vitamin D–refractory rickets; *see* Vitamin D–resistant rickets
Hypophosphatemic vitamin D–resistant rickets, 142
Hypophyseal infantilism, *103*
Hypopituitarism, 102-104
Hypothyroidism, 104-105

I

Idiocy, amaurotic, 119
Immobilization, inadequate, as cause of nonunion, 6
Inclusion cysts, epidermoid, **258**, *258*
Incomplete fracture, fibrous repair of, *2*
Infantile cortical hyperostosis, 77-80, *78-79*
  skeletal changes in, 77-78
Infantilism, hypophyseal, *103*
Infarcts in bone, **234-239**, *235-238*
  in Gaucher's disease, *122*
Infected sequestrum, 57
Infections
  of bone, **52-80**
  of joints, **270-276**
    in Reiter's syndrome, 276
    in sarcoidosis, 276
  Nocardia, 64-65
  causing nonunion, 8
  Salmonella, 58, 60
  viral, skeletal changes in, **76-78**
Infectious arthritis, acute; *see* Pyogenic arthritis
Infectious hepatitis, joint changes in, 275
Injury to articular cartilage, 266, *268*
Insufficiency, renal, chronic; *see* Renal insufficiency, chronic
Intermittent hydrarthrosis, 292
Intermittent porphyria, acute, 132
Internal radiation, effect of, on bone, 216
Intervertebral discs
  in hereditary ochronosis, 128, *129*
  tissue of, herniation, **223-225**, *224*
Intoxication, fluoride, 212
Intraarticular fractures, 266
Intraosseous ganglion, 223
Involucrum, 52, *53*
Iodine deficiency, 134
Iproniazid for skeletal tuberculosis, 64

J

Jaundice, hemolytic, chronic; *see* Spherocytic anemia
Jaw, phossy, 211
Joint
  changes in
    in acromegaly, 102
    following trauma, **266-269**
  chondromatosis of, **294-295**, *294-295*
  coccidiomycosis of, 274-275, *274*
  damage to, from chronic hemarthrosis, **276-277**
  disease of, degenerative; *see* Osteoarthritis
  elbow, Charcot, *160*
  false; *see* Pseudoarthrosis
  hypersensitvity reactions affecting, **292**
  infections of, **270-276**
    in Reiter's syndrome, 276
    in sarcoidosis, 276
  knee, Charcot, *159, 161*
  in rheumatoid arthritis, 284-289, *285-288*
  synovial, disorders of, **265-300**
  syphilis affecting, 275
  systemic connective tissue diseases affecting, **290-291**
  tuberculosis of, 271-274
  viral diseases affecting, 275
Joint bodies, formation of, 266, 268, *269*
Joint mouse, 268, *269*
Juvenile osteochondritis, avascular necrosis in, **239-244**, *240-243*
Juvenile osteoporosis, 145
Juvenile rheumatoid arthritis; *see* Still's disease

K

Kerasin, 119-122
Kienböck's disease; *see* Juvenile osteochondritis
Klebsiella pneumoniae causing osteomyelitis, 58
Knee
  bucket-handle tear of meniscus, 218, 219, *219*
  Charcot, *159, 161*
  menisci of, pathology of, **218-219**
  osteoarthritis in, 279
  tuberculous synovitis of, 273
Köhler's disease; *see* Juvenile osteochondritis
Kümmell's disease, 244

L

Lacerated meniscus, 218-219, *219*
Late rickets, 92
Lathyrism, 214
Lead, effects of, on bone, 210, *211*
Lead lines, 210, *211*
Legg-Perthes' disease; *see* Juvenile osteochondritis
Leontiasis ossea, 193
Leprosy, skeletal changes in, **67-68**
Léri type of osteoporosis; *see* Melorheostosis
Letterer-Siwe syndrome; *see* Histiocytosis X, acute or subacute disseminated
Lignac-Fanconi disease; *see* Cystine storage disease

Index

Lipid gout; *see* Xanthoma tuberosum multiplex
Lipid metabolism, primary disorders of, **118-123**
Lipogranulomatosis, 133
Lipoid granulomatosis; *see* Histiocytosis X
Lobstein's syndrome; *see* Osteogenesis imperfecta
Localized gigantism causing hyperostoses, 192
Looser zone in osteomalacia, *94*, 96
Lorain type of dwarfism, 102, *103*
Lues, congenital, 68
Lupus erythematosus, disseminated, 290-291

M

Macrogenitosomia praecox, 106
Madura foot, 64-67, *66*
Maduromycosis, 65-67, *66*
Maffucci's syndrome, 28
Malignancy in Paget's disease, *188*, 189
Malignant tumor as sequel of chronic osteomyelitis, 61
Manganese deficiency, 134
Marble bone disease; *see* Osteopetrosis
Marie-Strümpell arthritis; *see* Rheumatoid spondylitis
Massive osteolysis, 244-245
Measles, German, skeletal changes in, 77
Mediterranean anemia, 169
Medullary osteosclerosis, monomelic, **47-48**, *48*
Melorheostosis, **44**, 47
Meningiomas causing hyperostoses of skull, 192
Meningococcus causing pyogenic arthritis, 270
Meniscus
 cysts of, 219, *220*, 222
 discoid, 219, *220*
 of knee, pathology of, **218-219**
 lacerated, 218-219, *219*
Mercury, effect of, on bone, 213
Mesothorium causing bone sarcoma, 216
Metabolic disorders
 arthritic manifestations of, **277**, 278-279
 skeletal changes in, **118-134**
Metabolic rickets, 142
Metabolism
 lipid, primary disorders of, **118-123**
 mucopolysaccharide, systemic disorders of, **132-133**
Metaphyseal dysostosis, 48
Metaphyseal dysplasia, familial, 48
Metaplastic ossification, **248-250**, *248-251*
Microabscess in chronic osteomyelitis, 58, *59*
Micromelia; *see* Achondroplasia
Milkman's syndrome, 96
Mithramycin for Paget's disease, 177
Möller-Barlow's disease; *see* Scruvy
Monomelic medullary osteosclerosis, **47-48**, *48*
Mononucleosis, infectious, joint changes after, 275
Monostotic lesions of fibrous dysplasia, *18*
Morquio syndrome, 43
Morquio-Brailsford syndrome; *see* Morquio syndrome
Morquio's disease, 37-39, *38*

MPS I; *see* Mucopolysaccharidosis
MPS II; *see* Hunter's syndrome
MPS III; *see* Sanfilipo syndrome
MPS IV; *see* Morquio syndrome
MPS V; *see* Scheie's syndrome
Mucopolysaccharide metabolism, systemic disorders of, **132-133**
Mucopolysaccharidosis, 43
Mutliple cartilaginous exostoses; *see* Hereditary multiple exostosis
Multiple diphyseal sclerosis, hereditary; *see* Progressive diaphyseal dysplasia
Multiple exostosis, hereditary, **24-28**, *25*
Mumps, joint changes in, 275
Mycetoma, 65-67, *66*
Mycobacterium leprae, 67, 68
Mycotic osteomyelitis, 75-76
Myositis ossificans, **245-247**, *246-247*
Myxedema, 104
Myxoid cysts, cutaneous, 223

N

Nanosomia pituitaria, 102
Necrosis, avascular, *10*, **234-239**, *235*, *238*
 in juvenile osteochondritis, **239-244**, *240-243*
Neuritis, leprous, 67
Neuroarthropathy, Charcot, 156
Neuroma, amputation, **230**, *230*
Neurotrophic disorders, skeletal changes in, 156-162
Neurotrophic foot in diabetes mellitus, 156, *157*
Nicotinic acid hydrazides, for skeletal tuberculosis, 64
Niemann-Pick disease, 118, 119
Nocardia infections of bone, 64-65
Nonarticular "rheumatism," **291-292**
Nonspecific villous synovitis, chronic, **266**, 267
Nonunion of fracture
 causes of, 6-8
 photomicrographs of, *9*

O

Ochronosis, hereditary, **127-132**
 skeletal changes in, *128-131*
Ochronotic ankylosing spondylitis, *128-129*, *130-131*
Ollier's disease; *see* Skeletal enchondromatosis
Orthopedic conditions, common and unusual, pathology of, **218-263**
Osgood-Schlatter's disease, *243*, 244
Ossification
 metaplastic, **248-250**, *248-251*
 periosteal, 248, *248*, *250*
Osteitis, radiation, 215
Osteitis deformans; *see* Paget's disease of bone
Osteitis fibrosa, 104, 107, *140*
Osteitis fibrosa cystica, generalized, 108
Osteoarthritis, **277-283**, *280-282*
Osteoarthropathy
 hypertrophic, 250, *251*
 xanthogranulomatous, 289
Osteoarthrosis; *see* Osteoarthritis
Osteocartilaginous exostosis, 24, *26*, *27*
 chondrosarcoma in, *26*, *27*

309

Index

Osteochondritis
 in congenial syphilis, 68-69, *69-70*
 juvenile, avascular necrosis in, **239-244**, *240-243*
Osteochondritis dissecans, 239, 240, *241-242*
Osteochondrodystrophia deformans; *see* Morquio's disease
Osteochondromas, 24, *26*
Osteodysplasia, familial, 194
Osteodystrophy
 renal, 92, *93*, 137, 143
 uremic or azotemic; *see* Renal insufficiency, chronic
Osteogenesis imperfecta, **32-35**, *33-35*
Osteogenesis imperfecta, congenita, 35
Osteogenesis imperfecta fetalis, 32
Osteogenesis imperfecta tarda, 34-35
Osteolysis, massive, 244-245
Osteomalacia, 93-97, *94-95*
 in chronic renal insufficiency, 141
Osteomata causing hyperostoses, 192
Osteomyelitis
 acute, 57, 58
 caused by *Brucella*, 58, 61
 chronic, 58, *59*
  sequelae of, 61
 as complication of fractures, 8
 Garré type of, 55
 Klebsiella pneumoniae causing, 58
 leprous, 67
 mycotic, 75-76
 Proteus causing, 58
 pyogenic, **52-61**
  antibiotics for, 52
 Salmonella causing, 58, *60*
 sclerosing, 55
 from smallpox, 77
Osteomyelitis variolosa, 77
Osteopathia condensans disseminata; *see* Osteopoikilosis
Osteopathia striata, 39, *41*
Osteopenia, 146; *see also* Osteoporosis
Osteoperiostitis
 in infantile cortical hyperostosis, 79
 in syphilis, 69
Osteopetrosis, **30-32**, *31*, *33*
Osteophytes in osteoarthritis, 283
Osteopoikilosis, **39-40**, *40*
Osteoporosis, 104, **145-154**, *147-153*
 in acromegaly, 150
 in biliary cirrhosis, 150
 causes of, 148-149
 gastrectomy causing, 149, *149*
 juvenile, 145
 mechanisms of, 148
 pathogenesis of, 146-151
 in scurvy, 150
Osteoporosis circumscripta cranii, 180, *180*
Osteopsathyrosis; *see* Osteogenesis imperfecta
Osteosclerosis
 in fluoride poisoning, *213*
 monomelic medullary, **47-48**, *48*
 renal, 138
Osteosclerosis fragilis; *see* Osteopetrosis

Osteosi eburnizzante monomelica; *see* Melorheostosis
Ovarian agenesis, 106
Oxalosis; *see* Primary hyperoxaluria
Oxycephaly in spherocytic anemia, 171

P

Paget's disease of bone, **173-194**
 clinical considerations in, 174, 176
 causing hyperostosis, 192
 malignant change in, *188*, 189
 pathologic changes in, 180-189
 treatment of, 176-178, *179*
Pancreas, skeletal changes caused by diabetes mellitus, 106
Parameniscal cysts, 219
Parasitic disease, bone lesions caused by, **76**
Parathormone, 107
Parathyroid adenomas, 107
Parathyroid glands
 in chronic renal insufficiency, **138-142**, *139-141*
 skeletal changes caused by, **107-115**
Parrot's pseudoparalysis, 275
Patella, chondromalacia of, 280
Pathologic changes in tendons and their sheaths, **225-229**
Pathologic fracture, *11*, *12*, *13*
 causes of, 11, 14-15
 definition of, 1
Pathology of common and unusual orthopedic conditions, **218-263**
Pelvospondylitis ossificans; *see* Rheumatoid spondylitis
Pendohyperparathyroidism, 111, 114
Penicillin
 for gonococcal arthritis, 271
 causing joint manifestations, 292
 for pyogenic arthritis, 270
 for syphilis, 68
Periarteritis nodosa, 291
Perineuritis, leprous, 67
Periosteal ossification, 248, *248*, 250
Periostitis in syphilis, 69
Phantom bones, 244-245
Phenylbutazone for gout, 125
Phosphorus, effect of, on bone, 211
Phossy jaw, 211
Pigmented villonodular synovitis, **296-300**, *296-300*
Pineal gland, skeletal changes caused by tumor of, **106**
Pituitary basophilism, 100
Pituitary gigantism, 101, *101*
Pituitary gland, skeletal changes caused by, **100-104**
Plumbism, 210
Plutonium causing osteogenic sarcoma, 216
Poisoning
 beryllium, 213
 bismuth, 210-211
 cadmium, 213
 fluoride, 211-213, *213*

310

Index

Poisoning—cont'd
   hypervitaminosis A, **84-85**, *84*
   hypervitaminosis D, **96-97**
   lead, 210, *211*
   mercury, 213
   phosphorus, 211
Poker back, 289; *see* ankylosing spondylitis
Polyarteritis nodosa, 291
Polychondritis, relapsing, **293-294**
Polyostotic fibrous dysplasia, 17, *20*
Porphyria, **132**
   acute intermittent, 132
Porphyria cutanea tarda, 132
Porphyria erythropoietica, congenital, 132
Porphyria hepatica, 132
Posttraumatic rarefaction of bone, **244-245**
Posttraumatic synovitis, 266
Pott's disease; *see* Tuberculous spondylitis
Primary disorders of lipid metabolism, **118-123**
Primary hyperoxaluria, 131-132
Primary hyperparathyroidism, 107-111, *109-113*
Primary hypogonadism, 106
Probenecid for gout, 125
Progressive diaphyseal dysplasia, **47**
   skeletal changes in, *46*
Proliferative arthritis; *see* Rheumatoid arthritis
Proteus causing osteomyelitis, 58
Pseudoarthrosis, 8, *10*
   of tibia, congenital, **233-234**, *234*
Pseudogout; *see* Chondrocalcinosis
Pseudo–hypo-hyperparathyroidism, 115
Pseudohypoparathyroidism, 115
Pseudoparalysis, Parrot's, 275
Pseudo-pseudohypoparathyroidism, 115
Psoriasis, association of, with rheumatoid arthritis, 289
Psoriatic arthritis, 289
Pyogenic arthritis, 270-271, *271*
   antibiotics for, 53
Pyogenic osteomyelitis, **52-61**
   antibiotics for, 52

R

Radiation, effects of, on bone, **214-217**, *215*
   external, 214-216
   internal, 216
Radiation osteitis, 215
Radium causing osteogenic sarcoma, 216
Rarefaction of bone, posttraumatic, **244-245**
Reabsorption defects, renal tubular, bone disease associated with, **142-143**
Reactions, hypersensitivity, joint manifestations in, **292**
Regional angiomatosis, 244-245
Reilly bodies, 39
Reiter's syndrome, joint inflammation in, 276
Relapsing polychondritis, **293-294**
Renal diabetes, 142
Renal disease, skeletal changes in, **137-144**
   hyperparathyroidism in, 137
   vitamin D deficiency in, 137-138
Renal dwarfism, 141
Renal excretion, failure of; *see* Renal insufficiency, chronic

Renal insufficiency, chronic
   bone disease associated with, **138-142**
   chronic acidosis in, 138-139
   osteomalacia in, 141
   parathyroid glands in, 138-139
   resorptive skeletal changes in, 138, *139-140*
   secondary hyperparathyroidism in, 139, *140*
Renal osteodystrophy, 92, *93*, 137, 143
Renal osteosclerosis, 138
Renal rickets, 92, *93*, *141*
Renal tubular acidosis, 142
Renal tubular reabsorption defects, bone disease associated with, **142-143**
Resorption of bone by parathormone, 107
Rheumatic fever, 290
Rheumatism
   desert, 274
   nonarticular, **291-292**
Rheumatoid arthritis, **283-289**, *285-288*
   association of, with psoriasis, 289
   with hypersplenism; *see* Felty's syndrome
   juvenile; *see* Still's disease
Rheumatoid spondylitis, 289
Rice bodies, in rheumatoid sinovitis, 286
Rickets, 88-92
   late, 92
   metabolic, 142
   renal, 92, *93*, *141*
   skeletal changes in, 90, *91*
   vitamin D–resistant, *91*, 92
      hypophosphatemic, 142
Rickets tarda, 92
Rubella
   joint changes from, 275
   skeletal changes in, 77
Rupture of tendons, traumatic, 229

S

Salmonella infections, 58, *60*
Salmonella osteomyelitis in sickle cell anemia, 168, *169*
Sanfilipo syndrome, 43
Sarcoid of tendon sheaths, 226
Sarcoidosis, joint involvement in, 276
Sarcoma
   following irradiation, 214-217
   in Paget's disease, 189, *188-189*
Scheie's syndrome, 43
Schmorl's node, *224*, 225
Schüller-Christian disease; *see* Histiocytosis X, chronic disseminated
Scleroderma, 291
Sclerosing osteomyelitis, 55
Scorbutus; *see* Scurvy
Scurvy
   osteoporosis in, 150
   skeletal changes in, 85-88, *86-87*
Seabright bantam syndrome; *see* Pseudohypoparathyroidism
Secondary hyperparathyroidism in chronic renal insufficiency, 139, *140*
Senescent arthritis; *see* Osteoarthritis
Septic arthritis; *see* Pyogenic arthritis

311

Index

Sequestrum, 52, 53
  infected, 57
Serum sickness causing joint hypersensitivity, 292
Sheaths, tendon
  pathologic changes in, **225-229**
  sarcoid of, 226
Sickle cell anemia, 167-168, *169*
  Salmonella osteomyelitis in, 168, *169*
Sickle cell dactylitis, 168
Sicklemia, 167, 168
Simmond's disease, 104
Skeletal changes
  caused by adrenal glands, **104**
  in blood diseases, **164-171**
  in cat-scratch fever, 77
  in chickenpox, 78
  in cleidocranial dysostosis, 42
  in enchondromatosis, **28-30**, *28-30*
  in endocrine disorders, **100-115**
  in gargoylism, 45
  in Gaucher's disease, 120-121
  caused by gonads, **106**
  in hereditary ochronosis, 128-131
  in infantile cortical hyperostosis, 77-78
  in leprosy, **67-68**
  in metabolic disorders, **118-134**
  in Morquio's syndrome, 38
  in neurotrophic disorders, 156-162
  with osteopetrosis, 31
  caused by pancreas, 106
  caused by parathyroid glands, **107-115**
  caused by pineal gland, **106**
  caused by pituitary gland, **100-104**
  in progressive diaphyseal dysplasia, 46
  in renal disease, **137-144**
  resorptive, in chronic renal insufficiency, 138, *139-140*
  in rickets, 90, *91*
  in rubella, 77
  in scurvy, 85-88, *86-87*
  in smallpox, 76-77
  caused by thymus, **106**
  caused by thyroid gland, **104-106**
  in vaccinia, 77
  in viral infections, **76-78**
  in vitamin A deficiency, **83-84**
  in vitamin A excess or poisoning, **84-85**, *84*
  in vitamin C deficiency, **85-88**, *86-87*
  in vitamin D deficiency, **88-96**, *89*
  in vitamin D excess or poisoning, **96-97**
Skeletal development, systemic anomalies of, **16-49**
Skeletal enchondromatosis, **28-30**, *28-30*
Skeletal involvement
  in fungal infections, **72-76**
  in granuloma inguinale, 68
Skeletal manifestations of syphilis, **68-72**
Skeletal tuberculosis, **61-67**
Skeleton, influence of trace elements on, 134
Skull
  changes in, in gargoylism, 43
  hyperostoses affecting, **190-194**

Slipped capital femoral epiphysis, **233**, *233*
Smallpox
  joint changes in, 275
  skeletal changes in, 76-77
Soft tissues, calcification of, 227, 228-229
Solitary lesions of fibrous dysplasia of bone, 17, 19, 22
Solitary unicameral bone cyst, 251-252
Spherocytic anemia, 170-171
Spherocytosis, hereditary; *see* Spherocytic anemia
Spine
  bamboo, 289
  Charcot, *159*
Spondylitis
  ochronotic ankylosing, *128-129*, 130-131
  rheumatoid, 289
  tuberculous, 61, 64
Spondylitis rhizomelic; *see* Rheumatoid spondylitis
Sporotrichosis, bone involvement in, 75
Spotty bones; *see* Osteopoikilosis
Staphylococcus aureus causing pyogenic arthritis, 270
Stenosing tenovaginitis, 229, *229*
Steroids
  for acute or subacute disseminated histiocytosis X, 205, 206
  for histiocytosis X, 209
  for Reiter's syndrome, 276
Still's disease, 289
Streptococcus hemolyticus causing pyogenic arthritis, 270, *271*
Streptomycin
  for brucellosis, 61
  for skeletal tuberculosis, 64
Stress fracture, 3
Strontium 90 causing osteogenic sarcoma, 216
Subcutaneous nodule in rheumatoid arthritis, 287-288, *288*
Subungal exostosis, 249, 250
Sudeck's atrophy, 244
Sulfanilamides causing periarteritis nodosa, 291
Sulfinpyrazone for gout, 125
Sulfonamides causing joint hypersensitivity, 292
Suppurative arthritis; *see* Pyogenic arthritis
Syndrome
  Albright's 19; *see also* Fibrous dysplasia of bone
  Cushing's, 100, 104
  de Toni-Debré-Fanconi; *see* Vitamin D–resistant rickets
  Fanconi, 94
  Felty's, 289
  Gardner's, 193
  Hunter's, 43
  Hurler's; *see* Gargoylism
  Letterer-Siwe; *see* Histiocytosis X, acute or subacute disseminated
  Lignac-Fanconi, 142
  Lobstein's; *see* Osteogenesis imperfecta
  Maffucci's, 28
  Milkman's, 96

Morquio, 43
Morquio-Brailsford; *see* Morquio syndrome
Reiter's, joint infections in, 276
Sanfilipo, 43
Scheie's, 43
van der Hoeve's; *see* Osteogenesis imperfecta
Synovectomy
   for joint chondromatosis, 295, *295*
   for pigmented villonodular synovitis, 300
Synovial cyst, 223; *see also* Intraosseous ganglion
Synovial joints, disorders of, **265-300**
Synovitis
   chronic nonspecific, villous, **266**, *267*
   pigmented villonodular **296-300**, *296-300*
   posttraumatic, 266
   in rheumatoid arthritis, 284-286, *285*
   tuberculous, of knee, *273*
Synovium, changes in, from trauma, 266
Syphilis
   acquired, 70-72, *71*
   congenital, 68-70
      causing hyperostosis, 192
      manifestations of, 70
   joint manifestations in, 275
   skeletal manifestations of, **68-72**
Syringomyelia, 156-162, *161-162*
Systemic anomalies of skeletal development, **16-49**
Systemic connective tissue dieseases, joint manifestations in, **290-291**
Systemic disorders of mucopolysaccharide metabolism, **132-133**

T

Tabes dorsalis, skeletal changes in, 156, 160, *160*
Taenia echinococcus, causing lesions of bone, 76
Tay-Sachs disease, 119
Tear of meniscus of knee, bucket-handle, 218, 219, *219*
Tendon sheaths
   pathologic changes in, **225-229**
   sarcoid of, 226
Tendons
   calcification of, 226-229, *228-229*
   degeneration of, *228*, 229
   pathologic changes in, **225-229**
   traumatic rupture of, 229
Tenovaginitis, stenosing, 229, *229*
Tetracycline
   for brucellosis 61
   for pyogenic arthritis, 270
Thalassemia, 169-170, *171*
Thalassemia major, 169-170, *170*
Thymus, skeletal changes caused by, **106**
Thyrocalcitonin, 105
Thyroid gland, skeletal changes caused by, **104-106**
Tibia, pseudoarthrosis of, congenital, **233-234**, *234*
Tophaceous gout, chronic, 125-127, *125-126*
Torticollis, congenital, 232

Torulosis, 75-76
Trace elements, influence of, on skeleton, 134
Trauma
   joint changes following, **266-269**
   synovial changes from, 266
Traumatic rupture of tendons, 229
Treatment of Paget's disease of bone, 176-178, *179*
Trident hands, 35, *36*
Trigger finger, 229, *229*
Tuberculosis
   of joints, 271-274
   skeletal, **61-67**
Tuberculous dactylitis, 63, *64*
Tuberculous spondylitis, 61, *64*
Tuberculous synovitis of knee, *273*
Tubular acidosis, renal, 142
Tubular reabsorption defects, renal, bone disease associated with, **142-143**
Tumors
   of adrenal cortex, 104
   brown, 108, *110*, *111*, *113*
   causing hyperostosis of skull, 192
   caused by irradiation, 214, *216*
   malignant, as sequela of chronic osteomyelitis, 61
Zollinger-Ellison, 114

U

Unicameral bone cyst, **250-258**, *252-255*
   solitary, 251-252
Urate deposits in gout, 125, *125-126*, 127, *278*
Uremic osteodystrophy; *see* Renal insufficiency, chronic

V

Vaccinia, skeletal changes in, 77
van der Hoeve's snydrome; *see* Osteogenesis imperfecta
Vanishing bone disease, 244-245
Varicella, joint changes after, 275
Villonodular synovitis, pigmented, **296-300**, *296-300*
Villous synovitis, chronic nonspecific, **266**, *267*
Viral diseases, joint manifestations in, 275
Viral infections, skeletal changes in, **76-78**
Vitamin A
   deficiency of, skeletal changes in, **83-84**
   excess of or poisoning by, skeletal changes in, **84-85**, *84*
Vitamin C, deficiency of, skeletal changes in, **85-88**, *86-87*
Vitamin D
   deficiency of
      in renal disease, 137-138
      skeletal changes in, **88-96**, *89*
   excess of or poisoning by, skeletal changes in, **96-97**
Vitamin D–resistant rickets, *91*, 92
   hypophosphatemic, 142
Volkmann's contracture, **230**, *231*
von Bechterew's arthritis; *see* Rheumatoid spondylitis
Voorhoeve's disease, 39, *41*

Index

W

Wryneck, 232

X

Xanthogranulomatous osteoarthropathy, 289
Xanthoma tuberosum multiplex, 122-123, *123*

Y

Yaws, skeletal lesions in, 68, *69*
Yellow phosphorus, causing osteomyelitis, 211

Z

Zinc deficiency, 134
Zollinger-Ellison tumors, 114